Concepts in Sterile Preparations and Aseptic Technique

Pamella S. Ochoa, PharmD
Assistant Professor
School of Pharmacy
Texas Tech University Health Sciences Center
Abilene, Texas

José A. Vega, PharmD
Assistant Professor
School of Pharmacy
Texas Tech University Health Sciences Center
Abilene, Texas

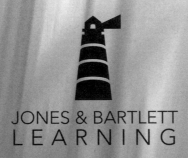

JONES & BARTLETT
LEARNING

World Headquarters
Jones & Bartlett Learning
5 Wall Street
Burlington, MA 01803
978-443-5000
info@jblearning.com
www.jblearning.com

Jones & Bartlett Learning books and products are available through most bookstores and online booksellers. To contact Jones & Bartlett Learning directly, call 800-832-0034, fax 978-443-8000, or visit our website, www.jblearning.com.

Substantial discounts on bulk quantities of Jones & Bartlett Learning publications are available to corporations, professional associations, and other qualified organizations. For details and specific discount information, contact the special sales departmer at Jones & Bartlett Learning via the above contact information or send an email to specialsales@jblearning.com.

The content, statements, views, and opinions herein are the sole expression of the respective authors and not that of Jones & Bartle Learning, LLC. Reference herein to any specific commercial product, process, or service by trade name, trademark, manufacturer, otherwise does not constitute or imply its endorsement or recommendation by Jones & Bartlett Learning, LLC and such reference not be used for advertising or product endorsement purposes. All trademarks displayed are the trademarks of the parties noted her *Concepts in Sterile Preparations and Aseptic Technique* is an independent publication and has not been authorized, sponsored, or otherwise approved by the owners of the trademarks or service marks referenced in this product.

There may be images in this book that feature models; these models do not necessarily endorse, represent, or participate in the activities represented in the images. Any screenshots in this product are for educational and instructive purposes only. Any individ and scenarios featured in the case studies throughout this product may be real or fictitious, but are used for instructional purposes

The authors, editor, and publisher have made every effort to provide accurate information. However, they are not responsible for errors, omissions, or for any outcomes related to the use of the contents of this book and take no responsibility for the use of the products and procedures described. Treatments and side effects described in this book may not be applicable to all people; likewise some people may require a dose or experience a side effect that is not described herein. Drugs and medical devices are discussed th may have limited availability controlled by the Food and Drug Administration (FDA) for use only in a research study or clinical trial Research, clinical practice, and government regulations often change the accepted standard in this field. When consideration is bei given to use of any drug in the clinical setting, the health care provider or reader is responsible for determining FDA status of the d reading the package insert, and reviewing prescribing information for the most up-to-date recommendations on dose, precautions, contraindications, and determining the appropriate usage for the product. This is especially important in the case of drugs that are or seldom used.

Production Credits

Executive Publisher: William Brottmiller
Executive Editor: Rhonda Dearborn
Editorial Assistant: Sean Fabery
Associate Production Editor: Sara Fowles
Marketing Manager: Grace Richards
VP, Manufacturing and Inventory Control: Therese Connell

Composition: Laserwords Private Limited, Chennai, India
Cover Design: Michael O'Donnell
Director of Photo Research and Permissions: Amy Wrynn
Cover Image: © Taiga/Shutterstock, Inc.
Printing and Binding: Edwards Brothers Malloy
Cover Printing: Edwards Brothers Malloy

To order this product, use ISBN: 978-1-284-03572-8

Library of Congress Cataloging-in-Publication Data
Concepts in sterile preparations and aseptic technique / [edited by] Pamella S. Ochoa, José A. Vega.
   p. ; cm.
Includes bibliographical references and index.
ISBN 978-1-4496-7863-0 (pbk.) — ISBN 978-1-284-03572-8
I. Ochoa, Pamella S., editor of compilation. II. Vega, Jose A. editor of compilation.
[DNLM: 1. Infusions, Parenteral—methods. 2. Infusions, Parenteral—standards. 3. Drug Compounding—methods.
4. Drug Compounding—standards. 5. Sterilization--methods. 6. Sterilization—standards. WB 354]
RM170
615'.6—dc23
                                                                                                2013050989
6048

Printed in the United States of America
18 17 16 15 14   10 9 8 7 6 5 4 3 2

Dedication

To our children, Anthony, Daniel, and Natalie—you inspire me to be the best that I can be for you. I love you all forever. And yes, my dear children, I am finally finished writing my book and now we can go play. To my husband, who has been my continuous pillar of support. You are my best friend and the love of my life. To my parents, Tina and Al, who both instilled in me the desire to never stop learning, to expand my horizons, and to always persevere. Thank you for teaching me that anything is possible. To my mentors and colleagues, who have helped me learn, understand, and shape me into the professional that I am today. Especially for those who have dedicated themselves to paving the road for our profession. To my students and residents, for the hope you bring me for the bright future of our treasured profession.

For all the sacrifices endured by my family, and for the unwavering support and encouragement of my friends, colleagues, and relatives. Thank you. "The book" is done.

And—most importantly—for Your Glory, Lord. Without You, none of this would have been possible.

Pamella S. Ochoa

I dedicate this book to my brilliant and beautiful wife who has been my inspiration, and without whom this book would have not been completed. I also dedicate this book to my parents who overcame great hardships and sacrifices to provide me the opportunity to pursue my dreams.

José A. Vega

Contents

**Chapter 9   Multiple Product Preparations for Parenteral
Nutrition   289**

**Chapter 10 Considerations for Intravenous Drug Therapy
in Infants and Children   313**

Preface

This is an interesting time in the evolution of sterile compounding. The recent past has revealed many changes and standards in regard to compounding sterile preparations. While much progress has been made, there is still more that needs to be accomplished as we continue to recognize the need for further changes for the safety of our patients. Our generation has been unfortunate in witnessing landmark events related to adverse patient outcomes—from contamination of medications to compatibility misadventures and errors in dosing related to compounded sterile preparations. This has fueled the need to immediately address specifics of sterile compounding such as the training of persons compounding sterile preparations, current verification processes, environmental controls, and much more.

The content of this book is derived from current practice, current standards and regulations, literature, and best practice. Information from USP Chapter <797> is included throughout the book. To emphasize the application of these USP standards, specific content from the standards has been strategically placed based on the content of the chapter.

It is the goal of the authors to bring attention to the patient. Concern for the patient must be at the forefront of our thoughts and actions as we consider the terminal purpose of our preparations. In addition to descriptions and alerts for patient safety issues, historical examples are included in an effort to connect sterile compounding to real life situations.

It is important that pharmacists understand fundamentals of aseptic technique, as well as current standards and best practices as they relate to sterile compounding. The intent of this book is to provide a source of information for these topics. Our hope is that this book will prove useful in the education of pharmacy students as part of their coursework and in the training of pharmacists and pharmacy technicians who will be involved in sterile compounding. For those who are already compounding sterile preparations, we hope that this book will serve as a valuable resource to enhance current practice.

How to Use this Book

This book provides a comprehensive overview of the fundamentals of aseptic technique and sterile compounding. The book includes the following pedagogical features:

- **Videos**: Instructional videos are included on the Navigate Companion Website to demonstrate important techniques that are common with sterile compounding. These videos provide verbal step-by-step instructions with a visual depiction of various techniques. To facilitate a comprehensive review of techniques and processes, the video content correlates with the content of each chapter.
- **Tips**: Techniques and practices that are helpful for compounding sterile preparations are included throughout the book. These tips are intended to provide guidance based on current practice, literature, and the experiences of those who have compounded sterile preparations.
- **Alerts**: Important information that may relate to patient safety, operator safety, or current regulations and standards is highlighted throughout the book. Not only are

these alerts intended to draw the attention of the reader to the importance of the information, but they also serve as a helpful tool for remembering important information.

- **Case Studies**: While the information presented in the book is useful, its application is of utmost importance. For this reason, the authors have included case studies for each chapter. The case studies provide realistic scenarios that provide an opportunity to apply the content from the chapter. The case studies enhance learning by requiring the reader to synthesize answers.
- **Review Questions**: Each chapter includes a series of review questions that provide an opportunity for the reader to assess knowledge of important information. The review questions also serve as useful tools for the application of content presented in the chapter.
- **Additional Features**: A glossary of terms appears at the end of the book. Each chapter begins with an overview of its content and its relevance to current practice, while end-of-chapter summaries are also included. References are included for each chapter.

With the use of videos, tips, alerts, case studies, and review questions, the reader is provided with numerous methods to enhance their learning and assess their understanding.

Student Resources

The Navigate Companion Website features useful study activities, including Videos, Chapter Quizzes, Crossword Puzzles, Interactive Flashcards, an Interactive Glossary, Matching Exercises, and Web Links. To redeem the Access Code Card available with your new copy of the text, or to purchase access to the website separately, call 800-832-0034 and request ISBN-13: 9781449693381, or visit go.jblearning.com/OchoaCWS.

Navigate Companion Website features:

Videos

These exclusive videos demonstrate important techniques.

Chapter Quizzes

Complete a quiz at the end of each chapter to assess your knowledge of key concepts. Results can be emailed to your course instructor.

Crossword Puzzles

Enjoy an interactive overview of terms from each chapter with real crossword puzzles made up of terms from the text.

Interactive Flashcards

Enhance retention as these helpful tools guide you through the key terms vital to understanding important topics.

Interactive Glossary

Search for key words and terms and their definitions alphabetically or by chapter.

Matching Exercises

Engage in an enjoyable online activity to connect concepts and terms with their meanings.

Web Links

Explore external sites that provide additional information about topics covered in the textbook.

Instructor Resources

Qualified instructors can also receive the full suite of Instructor Resources, including PowerPoint Presentations, a Test Bank, an Instructor's Manual, and an Answer Key. To gain access to these valuable teaching materials, contact your Health Professions Account Specialist at go.jblearning.com/findarep.

PowerPoint Presentations featuring more than 375 slides
Test Bank containing more than 175 questions
Instructor's Manual including lab exercises and supplies list
Answer Key containing answers for the end-of-chapter Review Questions

Acknowledgements

We are immensely grateful to all of the contributors of this book for their dedicated efforts and for sharing their expertise for the purpose of this book. A special thanks to Dr. Gordon Sacks for his contribution to laboratory ancillary materials.

The authors would like to acknowledge and thank the editorial, marketing, and acquisitions team at Jones & Bartlett Learning for their professionalism as well as for their continuing vision and commitment to this book, including Sean Fabery, Rhonda Dearborn, Sara Fowles, Maria Leon Maimone, Grace Richards, Teresa Reilly, and Katey Birtcher.

The authors would also like to thank the pharmacy students who volunteered in various respects for the purpose of this book, including Rebecca Koch, Landon Schwartz, and Louis Robison for their assistance with videos and images.

About the Authors

Dr. Pamella S. Ochoa is originally from Portland, Texas. The idea of becoming a pharmacist originated during a conversation with her father about potential careers. After graduating from high school, Dr. Ochoa attended Texas A&M University in College Station, Texas, where she obtained a Bachelor of Science degree in Biochemistry with a minor in Genetics. She then attended Texas Tech University Health Sciences Center School of Pharmacy, where she earned a Doctor of Pharmacy degree. Following graduation, Dr. Ochoa completed a PGY1 Pharmacy Practice residency at the University of Texas Health Center in Tyler, Texas. Dr. Ochoa's professional experience includes working as a clinical pharmacist, hospital pharmacist, pharmacy technician, and pharmacy intern in various hospital settings. She underwent training as a pharmacy technician for compounding of sterile preparations, including chemotherapy, and performed aseptic parenteral compounding thereafter. Dr. Ochoa has assisted in training pharmacy technicians, pharmacy students, and pharmacists as it relates to sterile compounding. She is a team member of the Sterile Compounding course, teaching both in laboratory and didactic portions of the course. She continues to provide education through the delivery of a Sterile Preparations Certification course and other continuing education in the field of sterile compounding for pharmacists and pharmacy technicians. Dr. Ochoa currently practices as a clinical pharmacist in a hospital setting.

Dr. José A. Vega is originally from Friona, Texas. He established an interest in the field of Pharmacy early in his studies. To pursue this goal, he first attended West Texas A&M where he earned a degree in Biochemistry. His education extended to include a Doctor of Pharmacy degree from Texas Tech Health Sciences Center School of Pharmacy. He completed a PGY1 Pharmacy Practice residency at the University of Texas Health Center at Tyler. Dr. Vega worked in the community setting as a pharmacy technician, followed by professional experience as both a clinical and hospital pharmacist. He is involved in the training of pharmacy students, pharmacy technicians, and pharmacists in the area of sterile compounding. His involvement in providing education also includes the development and delivery of continuing education for sterile compounding, as well a Sterile Preparations Certification course for pharmacists. Dr. Vega serves as the course team leader for the Sterile Compounding course in which didactic and laboratory experiences provide education to pharmacy students. He currently practices as a clinical pharmacist in a hospital setting.

Contributors

Paul Holder, PharmD
Assistant Director of Enforcement
Texas State Board of Pharmacy

Patricia C. Kienle, RPh, MPA, FASHP
Director, Accreditation and Medication Safety
Cardinal Health Innovative Delivery Solutions

Sherry Luedtke, PharmD, FPPAG
Associate Professor, Pediatrics
School of Pharmacy
Texas Tech University Health Sciences Center

Gordon Sacks, PharmD, BCNSP, FCCP
Professor, and Department Head, Pharmacy Practice
James I. Harrison School of Pharmacy
Auburn University

Hardeep Singh Saluja, PhD
Assistant Professor of Pharmaceutical Sciences
College of Pharmacy
Southwestern Oklahoma State University

Helen T. Wu, PharmD, BCOP
Pharmacy Senior Supervisor, Adult Hematology/Oncology
Associate Clinical Professor
School of Pharmacy
University of California—San Francisco

Reviewers

Shuhua Bai, PhD
Assistant Professor
School of Pharmacy
Husson University

Charles C. Collins, RPh, PhD
Professor
Bill Gatton College of Pharmacy
East Tennessee State University

Anthony Corigliano, RPh
Assistant Professor
Wegmans School of Pharmacy
St. John Fisher College

Duc P. Do, PhD
College of Pharmacy
Chicago State University

Tony Guerra, PharmD
Chair
Pharmacy Technician Program
Des Moines Area Community College

William J. Havins, BUS, CPhT
Clinical Coordinator
Pharmacy Technician Program
Central New Mexico Community College

Jason L. Iltz, PharmD
Director of Pharmacy, Home and Ambulatory Infusion
Integrated Health Professionals
Clinical Associate Professor of Pharmacotherapy
College of Pharmacy
Washington State University

Tracy Kosinski, PharmD
Assistant Professor
School of Pharmacy
Concordia University Wisconsin

P. L. Madan, PhD
Professor
College of Pharmacy and Health Sciences
St. John's University

Anita Mosley, PhD, PharmD
Assistant Professor
Feik School of Pharmacy
University of the Incarnate Word

S. Narasimha Murthy, PhD
Associate Professor
School of Pharmacy
University of Mississippi

CHAPTER 1

Introduction to Parenteral Preparations

José A. Vega, Pamella S. Ochoa, and Paul Holder

Chapter Objectives

1. Define a parenteral preparation.
2. List various routes of parenteral administration.
3. Describe advantages and disadvantages of the parenteral route of administration.
4. Discuss the role of safety, accuracy, and attitude in risk prevention associated with parenteral preparation.
5. Discuss United States Pharmacopeia chapters applicable to pharmaceutical compounding of sterile preparations.

Key Terminology

Hazardous agent
Pyrogen
Sterility
Particulate matter
Isotonicity
Normal saline
United States Pharmacopeia

Compounded sterile preparations
Automated compounding devices
Radiopharmaceutical
Parenteral nutrition
Accreditation Council for Pharmacy Education (ACPE)
Precipitate

Overview

Compounded sterile preparations (CSPs) are often prepared for parenteral administration from manufactured sterile products. Patients frequently require administration of parenteral preparations as a means of drug delivery. This mode of delivery provides both benefits and risks compared to other forms of drug delivery. Pharmacists and pharmacy technicians assume various roles in the preparation and verification of parenteral preparations. Understanding the basics of parenteral preparation is the beginning of building the knowledge and skills needed as part of required personnel training. Patient and personnel safety related to the preparation and administration of parenteral preparations depends on many factors, including accuracy, safety, and the attitude of those involved in the compounding process.

[handwritten margin notes: preparation made by RPh / product made by manufacturer / needs unique set of skills, knowledge]

Parenteral Administration

Medications can be delivered into the body through a variety of routes. Drug delivery characteristics and pharmacodynamic properties vary depending on the route of administration chosen for the drug. Parenteral preparations circumvent the intestinal tract and, therefore, are not subject to pharmacodynamic properties associated with oral or other formulations. While many routes of parenteral administration are available, all of which bypass the intestinal tract, the intravenous, intramuscular, and subcutaneous routes of administration are the most commonly used. **Table 1-1** lists various routes and locations of delivery of parenteral administration. **Figure 1-1** illustrates the locations utilized in intravenous, intradermal, intramuscular, and subcutaneous parenteral

[handwritten margin notes: Enteral: intestinal or digestive tract / oral, SL, buccal, rectal]

Table 1-1 Parenteral Routes

Route	Injection Site
Intravenous (IV)	Vein
Intramuscular (IM)	Muscle tissue
Intradermal (ID)	Dermis of the skin
Subcutaneous (subcut; SQ)	Subcutaneous tissue of the skin
Intrathecal (IT)	Subarachnoid space of the spinal cord
Epidural	Epidural space of the spinal cord
Intra-arterial	Artery
Intra-articular	Joint space
Intracardiac	Heart
Intraocular	Eye
Intraperitoneal	Peritoneal cavity

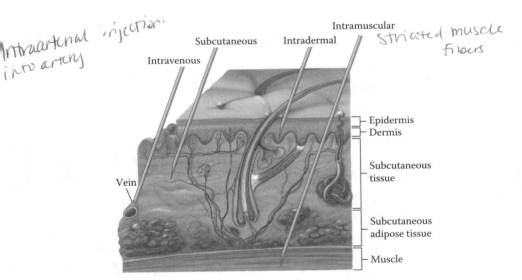

Intraarterial injection: into artery

Striated muscle fibers

Figure 1-1 Routes of Parenteral Administration

administration. Intrathecal and epidural administration of medications offer additional routes of administration within the spinal cord; **Figure 1-2** depicts the location of drug delivery with these routes of administration. Because medications administered parenterally bypass the intestinal tract, the pharmacodynamic properties of such medications will differ depending on the site

[handwritten annotations:]
3 membranes that coat
brain
outside dura mater
arachnoid mater
pia mater

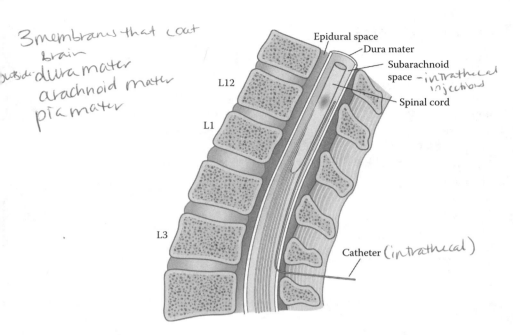

Epidural space
Dura mater
Subarachnoid space *—intrathecal injection*
Spinal cord
L12
L1
L3
Catheter *(intrathecal)*

Figure 1-2 ~~Epidural~~ administration
[handwritten:] Intrathecal

of administration. This can result in advantages—and sometimes disadvantages—that are unique to the parenteral formulation.

The United States Pharmacopeia (USP) defines five main types of preparations intended for parenteral administration:

- Injection: liquid preparations that are drug substances or solutions thereof
- *(powder—all diluent below)* For injection: dry solids that, upon addition of suitable vehicles, yield solutions conforming in all respects to the requirements for injections
- Injectable emulsion: liquid preparations of drug substances dissolved or dispersed in a suitable emulsion medium
- Injectable suspension: liquid preparations of solids suspended in a suitable liquid medium
- For injectable suspension: dry solids that, upon addition of suitable vehicles, yield preparations conforming in all respects to the requirements of injectable suspensions

Advantages and Disadvantages of Parenteral Administration

While many drugs are available only for parenteral administration, the parenteral route is often chosen as the preferred method of administration in certain circumstances. It provides advantages in circumstances in which multiple medications need to be administered simultaneously, in emergent situations, and for specialized dosing regimens. Often, patient-specific dosing is needed to achieve optimal drug levels, as with medications needing monitoring for narrow therapeutic windows. Additionally, continuous infusions and unique titrations can be achieved conveniently with parenteral administration of certain medications.

Patients who are unable to tolerate oral medications or are unconscious may be limited to receiving medications parenterally. Examples include patients who do not have a functioning gastrointestinal tract, who have restricted oral intake, and who may be experiencing nausea or vomiting. For these patients, parenteral preparations can be a means of effective drug delivery.

Further, bypassing the gastrointestinal tract can provide an immediate physiological response and complete systemic circulation of a drug, resulting in increased serum concentration of the drug. For example, many antibiotics achieve higher serum peak concentrations with IV delivery compared to the oral route, due to the limited bioavailability of some oral antibiotics. In addition, parenteral CSPs offer benefits to patients such as quick onset of action, providing rapid availability of the drug to the body. Pain medications and emergent situations are examples of situations in which the quick onset of action provided by parenteral preparations represents a key advantage over oral or other formulations. Parenteral CSPs also offer the advantage of localized delivery of drugs, as with intra-articular administration of corticosteroids in patients with rheumatoid arthritis.

Finally, the potential for an extended duration of effect is a key consideration when choosing drug formulations. For example, depot injection of certain drugs, such as contraceptives, can provide an extended effect with a single injection.

While the benefits of parenteral administration of drugs are many, use of this route also poses some potentially significant risks to the patient. Disadvantages of parenteral preparations to the patient include lack of drug reversal, risk of infection and emboli, risk of hypersensitivity reactions, and cost. In particular, because parenteral drugs may be introduced into the systemic circulation of the body, as with the IV route, drugs administered parenterally may not be able to be readily removed or their effects easily reversed. This is an important point of consideration, and it explains why any drug delivered parenterally must be prepared and verified in such a manner to ensure complete accuracy and sterility. Proper preparation and verification of CSPs can prevent misadventures in dosing and potential risks, including death, to the patient.

If contamination of the preparation occurs, such as with bacteria, fungi, or viruses, the contaminants will be directly administered to the patient—an outcome that will likely result in infection or even potentially death of the patient. Physical contamination of a parenteral preparation, such as with microscopic shards of glass or precipitates, can cause an embolus if administered into the vein or artery.

In addition, compared to other formulations, administering drugs parenterally may increase the risk of hypersensitivity reactions. While other routes of administration also pose the risk of hypersensitivity reactions, the parenteral route is believed to be the most immunogenic.[1, 2]

Finally, the overall cost of parenteral administration can often exceed the cost of other formulations. This cost is not limited to the drug alone, which is typically more expensive than medications delivered via other routes.[3] Increased costs incurred with parenteral administration of medications may include the cost of supplies and preparation, such as tubing and syringes, and the cost of personnel time to prepare the CSP. Additionally, parenteral medications may require dedicated (and costly) equipment and personnel—only personnel with specialized training can administer parenteral preparations. Because of the increased potential for adverse effects associated with parenteral administration of medications, mitigation of such adverse effects can add even more costs.

Table 1-2 lists various advantages and disadvantages of administering drugs parenterally.

Table 1-2   Advantages and Disadvantages of Parenteral Products

Advantages	Disadvantages
Provides drug and nutritional options for patients unable to tolerate oral therapy	Difficulty/impossibility of drug removal/reversal
Circumvents absorption limitations of gastrointestinal tract	Risk of infection
Quick onset of action	Risk of emboli (thrombus *lclot that breaks off & travels -ie to brain, heart, lung*)
(IA) Localized delivery (*not IV, IM, sa, IP*)	Risk of hypersensitivity reactions
Prolonged duration of effect	Higher costs

not all contraceptives ✓   *training, equipment*

Safety, Accuracy, and Attitude

Safety is an important consideration when preparing parenteral medications, both for the patient and for the personnel involved in compounding. Because of the significant risks that this route of administration may pose to the patient, such as emboli and infection, patient safety must be a primary focus during the preparation process. Quality measures and preparation practices utilized on a consistent basis will provide aseptic preparations that are safe for patient administration. Risks also exist to the personnel involved in compounding. Exposure to certain types of hazardous agents and injuries resulting from needle sticks are examples of these risks. In addition to measures that ensure patient safety, measures should be incorporated into each preparation process that lead to increased personnel safety.

Due to the nature of the delivery method, parenteral medications must be prepared in a manner so as to ensure their accuracy. Owing to the inability to reverse the effects and quick onset of action with many medications when administered parenterally, there is no leniency regarding accuracy of the preparation. Accuracy is important for selection of products, calculations, and preparation technique. For example, an error of one decimal point when calculating the amount of product to use may result in serious harm or death, depending on the medication being administered. Thus verification processes must be integrated into the preparation process and consistently utilized to ensure accuracy. Importantly, personnel involved in compounding must accept responsibility for ensuring accuracy and systematic measures must be in place to support personnel with such responsibility.

Developing and maintaining an attitude of safety and accuracy is the core of parenteral preparation and administration. The level of attentiveness by each individual in the preparation, verification, and administration of parenteral medications is an important component of ensuring patient and personnel safety. It must be emphasized that the ultimate responsibility for care of the patient and prevention of risks related to parenteral preparations is directly in the hands of those personnel involved in compounding and administering the CSP. At all points in time, techniques to ensure safety and accuracy must be utilized. As discussed earlier in the chapter, parenteral administration does not allow for easy removal of the drug and poses multiple risks to the patient. Thus safety and accuracy are of utmost importance.

While certain risks may inevitably be associated with parenteral administration, processes and techniques can be employed to mitigate those risks:

- Proper training of all personnel involved in compounding and administering parenteral preparations
- Maintaining a proper environment for compounding sterile preparations
- Using aseptic techniques and manipulations while compounding
- Implementing systems to ensure accuracy and quality of the preparation prior to patient administration

It is the responsibility of all persons involved in the preparation and verification processes to ensure that methods to prevent risks to patients are utilized with each preparation. Ensuring that such risk prevention strategies are utilized can prevent harm to both the patient and the personnel compounding parenteral preparations.

Because of the potentially significant risks to the patient in the event of error or contamination, stringent parameters must exist regarding the quality of the final preparation. Preparations not only need to meet standards for accuracy, potency, and stability, but also need to meet standards for microbial (pyrogens and sterility), physical (particulate matter), and chemical (isotonicity) parameters.[5]

United States Pharmacopeia Chapters

The USP is an independent organization that provides definitions, descriptions, and requirements for multiple pharmaceutical settings. In particular, this organization publishes standards for identity, quality, strength, purity, packaging, and labeling. Standards provided by the USP provide guidance as to processes and conditions for sterile compounding.

USP standards are organized into chapter numbers. Chapters numbered from <1> to <999> are considered enforceable, whereas chapters numbered from <1000> to <1999> are not enforceable. USP Chapter <797> provides procedures and requirements for all persons who transport, store, and prepare CSPs, as well as all places where CSPs are prepared. Locations where CSPs may be prepared include hospitals, pharmacies, treatment clinics, and physicians' offices. Personnel who may transport, store, and prepare CSPs include pharmacists, pharmacy technicians, nurses, and physicians. The objective of the <797> chapter is to prevent harm to patients by preventing exposure to microorganisms or bacterial endotoxins as well as to provide patients with sterile, stable, and accurate CSPs.[5, 6]

The USP Chapter <797> was first introduced on January 1, 2004. The original version underwent extensive revision following considerable feedback from the public. The revised standard was released in December 2007 and became official on June 1, 2008. The chapter is enforceable by the Food and Drug Administration (FDA), although the enforcement is typically deferred to state boards of pharmacy.[5]

State boards of pharmacy are empowered by the individual state legislatures to promulgate rules designed to ensure the health and safety of the citizens residing within their specific states. Therefore, state boards of pharmacy can deviate somewhat from the standards set forth in USP chapter <797>. For instance, a given state board of pharmacy may require training for personnel who are compounding sterile preparations that is more stringent than the training requirements provided in chapter <797>. Through the rules-making process, a board of pharmacy may require proof of completion of an Accreditation Council for Pharmacy Education (ACPE)–certified course providing a specified number of didactic and experiential hours in compounding sterile preparations. In addition, a state board of pharmacy may require more training, provided by the individual pharmacy in which the pharmacist or pharmacy technician works, before that person is allowed to compound a CSP intended for administration to a patient. Moreover, a state board of pharmacy may require proof of sterile compounding competencies and demonstration of aseptic technique for all pharmacy compounding personnel. This assurance could be provided through written and/or practical examinations and completion of media-fill testing, followed by a waiting period for sterility results, before allowing the individual compounder to prepare patient-specific CSPs.

State boards of pharmacy may also require stricter environmental controls, quality assurance, and quality control procedures than those required in USP Chapter <797>. Likewise, a state may develop specific requirements for recall procedures, if it is discovered that a compounded sterile preparation or a batch of compounded sterile preparations has been identified as exhibiting the potential for, or confirmed, harm to a patient or patients. Thus it is incumbent upon all personnel involved in any aspect of the compounding of sterile preparations to be familiar with the contents of <797>, as well as the rules pertaining to sterile compounding set forth by the state's board of pharmacy.

Essential USP Chapter <797> procedures and requirements have been incorporated throughout this text to provide a general understanding of safe transport, storage, and preparation of CSPs, but the information presented here is not intended to serve as an alternative to the actual USP Chapter <797> publication. All personnel who prepare CSPs should at a minimum read the full USP Chapter <797> to fully understand the fundamental practices discussed in this text; they should also familiarize themselves with local state board of pharmacy rules. In addition to USP Chapter <797>, other USP chapters provide specific content that may be relevant to those involved in specific types of compounding, such as high-risk compounding. Other USP chapters that may serve helpful include: USP Chapter <71> on sterility tests, USP Chapter <85> on bacterial endotoxin tests, USP Chapter <788> on particular matter in injections, USP Chapter <1075> on good compounding practices, USP Chapter <1116> on microbiological evaluation of cleanrooms and other controlled environments, and USP Chapter <1191> on stability considerations. USP Chapter <823> provides useful information for those involved in compounding radiopharmaceuticals. The following outline describes the major sections of the USP Chapter <797>:[6]

- Definitions
- Responsibility of Compounding Personnel
- CSP Microbial Contamination Risk Levels
- Personnel Training and Evaluation in Aseptic Manipulation Skills
- Immediate-Use CSPs
- Single-Dose and Multiple-Dose Containers
- Hazardous Drugs and CSPs
- Radiopharmaceuticals and CSPs
- Allergen Extracts and CSPs
- Verification of Compounding Accuracy and Sterility
- Environmental Quality and Control
- Suggested Standard Operating Procedures
- Elements of Quality Control
- Verification of Automated Compounding Devices for Parenteral Nutrition Compounding
- Finished Preparation Release Checks and Tests
- Storage and Beyond-Use Dating
- Maintaining Sterility, Purity, and Stability of Dispensed and Distributed CSPs
- Patient or Caregiver Training
- Patient Monitoring and Adverse Events Reporting
- Quality Assurance Program
- Abbreviations and Acronyms

Responsibilities of Compounding Personnel

Throughout this text, the responsibility of compounding personnel will be discussed. It is important to understand the role and accountability that each individual has in compounding a sterile preparation that is sterile, accurate and safe for patients. USP Chapter <797> defines the responsibility that all personnel involved in compounding share, as listed here. These responsibilities will be expanded upon and discussed further in the textbook.

Personnel Responsibilities[6]

- Perform antiseptic hand washing and maintain good hand hygiene
- Disinfection of critical areas, such as non-sterile compounding surfaces
- Proper selection and donning of personal protective equipment
- Maintenance or achievement of sterility of CSPs in appropriate compounding devices
- Protect personnel and compounding environments from contamination by radioactive, cytotoxic, and chemotoxic drugs
- Accurately identify, weigh, and measure ingredients
- Manipulate sterile products aseptically
- Sterilize high-risk level CSPs, while maintaining integrity and strength of active ingredients
- Label and quality inspect CSPs

The Role of the Pharmacist

State boards of pharmacy are often asked why an individual pharmacist who only "checks" the final preparation should receive the same training in sterile compounding as the pharmacists or pharmacy technicians who actually compound the preparations. As has already been stated, the most important consideration in compounding of sterile preparations is the safety of the patient for whom the preparation is intended. The pharmacist who provides the final verification of a compounded sterile preparation is usually the last person with pharmacy expertise who sees the preparation prior to its administration to the patient. Thus this person must be fully familiar with all aspects of the compounding of sterile preparations, including drug–diluent incompatibilities, physical characteristics of the finished preparation, proper dosing and calculations associated with the preparation, methods for determining whether precipitants exist in the preparation, and so on. For example, certain chemotherapeutic preparations are very highly colored. If a sterile doxorubicin preparation is being verified, the pharmacist verifying the preparation should expect to see a final preparation that is a shade of red and not dark blue, which could indicate that mitomycin was added to the diluent by mistake.

In particular, the pharmacist should verify the following items before releasing the CSP to leave the pharmacy:

■ Incompatibilities and/or particulate matter is not present in the CSP.
■ All calculations involved in preparation of the CSP were performed correctly.
■ The right drug was used.
■ The right volume of drug was used.
■ The right diluent was used.
■ The right volume of diluent was used.
■ The expiration date of drug(s) used is in-date.
■ The expiration date of diluent(s) used is in-date.
■ Labeling accurately reflects contents.
■ Auxiliary labels are included and are appropriate.
■ Instructions for administration are correct.

Pharmacists involved in the preparation and distribution of CSPs should consider the preceding list to be the minimum components that should be verified. Verification methods will vary by organization as well as by the type of preparation. For example, some organizations may utilize procedures that involve weighing the final preparation to verify the volume of contents added

Table 1-3 The Five Rights of Medication Administration

1. The right medication
2. The right dose
3. The right time
4. The right route
5. The right patient

to the CSP. Other preparations may require that two pharmacists are involved in the verification process.

Once the CSP has been distributed, those involved in administration of that CSP should utilize the "Five Rights" of medication administration—a patient safety measure that is completed prior to administering a medication to a patient (**Table 1-3**).

Conclusion

CSPs are an important mode of drug delivery for patients who may benefit from advantages that parenteral preparations provide. While risks are associated with administration of CSPs, it is the responsibility of all persons involved in the preparation and administration of CSPs to ensure that such risks are mitigated to the greatest extent possible by using proper techniques and having systems in place to ensure accuracy and sterility of the preparation. Personnel involved in the preparation process must unfailingly consider the patient who will be receiving the preparation and attitudes of patient safety must consistently and uniformly be employed.

Review Questions

1. List advantages and disadvantages of parenteral administration.
2. List circumstances in which parenteral administration may be preferred.

3. What is the role of attitude in parenteral product preparation?
4. Which methods can be utilized to increase safety and accuracy of parenteral preparation and administration?
5. Which USP chapters provide recommendations regarding the transport, storage, and preparation of compounded sterile preparations?

References

1. Thong B, Tan TC. Epidemiology and risk factors for drug allergy. *Br J Clin Pharmacol.* 2011;71(5):684–700.
2. Gomes ER, Demoly P. Epidemiology of hypersensitivity drug reactions. *Curr Opin Allergy Clin Immunol.* 2005;5:309–316.
3. Parker SE, Davey PG. Pharmacoeconomics of intravenous drug administration. *Pharmacoeconomics.*1992;1(2):103–115.
4. Williams KL. *Microbial contamination control in parenteral manufacturing.* New York, NY: Marcel Dekker; 2005:61.
5. American Society of Health System Pharmacists discussion guide on USP Chapter <797> for compounding sterile preparations. Available at: http://www.ashp.org/s_ashp/docs/files/discguide797-2008.pdf. Accessed May 5, 2013.
6. USP/NF Chapter <797>. Pharmaceutical compounding: sterile preparations. Available at: http://www.pharmacopeia.cn/v29240/usp29nf24s0_m88870.html. Accessed February 8, 2013.

Supplies and Equipment for Compounding and Administering Sterile Preparations

José A. Vega and Pamella S. Ochoa

Chapter Objectives

1. Review supplies used for compounding sterile preparations.
2. Differentiate open and closed systems.
3. Describe supplies and equipment utilized to administer compounded sterile preparations.
4. Identify factors that influence selection of supplies.
5. Describe important safety considerations with supplies used in preparation and administration of compounded sterile preparations.

Key Terminology

Gauge
Spike
Microns
Solutions
Reconstitute
Leaching

Adsorption
Absorption
Diluent
Admixture
Open system
Closed system
Diaphragm
Piggyback
Coring
Crystalloid solutions

Overview

Certain supplies are essential to conduct the necessary processes and techniques used for compounded sterile preparations (CSPs). This chapter introduces the supplies used in parenteral preparations and provides foundational knowledge that will be referenced in subsequent chapters.

A variety of supplies are used in the preparation process, each with a specific function, and understanding their role is important to be able to effectively prepare CSPs using sterile technique. Moreover, each category of these items often comes in a variety of types. The benefit of such variety is that the operator is able to select the most appropriate supplies during parenteral compounding to best facilitate an accurate preparation and efficient process. If inappropriate supplies or equipment are chosen, this can result in excess time consumption, errors in measurement, loss of product, or inability to effectively and properly prepare the CSP.

Needles and Syringes

Needles and syringes are used during the preparation process to facilitate manipulations. These supplies are fundamental for transferring of medications to and from a variety of containers. Both needles and syringes are manufactured in many different sizes and types, depending on the type of manipulation necessary.

NEEDLES · *attach to syringe*

Needles, made of aluminum or stainless steel, are utilized to transfer solutions and are fundamental in preparing CSPs. They are packaged individually by the manufacturer in a plastic or paper overwrap that guarantees sterility of the needle until the package has been opened or is no longer fully intact.

The parts of a needle are illustrated in **Figure 2-1**. The main parts of a needle are the bevel, hub, heel, shaft, and lumen. The bevel of the needle is the slanted portion of the needle that exposes the opening of the needle. It gives way to the sharp, pointed end of the needle, referred to as the bevel tip, which is intended to enter a vial or container. The heel of the needle is the short end of the bevel and is opposite from the sharp, pointed tip. The lumen, or

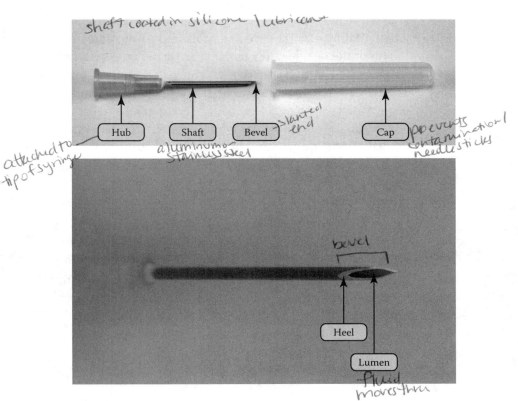

shaft coated in silicone lubricant

Hub — *attached to tip of syringe*
Shaft — *aluminum stainless steel*
Bevel — *slanted end*
Cap — *prevents contamination/needlesticks*

bevel

Heel

Lumen — *fluid moves thru*

Figure 2-1   Parts of a Needle

bore, of the needle is the inner portion of the needle that allows for the flow of liquid from a syringe into a container or vial. The shaft of the needle is composed of aluminum or stainless steel with an outer surface coated with a silicone lubricant to facilitate smooth penetration through the closures of containers. It is important never to wipe the outer surface of the needle with alcohol, as this action will remove the coating, making entries and exits of the needle through the rubber closures difficult. As the number of manipulations increases, the coating will gradually wear off. This becomes easy to identify during compounding because the entry into closures gradually becomes more difficult as the needle loses its gliding effect from lack of coating. The number of punctures, or entries into closures, per needle should not exceed five.

Needles vary in their length and lumen diameter, and both characteristics should be selected based on the intent of use. The length of the needle is the distance from the hub of the needle to the tip of the needle. The diameter of the lumen is referred to as the needle gauge and comes in different sizes, ranging from 13 to 31. Gauge is a unit of measurement developed early in the 19th century as a way to measure medical equipment and catheters. It was originally developed by the iron wire industry to standardize sizing of wiring, with its use to size needles evolving in the 20th century.[1,2] Besides needle hubs being color coded based on gauge size, needles are also labeled with a number, followed by a G, followed by yet another number. In the example 22 G ½, the "22" references the gauge (G), or outer diameter, of the needle; "G" is an abbreviation for "gauge"; and "½" refers to the length of the needle, in inches. As the number referring to the gauge of the needle increases, the lumen diameter decreases, and vice versa. For example, a 22-G needle will have a smaller lumen diameter than an 18-G needle. Examples of different gauges can be seen in **Figure 2-2**.

TIP: *As the gauge of the needle increases, the diameter of the needle lumen decreases.*

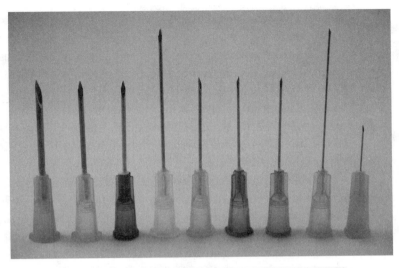

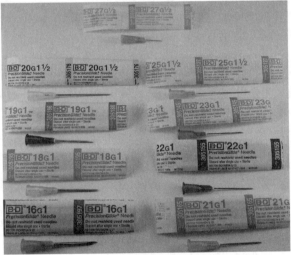

Figure 2-2 Needle Gauges

Selection of the proper gauge depends on the type of solution being transferred. For example, thick or viscous solutions should be transferred using small-gauge needles, such as 19–20, to allow for easier flow of the solution through the needle. Larger-gauge needles can be used for aqueous-based solutions. A needle with a smaller gauge may also serve best when penetrating thick rubber

SQ 5/8"

IM 1-1'/2"

closures, which will make entries easier. Although use of smaller-gauge needles allows for easier and quicker flow of solutions, the risk of coring increases as the gauge of the needle decreases. Thus smaller-gauge needles should be chosen only when needed and should not be utilized routinely. An 18-gauge needle is most commonly utilized for sterile compounding. Needle gauge is also a factor when administering CSPs. Gauges of 22–25 should be used to deliver IM injections, while gauges 23–25 are best suited for subcutaneous injections.

Needle lengths vary from ⅜ inch to 2 inches. A longer needle should be chosen when working with thick closures or lengthy entry ports on containers. When transferring solutions into a container through the entry port, using a longer needle will allow the contents of the syringe to be transferred directly into the container and prevent accumulation of solution within the entry port. Insulin needles with short needle lengths, for example, will deposit solutions into the entry port of large container bags, requiring subsequent flushing of the port. Needle length also becomes a consideration when administering medications to patients. Longer needles are required for intramuscular injections and shorter needles for subcutaneous and intradermal injections. For example, a needle length of 1–1.5 inches is typically chosen for IM injections in adults, while a needle length of ⅝ inch is typically used for subcutaneous injections in adults.

The gauge and length of the needle selected should also factor into the size of the syringe used. **Table 2-1** offers some guidelines for selecting the type of needle for routine manipulations based on the syringe size or solution type.

Several types of needles are available to facilitate different types of transfers and manipulations, including double-ended needles, filter needles, and vented needles. Also within a similar category, although not necessarily considered needles, are filter straws.

Double-Ended Needles and Transfer Sets

As the name describes, a double-ended, or double-sided, needle has two needles adjoined with a plastic center hub (**Figure 2-3**).

Table 2-1 Selecting Syringe and Needle Sizes[1]

Syringe Size	Needle Gauge	Needle Length
1 mL 3 mL 5 mL	20 gauge	1 inch
10 mL 20 mL 30 mL 60 mL	18 gauge	1½ inch
Large volume Viscous solutions	16 gauge	1½ inch
Ampule	Filter needle	

Source: Adapted from Aseptic technique: using needles, syringes, and filters. In: *Basics of aseptic compounding technique.* Bethesda, MD: American Society of Health-System Pharmacists; 2006:39.

The needle can be handled only from the center hub to avoid touching the metal portion of the needle, which would result in contamination. Double-ended needles are useful when transferring solutions directly from one container to another. When using a double-ended needle, one side of the needle is inserted into one container and the other side of the needle is inserted into a different container. The container into which solution is being transferred should be on the bottom during this process. This allows the content to flow directly from one container into the container on the bottom. Because these types of needles do not attach to a syringe, the volume of the contents cannot be measured. Thus double-ended needles are intended to be used when the entire contents of one container need to be transferred to another container.

Transfer sets are also used to transfer solutions directly from one container to another. Transfer sets consist of plastic tubing with a spike at one end, a syringe connection with a two-way valve at the other end, and a clamp in the middle (**Figure 2-4**). Because a syringe can be connected to one end of the transfer set, the flow

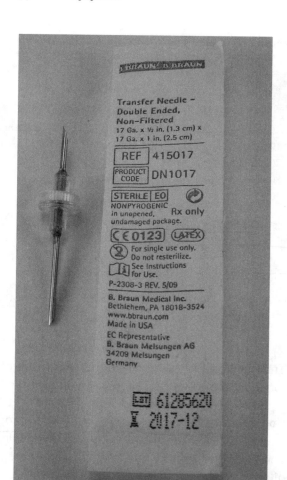

Figure 2-3 Double-Ended Needle

can be controlled and the volume of solution being transferred from one container to another can be measured.

Filter Needles and Filter Straws

Needles are available that contain a filter embedded within the hub of the needle and that attach to the syringe in a typical manner. The filter is typically 5 microns, which is the maximum pore size necessary to prevent particulate matter from passing through the needle. Although the filter cannot be seen, it plays an important role when transferring solutions from ampules. Fragments

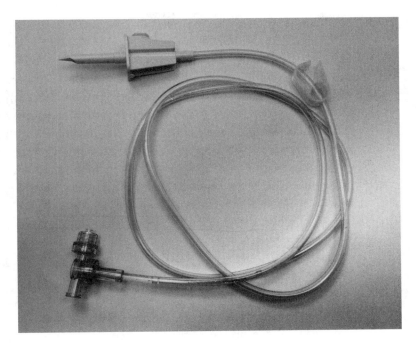

Figure 2-4   Transfer Set

of glass—some microscopic—can result from breaking an ampule and cause serious patient harm or death if infused. To prevent pieces of glass and other unwanted material from being transferred into the final preparation when withdrawing a solution from an ampule, a filter needle must be used every time. When using a filter needle to withdraw solution from an ampule into a syringe, particles are trapped on the underside of the filter. In contrast, solutions expelled from a syringe through a filter needle will result in particles being trapped on the upper side of the filter. Thus it is essential that filter needles be used only one time and used in only one direction. Using a filter needle to both withdraw and expel solution will cause any material trapped in the filter to be expelled into the final preparation.

ALERT: *Always use a filter needle when withdrawing solution from an ampule into a syringe. The needle should then be changed prior to expelling the contents from the syringe.*

If the contents of a syringe will be used for direct patient administration, a filter needle should be used to draw the solution into the syringe, and then the filter needle should be removed and replaced with a regular needle. Filter needles cannot be used with certain medications, such as suspensions and liposomal formulations, as the filter can remove important active ingredients.

Similar to filter needles, filter straws utilize filters within the hub to prevent passage of unwanted material. Filter straws are utilized for purposes similar to those for which filter needles are used. Because a filter straw has plastic tubing in place of the metal needle, it offers the benefit of flexibility and length, which can be useful when drawing up solutions from the bottom of large ampules.

Vented Needles

Vented needles are plastic spikes that are thicker in diameter than the typical needle (**Figure 2-5**). During preparation of CSPs, positive and negative pressure must be accounted for during withdrawal of solutions. Vented needles allow air to pass in and out of a "vent," thereby preventing pressure differences. These types of needles are useful whenever pressure effects are unwanted, but are particularly beneficial for reentering multiple-use vials or when preparing chemotherapy. Attaching a vented needle into a large-volume solution or multidose vial allows reentry multiple times without compromising the integrity of the closure of the container from multiple penetrations. When preparing chemotherapy, positive pressure can result in spraying of vial contents, putting the operator at risk of exposure. Vented needles alleviate the need to account for positive and negative pressures and result in better protection of the operator from spraying of hazardous drugs.

SYRINGES

Syringes attach to a needle and house solutions that are to be administered to a patient or transferred from one container to another. Traditionally, glass syringes were used, but have been almost completely replaced with plastic syringes. Glass syringes

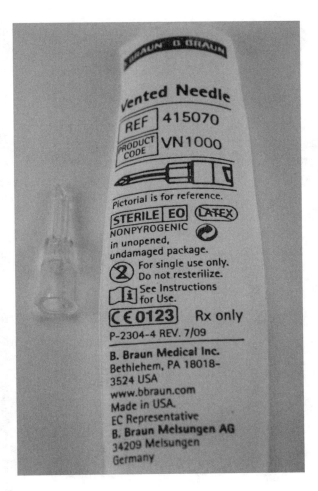

Figure 2-5   Vented Needle

are still used for patients with a plastic allergy and offer the advantage of being able to be sterilized and reused. While plastic syringes offer advantages in terms of less cost, less risk of breaking, and disposability, resulting in decreased risk of contamination, their increased use has also created minor issues with medications that are not compatible with plastic. Because of the short amount of time that the contents remain within the syringe when being transferred, this issue only rarely becomes a problem, such as with medications in which a direct incompatibility may exist. In these situations, using a glass syringe will circumvent compatibility issues arising from exposure to plastic.

Parts of a Syringe

The parts of a syringe are illustrated in **Figure 2-6**. These parts include the tip, barrel, plunger, top collar, and flange. Syringes are packaged by the manufacturer in an individually sealed paper or plastic overwrap and are intended for a single use. Sterility of the syringe is guaranteed until the package has been opened or has been compromised.

Syringes are available with a Luer Lock tip or a slip-tip (**Figure 2-7**). The tips of Luer Lock syringes contain threads that allow the needle hub to fasten onto the syringe by twisting the

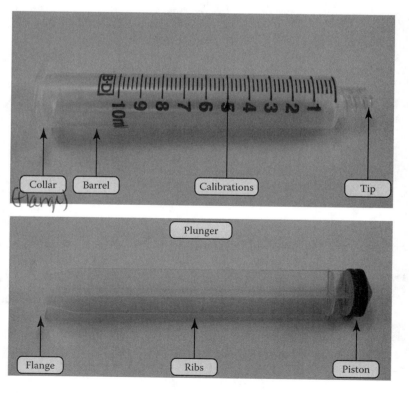

Figure 2-6   Parts of a Syringe

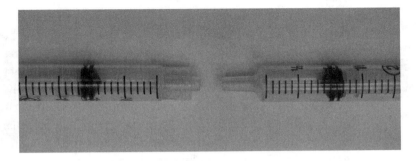

Figure 2-7   Luer Lock (l) and Slip-tip Syringes

hub onto the syringe tip. When using a Luer Lock syringe, the needle should be secured firmly, while taking care not to excessively tighten it. Luer Lock syringes are also available with a needle already attached. When using these types of syringes, the needle should be tightened slightly, prior to its use, by rotating the needle until firmly secured.

Slip-tip syringes do not contain threading; instead, they have a smooth surface upon which tension and friction allow the needle hub to stay attached to the syringe. A disadvantage of slip-tip syringes is the tendency of the needle to disengage from the syringe if not properly attached. When attaching a needle to a slip-tip syringe, the operator should press the hub of the needle firmly on the tip while using a slight twisting motion. Disengagement is most likely to occur when removing the needle cap from a needle attached to a slip-tip syringe. To avoid this problem, the syringe and needle can be slightly bent so as to provide tension at the point where the needle attaches to the syringe. When removing the cap, push the needle cap toward the syringe tip and then quickly pull the cap off while maintaining a slight bend. This should be done in one continuous motion. Because of the potential for needles to disengage from a slip-tip syringe, these types of syringes should not be used to prepare chemotherapy or other hazardous agents.

The barrel of the syringe holds the solution that is to be transferred. Calibration marks are found on the barrel that permit volume measurement. As the size of the syringe increases, the increments of the calibration marks become larger.

divide smallest increment of calibration marks in half to determine accuracy of syringe

The syringe plunger consists of the plunger piston, ribs, and flange. The flange is also referred to as the lip or flat end of the plunger. The ribs of the plunger are located between the flange and the plunger tip. This portion of the plunger comes in contact with the inside of the barrel when the plunger is pushed in fully; thus the inside of the barrel may become contaminated if the ribs are touched. The flange provides a flat surface that facilitates manipulation of the syringe. The tip of the plunger piston is pointed and resembles a triangle. The plunger piston comes in direct contact with the solution being transferred and is used to measure the syringe's contents along the calibration marks. The base, or flat, part of the triangular portion is referred to as the final edge and should be used to align with the calibration marks to measure the desired volume. **Figure 2-8** illustrates the final edge of the piston plunger that is aligned using the calibration marks to ensure accurate measurements; this figure depicts a measurement to 10 mL.

TIP: *The final edge of the plunger piston should be aligned with the calibration marks on a syringe to measure the desired volume.*

Syringe Size

Syringe sizes vary from 0.5 mL to 60 mL, indicating the maximum volume that can be drawn up into the syringe. As the size of the syringe increases, the length and diameter of the syringe also increase. As mentioned previously, calibration marks vary with syringe size. For example, a 1-mL syringe will have calibration marks in increments of 0.01 mL, beginning with 0.01 mL and increasing to 1 mL.

It is important to consider accuracy of measurement when selecting a proper syringe size. A large syringe, for instance, should not be selected to draw up a small volume. Literature substantiates the relationship between syringe size and accuracy. One study found that both accuracy and reproducibility of 0.5 mL of volume decreased as the syringe size increased from 1 mL to 5 mL, with an error toward overdelivery of volume as the

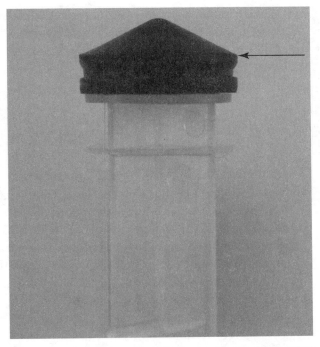

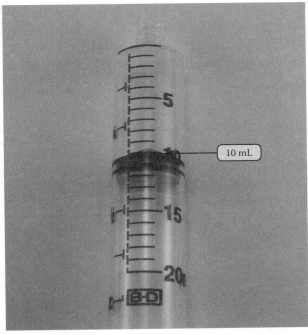

10 mL

Figure 2-8   Final Edge of Piston Plunger Used for Measuring

syringe size increased.[3] Thus small syringes will have the greatest accuracy compared to other sizes due to the small increments of the calibration marks. As a rule of thumb, the smallest syringe size that can accommodate the desired volume should be chosen.

> **TIP:** *The smallest syringe size that can accommodate the desired volume should be used.*

Accuracy of a syringe can be determined by dividing the smallest increment of the calibration marks in half. For example, a 10-mL syringe with 0.2-mL increments will be accurate up to 0.1 mL. Therefore, measurements of 3.2 mL and 5.1 mL could all be measured with confidence in accuracy. In contrast, measurements of 3.25 mL or 5.09 mL could not be accurately measured in a 10-mL syringe. Calibration increments for common syringe sizes can be found in **Table 2-2**.

Mistakes during measurement may arise secondary to confusion created by the calibration markings of insulin syringes and 1-mL syringes. Calibration marks on an insulin syringe are in units, the standard measurement of insulin. Because most

Table 2-2 Calibration Mark Increments for Common Syringe Sizes

Syringe Size	Calibration Graduations
Insulin syringes:	
Standard U-100 (holds 1 mL or 100 units)	2 units (dual scale with numerical markings for every 10 units—with even 2 unit increments on one side and odd 2 unit increments on the other)
U-50 (holds 0.5 mL or 50 units)	1 unit
U-30 (holds 0.3 mL or 30 units)	1 unit
1 mL (tuberculin syringe)	0.01 mL
3 mL	0.1 mL
5 mL	0.2 mL
10 mL	0.2 mL
20 mL	1 mL
30 mL	1 mL
60 mL	2 mL

manipulations involve measurements with calibration markings in milliliters, switching between insulin syringes and 1-mL syringes commonly results in a mistake in the volume of insulin withdrawn. With insulin being a high-risk medication, this type of error can result in great harm to the patient and even death.

Oral Syringes

Oral syringes allow medications to be administered directly to the patient, but the structure of the syringe tip will not accommodate attachment of a needle. In the inpatient setting, oral syringes can be available, but must be used only for oral administration of medications. Similarly, non-oral syringes should never be used for delivering oral medications. Using non-oral syringes to hold oral medications can result in accidental administration of an oral medication through a parenteral route. To prevent this possibility, oral medications must never be placed in a non-oral syringe. A multitude of incidents involving such accidental administration have been reported, with many resulting in irreversible patient harm and death of adults and children alike.[4] In an effort to increase patient safety, any medication to be administered orally should be prepared only in an oral syringe and should be clearly marked with an auxiliary label, such as "For Oral Use Only."

ALERT: *Oral medications must never be placed in a non-oral syringe.*

Prefilled Syringes

Often, medications may be drawn up into a syringe with the intention of delivering them via direct patient administration through parenteral routes. When preparing a syringe for direct patient administration, the needle can be removed from the syringe and a plastic syringe cap can be easily pushed or twisted onto the tip of a syringe to provide closure and maintain sterility until the contents are ready to be administered (**Figure 2-9**).

Prefilled syringes are also available; these syringes are provided by the manufacturer with a specific volume of medication

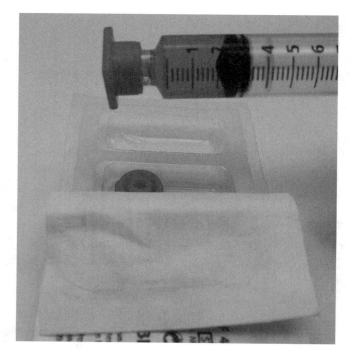

Figure 2-9 Syringe Cap

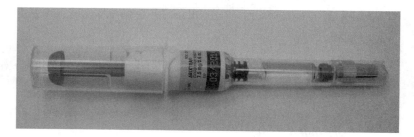

Figure 2-10 Prefilled Syringe

already present within the syringe and are intended for direct administration to a patient (**Figure 2-10**). These types of syringes are gaining popularity in the healthcare setting and their use is expected to increase over the next few decades. Such single-use syringes are provided by the manufacturer in either glass or plastic and come either as a needleless system that attaches directly to an access catheter or as a unit with a needle already attached. Glass prefilled syringes can be dual-chambered devices, with one chamber containing medication in a powder formulation and the other a diluent. The syringe can be activated and the contents of both chambers mixed just prior to administration.

Prefilled syringes accommodate volumes that typically range from 0.25 to 5 mL and are most suitable for solutions or medications that will be administered by subcutaneous or intramuscular injection. Antithrombotics, vaccines, and biotechnology-based drugs account for the majority of prefilled syringes currently available.[5] Some interferons, rheumatoid arthritis medications, and blood stimulants are also provided by the manufacturer in prefilled syringes.

Because these syringes are prefilled, and some are needle-less units, the operator does not need to withdraw medication from a vial, which in turn minimizes the potential for medication errors, contamination, and needle sticks. Besides improved accuracy and safety, prefilled syringes offer added convenience, efficiency, and ease of use. Disadvantages of these systems include their complexity as well as the potential for needle sticks with those that are not provided by the manufacturer as needleless devices. Additionally, problems with malfunction, breaking, or clogging with certain prefilled glass syringes have been reported in the past. Because of these limitations, in 2011 the FDA recommended the avoidance of needleless glass prefilled syringes in emergency situations.[6]

Safety Needles/Syringes   protect healthcare workers

Needle stick injuries from manipulation of needles introduce occupational hazards to healthcare personnel and introduce the potential for transmission of blood-borne pathogens. At an average-size hospital, approximately 30 needle stick injuries are reported by workers for every 100 beds every year.[7] Thus needle safety is of great concern in the healthcare setting.

To mitigate these risks, a variety of safety syringes are available with different mechanisms to shield the needle following use. One type, for instance, will inactivate the plunger of the syringe once the plunger is fully depressed, preventing reuse of

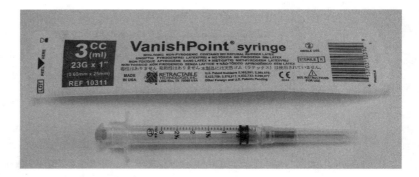

Figure 2-11   Safety Syringe

the syringe altogether. Another type of safety syringe shields the needle, either by retracting the needle into the syringe barrel when the plunger of the needle is pulled back or by deploying a protective shield over the needle. **Figure 2-11** depicts an example of a safety syringe. Safety syringes and needles are more expensive, but are much more effective at protecting the healthcare worker from needle sticks.

Types of Containers

Containers are used throughout the sterile compounding process to house solutions such as diluents and medications, as well as powders for reconstitution. Empty containers into which solutions are transferred or for mixing multiple product preparations are also available. Most solutions placed within containers will chemically interact with the container either minimally or to the point of incompatibility. The type of container used for storing CSPs needs to be considered so as to minimize any potential interaction between the container and the preparation. While the manufacturer provides medications in suitable containers, sometimes the operator must choose the container type when preparing CSPs. Therefore, the operator should be knowledgeable as to the various forms of containers and be able to select the proper container appropriately.

AMPULES

Ampules are glass containers that hold sterile injectable solutions (**Figure 2-12**). Ampules may be used to contain hazardous medications, diluents, and medications with volumes that can range from 1 mL to 50 mL. Often, medications that pose risk of chemical incompatibility with plastic are supplied in glass ampules. Ampules, which structurally consist of a neck and a body, must be broken at the neck prior to accessing their contents. Many ampules are scored or have pressure points located on the neck to facilitate breaking them at the desired point. If it proves difficult to break the ampule, it can be turned one-quarter turn, which may help with locating the pressure point. A polyethylene breaker/collar that slips over the neck of the ampule can be used

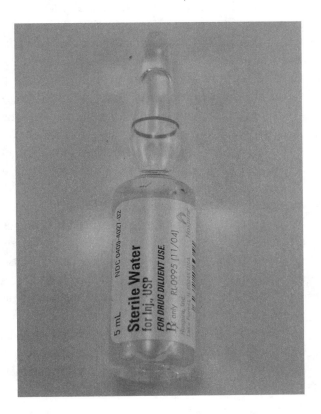

Figure 2-12 Ampule

to improve the operator's grip on the ampule neck, thereby facilitating breaking the ampule in a safe manner. Additionally, the barrel of a 10-mL sterile, clean syringe with the plunger removed can be slipped over the neck of the ampule, providing leverage and improving safety and ease of breaking.

As mentioned previously, because of the potential for glass to enter the solution being withdrawn, a filter needle or filter straw must be used when withdrawing or expelling contents from an ampule. All ampules are intended for single-dose only.

VIALS

Vials are made of either plastic or, more commonly, glass. Vials may contain medications in the form of a solution or a freeze-dried sterile powder that requires a diluent be added to form a solution, a process referred to as reconstitution. Because contents of glass vials are packed under a vacuum, some glass vials are equipped with venting tubing—that is, a small air tube located within the vial that facilitates removal of the solution without the need for venting by the operator. Glass vials typically have a rubber closure, also referred to as the rubber stopper or diaphragm, to prevent free passage of air or fluids in or out of the vial. An aluminum sealing ring along the circumference of the rubber closure secures it in place. A flip-top cap or aluminum cover protects the top of the rubber closure; it must be removed to access the contents of the vial. While these covers protect the otherwise exposed rubber closure, they do not guarantee sterility of the closure. Thus it is necessary to disinfect the rubber closure prior to puncturing it.

Plastic vials are available for some medications and are structured similar to the glass vials, with a rubber closure and flip-top cap. Other plastic vials are manufactured with a plastic pull ring that is removed in a circular manner to reveal a rubber plug that can be completely removed. This type of plastic vial is intended to be attached directly to a bag for intravenous infusion, and is commonly referred to as an adaptable system or adaptable container.

SINGLE-USE AND MULTIPLE-USE VIALS

Medications provided by the manufacturer in vials as solutions can be classified as single-use or multiple-use products, also referred to as single-dose and multidose vials. The differentiating factor is the addition of a preservative to the solution. When medications are manufactured with small amounts of preservatives, the length of time that the solution can be used is extended. The addition of preservatives impedes the growth of bacteria and other microorganisms within the solution. While the preservatives may retard the growth of bacteria, they will not ensure sterility if contamination occurs. Thus sterile techniques during the preparation process still need to be employed.

Vials that are intended for multiple uses contain preservatives and bear a label that identifies them as such. If the vial labeling does not state that it is a multiple-use product, then it should be considered to be for single use. Preservatives commonly used in multiple-use vials include phenol, benzalkonium chloride, benzyl alcohol, parabens, chlorobutanol, phenylmercuric salts, cresol, and thimerosal. Bacteriostatic water for injection contains preservatives, but addition of bacteriostatic water to reconstitute powders does not make the final solution appropriate for multiple uses. Because the addition of preservatives is in small amounts and safe for administration in normal doses, whenever large doses are used, the total amount of preservatives that will be administered to the patient needs to be considered.

It is imperative that medications containing preservatives never be used for epidural or intrathecal administration. Such administration can cause toxicity to the patient. In neonatal and pediatric patients, a small amount of preservative in medications can be significant relative to their size and, therefore, can also lead to toxicity. Given these considerations, preservative-free formulations should always be chosen, when available. When preparing preservative-free medications with the addition of bacteriostatic water for injection, the final solution will contain preservatives and should not be administered via epidural or intrathecal injection; its use should also be avoided in pediatric and neonatal populations.

ALERT: *Medications that contain preservatives or are prepared with bacteriostatic water for injection must never be used for epidural or intrathecal administration.*

ADAPTABLE SYSTEMS

ADD-Vantage, Vial-Mate, add-EASE, and Minibag Plus are all examples of adaptable systems (**Figure 2-13**). These systems facilitate direct attachment of a vial to a bag of diluent and are often referred to as ready-mix systems. Vial-Mate and add-EASE are binary connectors that allow the attachment of a vial and a bag together. ADD-Vantage and Minibag Plus systems utilize a special bag of diluent with three main components:

- Set port: for attaching tubing for administration to the patient
- Vial attachment port: for direct attachment of the vial to the bag
- Seal: to prevent the diluent from entering into the vial until the medication is ready to be administered

The ADD-Vantage system has a round plastic pull ring on the bag that is pulled and removed, allowing a vial to be securely screwed into the port. Plastic vials manufactured specifically for this type of system also have a plastic pull ring that can be removed in a circular fashion and is intended to allow attachment of the vial to the bag. The Vial-Mate system contains a plastic adapter with a spike that is covered for sterility and is directly attached to the bag. Once the spike cover is removed, the adapter can be firmly placed atop a compatible vial with a rubber closure and attached by pressing firmly on the plastic adapter, pushing the spike through the rubber closure of the vial.

When the medication is ready to be administered, tubing should be attached and the seal between the bag and the vial must be broken, which will allow the diluent from the bag to enter into the vial. The seal on the ADD-Vantage system consists of a rubber stopper located on the inner portion of the bag; this rubber stopper is cleaved to remove the seal. The seal on the Vial-Mate is a plastic cylinder between the bag and the vial. It can be "snapped" by applying inward pressure, similar to breaking a pencil. Once the seal is broken, the contents of the bag will move freely in and out of the vial. Slight pressure can then be applied to the bag to facilitate flow of the diluent into the vial. The vial and bag should

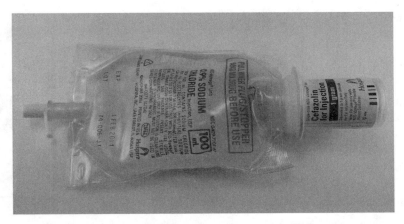

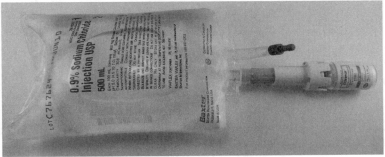

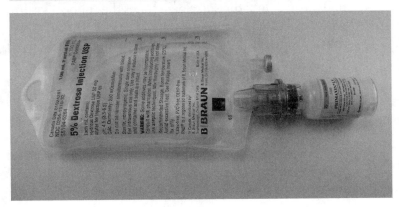

Figure 2-13 Adaptable Systems (ADD-Vantage®, Vial-Mate®, add-EASE®, and Minibag Plus: in order from top to bottom)

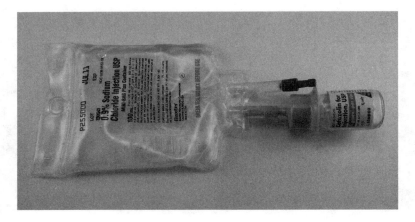

Figure 2-13   (*continued*)

be inverted several times to ensure that the contents of the bag and vial are well mixed prior to administration.

The add-EASE binary connector is plastic and structured similar to a cylinder with two spikes on either end, one for attaching to the vial and the other for attaching to a bag. To use this connector, the spike is centered on the rubber closure of the vial and pushed until the spike penetrates the rubber closure and the connector latches on to the top of the vial. The second spike, on the opposite end, is firmly pushed onto the medication port of the bag. When the medication is ready to be administered, the connector can be activated by folding the bag at the fluid line, which will deploy a plug from the connector into the medication vial. Squeezing the bag will result in flow of solution from the bag into the vial for mixing.

The Minibag Plus is similar to the Vial-Mate except the connector is already attached to the bag. The plastic connector spikes into the vial similarly to the Vial-Mate.

Several advantages and disadvantages are associated with adaptable systems. First, cost should be considered prior to adopting these systems, as the supplies are more costly than traditional supplies. Nevertheless, the faster preparation time, accuracy, reduction in drug wastage, and longer expiration dates help offset this increased cost. For example, adaptable systems facilitate direct attachment of the vial to a bag, while preparing the same medication without the adaptable system would require a syringe, needle, and personnel time and introduce the potential for errors in the measuring process. Additionally, because the medication in the vial and the solution in the bag remain separate until ready to be administered, the expiration dates are much longer compared to those observed when adding the medication from a vial directly into the bag. Adaptable systems also offer the advantage of convenience and improved efficiency, but come with the disadvantage of needing to store additional inventory, such as vials, that are specific to the system. *special equipment improper activation*

PREMIXED PARENTERAL MEDICATIONS

Many IV medications are available in an appropriate type and volume of diluent, ready for patient administration. Using premixed medications can circumvent problems often encountered with prepared admixtures, such as preparation errors and interruptions in pharmacy workflow. Delays in access to medications, resulting in delayed administration, is a consequence of preparing admixtures that can be improved with use of premixed medications. This is particularly beneficial in emergent situations requiring quick administration of medications. Use of premixed medications may be beneficial in preventing accidental misadventures related to standard and maximum allowed concentrations with high-risk medications. Use of premixed medications has also been found to improve time management and efficiency by saving time and labor, reducing turnaround time, eliminating admixture errors, and reducing drug waste.[8] Examples of premixed medications include metronidazole, theophylline, heparin, and amiodarone.

PLASTIC AND GLASS CONTAINERS

Containers for solutions used in parenteral preparations are made of either glass or plastic. Plastic containers are the most commonly used container for parenteral CSPs, storage of parenteral products, and patient administration. Plastics are mostly made of polymers, including polyethylene polypropylene, polyvinyl chloride (PVC), and polyolefin, some of which are not conducive to certain types of sterilization processes such as autoclaving.[9]

Table 2-3 Advantages and Disadvantages of Plastic and Glass Containers

	Advantages	Disadvantages
Glass	• Decreased chemical interactions between container and contents • Ability to sterilize	• Vacuum (in unvented bottles) • Breakability • Maximum volume of 1 L
Plastic	• Easy storage, including freezing • Flexibility of container • Disposability • Easily hung for IV administration	• Chemical incompatibilities • Easily punctured

Plastic containers offer many advantages over glass containers, as summarized in **Table 2-3**. Plastic containers tend to be less expensive than containers made of other materials and offer the convenience of easy storage and disposal. Despite their many advantages, use of plastic containers presents the most potential for problems with chemical reactions between the container and its contents—for example, leaching, absorption, and adsorption. Both leaching and adsorption are the result of chemical reactions that occur secondary to decreased chemical resistance with changes in pH levels of the contents. Other reactions, such as oxidation, can occur based on changes in temperature and pressure conditions and additives found in the container. Due to the permeable nature of plastic containers, medications that are easily oxidized cannot be stored in plastic containers; such is the case with nitroglycerin. Medications that are incompatible with plastic when in a solution are often stored in a powder formulation in glass containers, with the powder requiring reconstitution before its administration to a patient. Adding a solvent prior to administration minimizes the time that the medication spends as a solution and the contact time with the container. Examples of medications that are stored as powder formulations include vancomycin, penicillin, and ceftazidime.

Glass containers are less commonly used owing to the disadvantages listed in Table 2-3. Glass, which mostly consists of silicone dioxide, is used for ampules, vials, and large empty containers. While one of the most readily apparent disadvantages of glass is the risk of breaking, these containers offer the advantage of being less permeable and less likely to result in chemical reactions. The most likely reaction to occur with use of glass containers results from leaching of oxides from the glass into the solution, which can induce pH or other changes in the solution and give rise to additional chemical reactions. Different classifications of glass are available based on the chemical resistance of the glass to leaching and other chemical reactions. The United States Pharmacopeia (USP) provides a recommended maximum volume for glass containers and glass ampules, as well as overall requirements for glass containers.

When transferring medications into containers, the selection of glass or plastic should be considered. Manufacturer recommendations for the medication should be referenced to determine its potential incompatibility with plastic or glass.

Solutions or powders stored in plastic and glass containers are subject to light exposure, which can affect the integrity of some medications. Containment in amber glass can decrease the amount of light that enters the container. Certain medications that undergo chemical reactions secondary to light exposure are often provided by manufacturers in amber glass, such as multivitamins that degrade over time with light exposure. For certain CSPs, brown, green, or black plastic sleeves can be placed over the container to decrease light exposure. Some products include light-protective plastic sleeves in their packaging to ensure the preparation is light protected; **Figure 2-14** shows a sodium nitroprusside light-protective sleeve. Further information regarding compatibility and stability with glass and plastic will be discussed in a subsequent chapter of this text.

DILUENTS

Bags and bottles of solution are available as diluents for administration to patients for purposes of fluid and electrolyte replacement as well as for dilution of medications. An admixture is defined as a final solution resulting from medications, referred to as additives, being added to a bag or bottle of diluent.

The main parts of a plastic bag include an eyehole at the top of the bag for hanging the bag on an IV pole, a medication port, and

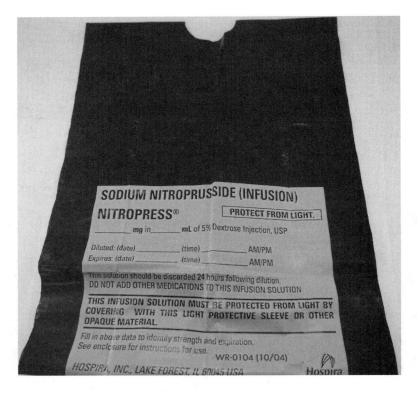

Figure 2-14   Light Protective Sleeve

an administration set port (**Figure 2-15**). Bags, which are more commonly used than bottles, are available for a variety of solutions with volumes ranging from 50 mL to 3000 mL. Bottles are available in a maximum size of 1000 mL, per USP requirements.

Most commonly, medications are added to bags or bottles containing either 0.9% sodium chloride, also called normal saline (NS), or 5% dextrose in water (D_5W). Compatibility, isotonicity, and patient-specific needs should all be considered when choosing the type of diluent; **Table 2-4** lists the types of diluents available. Many variations of NS, lactated Ringer's solution, and D_5W are available. While the majority of medications are compatible with NS, which is the most widely used diluent, some medications can be added only to D_5W due to compatibility limitations. For example, and in consideration of patient-specific factors, if a medication can be added to either D_5W or NS and the patient has diabetes with high blood glucose readings, NS may be the better choice for the patient. This decision is often left to the pharmacist's discretion but should be made in consultation with the prescribing physician.

Concentrated potassium chloride is often added to D_5W, NS, and parenteral nutrition for electrolyte replenishment.

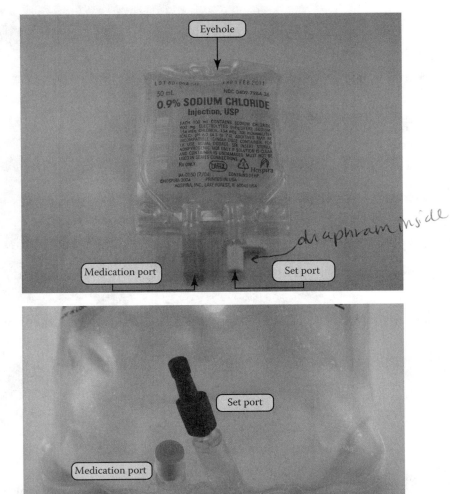

Figure 2-15   Parts of a Bag

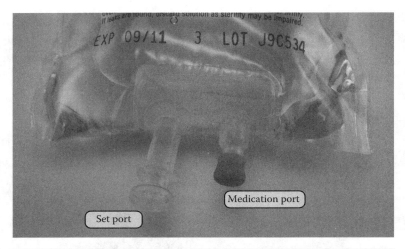

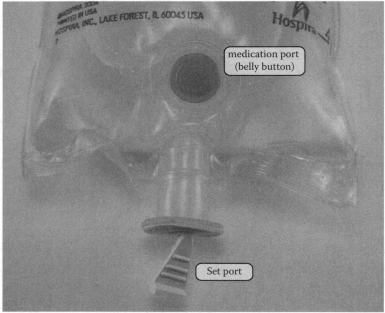

Figure 2-15   (*continued*)

Concentrated potassium chloride should be used only as an additive: It will cause patient death if injected directly or will cause serious patient harm, including cardiac dysfunction, with excessive doses or rates of infusion. Thus concentrated formulations of this high-risk medication should never be stored outside the

Table 2-4 Diluent Types

Diluent Type	Abbreviation	How Supplied	Parenteral Type
Sterile water	W or SWI	Sterile water for injection	LVP and SVP
Dextrose	D$_5$W	5% dextrose in water	LVP and SVP
	D$_5$NS	5% dextrose with 0.9% sodium chloride	LVP
	D$_{10}$W	10% dextrose in water	LVP
	D$_{10}$NS	10% dextrose with 0.9% sodium chloride	LVP
Saline	NaCl	3% sodium chloride	LVP
		5% sodium chloride	LVP
Normal saline	NS	0.9% sodium chloride	LVP and SVP
			LVP
Half-strength normal saline	½NS	0.45% sodium chloride	LVP
	D$_5$ ½NS	0.45% sodium chloride with 5% dextrose	
	¼NS	0.2% sodium chloride	LVP
Quarter-strength normal saline	D$_{10}$ ¼NS	0.2% sodium chloride with 5% dextrose	

(continues)

Table 2-4 Diluent Types (*continued*)

Diluent Type	Abbreviation	How Supplied	Parenteral Type
Lactated Ringer's (or Ringer's lactate)	LR	Ringer's injection	LVP
		Lactated Ringer's	
	D₅LR	Lactated Ringer's and 5% dextrose	LVP
Potassium chloride	KCl	Potassium chloride (as vial for additive only)	SVP
	NS with 20KCl	20 mEq/L potassium chloride with 0.9% sodium chloride	LVP
	NS with 40KCl	40 mEq/L potassium chloride with 0.9% sodium chloride	LVP
	½NS with 20KCl	20 mEq/L potassium chloride with 0.45% sodium chloride	LVP
	D₅W with 20KCl	20 mEq/L potassium chloride with 5% dextrose in water	LVP
	D₅W with 40KCl	40 mEq/L potassium chloride with 5% dextrose in water	LVP
	D₅ ¼NS with 20KCl	20 mEq/L potassium chloride with 5% dextrose and 0.2% sodium chloride	LVP
	D₅NS with 20KCl	20 mEq/L potassium chloride with 5% dextrose and 0.9% sodium chloride	LVP
	D₅NS with 40KCl	40 mEq/L potassium chloride with 5% dextrose and 0.9% sodium chloride	LVP

pharmacy, care should be taken while mixing preparations, and strict verification procedures should be in place.

> **ALERT:** *Concentrated potassium chloride is considered a high-risk medication and should be used only as an additive. Direct injection of potassium chloride and excessive doses can be fatal.*

Both NS and sterile water for injection (SWI) are considered the best diluents for reconstitution. NS is isotonic and can be used as IV fluid replacement for direct patient administration and as a diluent for medication reconstitution and dilution. SWI, in contrast, is hypotonic and should never be administered directly to a patient through the intravenous route. Such administration can cause hemolysis, resulting in serious patient harm. Confusion regarding the direct infusion of SWI may be influenced by the availability of this solution in a large IV bag that looks similar to IV bags of NS and D_5W. Error reporting programs have received multiple reports of direct IV administration of SWI, some of which resulted in patient death.[10] USP requires that bags of SWI be labeled with cautionary statements that sterile water "is not suitable for intravascular injection without first being having been made approximately isotonic by the addition of a suitable solute."[11] While the bags made available by the manufacturer are appropriately labeled, the text is often overlooked. Thus it is important to place the hospital patient label on the same side as the cautionary text, which may help alert personnel to the restrictions when reading the patient label. Reconstitution of powders for injection requires a relatively small volume of SWI, which should then be added to a larger volume of isotonic D_5W or NS for IV administration.

> **ALERT:** *Patient harm may result from direct injection or infusion of sterile water for injection. This diluent must first be made isotonic prior to intravascular injection.*

USP defines small-volume injections, also referred to as small-volume parenterals (SVPs), as those packaged and labeled with a volume of 100 mL or less.[11] Large-volume intravenous solutions, or large-volume parenterals (LVPs), are those labeled with a volume greater than 100 mL,[11] with typical sizes being 250 mL, 500 mL, and 1000 mL. LVPs are available in glass bottles, both vented and unvented, and in plastic bags. Plastic bags collapse when all air and fluid have been removed from the bag. Large-volume plastic bags are available as in 1 L, 2 L, and 3 L and are used for a variety of solutions, such as parenteral nutrition. Glass bottles are often packaged with a vacuum, requiring air to enter the bottle before the solution will flow out from the bottle. Vented glass bottles contain a small air tube that provides venting. Unvented bottles require administration using a special infusion set that supplies the bottle with air through an airway in the spike. SVPs include minibags, vials, ampules, and prefilled syringes.

Piggyback containers, also known as secondary infusion containers, are used to deliver a second infusion that "piggybacks" onto the primary administration set via a Y-site or medication port. These containers, which usually hold volumes of 50 mL to 250 mL in flexible bags, are manufactured with a base solution to which medications are added. Empty containers are also available for adding customized parenteral preparations.

The volume of diluent selected should be based on medication-specific concentration maximums and any patient-specific factors. For example, fluid-restricted or pediatric patients may require less total volume. In these situations, admixtures may be prepared with the smallest volume of diluent that is necessary to provide adequate stability of the medication in solution. Manufacturer recommendations, as well as compatibility resources, provide information on the maximum concentrations that are appropriate for parenteral medications. Certain medications that have a high likelihood of causing patient harm if infused at high concentrations or at too rapid an infusion rate are considered high-risk IV medications. In an effort to prevent patient harm, these high-risk medications should have standardized and maximum allowable concentrations and, without deviation, always be prepared at such concentrations that are established by the institution.

Open and Closed Systems

Containers can be classified as open or closed systems based on structural differences of the closure. Open systems refer to closures that expose the medication, solution, or powder to air when the container is opened. An example of an open system is an ampule. Once opened, air and fluid can freely move in and out of the ampule. In contrast, closed systems do not allow passage of air once opened. An example of a closed system is a vial in which, once the vial is opened or accessed, air does not pass in and out of the container. Plastic bags are also considered closed systems. The importance of understanding the distinction between open and closed systems derives from the differences in contamination risk between these two systems. As would be expected, as air exposure increases, the risk of contamination increases as well. Thus open systems have greater risk of contamination.

Supplies for Administration

Once a parenteral CSP is prepared and verified, it is ready to be administered to the patient. The final preparation will typically be in a bag, syringe, or glass container for direct administration. Certain administration supplies are needed to facilitate delivery of the medication from the container or syringe into the patient. A catheter is placed in the patient to whom the medication or solution will be administered. With intravenous administration, for instance, a catheter is placed within the vein and medications or solutions are dripped or pumped into the catheter for infusion into the vein.

Administration Sets

Intravenous administration of solutions or medications from a glass bottle or bag requires the use of an administration set.

Several types of administration sets exist, but most commonly such sets will include the following main parts:

1. Tubing: plastic tubing with two ends, one for attachment to the patient catheter and the other for attachment to the bag or bottle.
2. Needle adapter: located at the end of the tubing and structured to attach directly to the catheter.
3. Clamp: typically a roller or slide clamp. Increasing intensities of pinching will narrow the tubing to regulate the flow of the fluid through the tubing. The clamps can be loosened so that fluid freely moves through the tubing, can be completely clamped off, or can be manipulated for slower or faster flow of fluid.
4. Drip chamber: a plastic cylinder attached to the tubing, directly below the bag, into which the contents of the bag or bottle drip prior to flowing into the tubing. The drip chamber can be used to regulate the rate of infusion in drops per minute (gtt/min) or mL/hr, although regulation "by eye" is infrequently used with the advent of infusion pumps. Some drip chambers have graduated markings to allow for more accurate determination of the infusion rate.
5. Spike: located at the end of the tubing opposite the needle adapter. The spike is used to puncture the set port of the bag or rubber stopper of a bottle.
6. Proximal Y-site: located between the drip chamber and the clamp. This additive, or injection, port is used to attach secondary IV sets and contains a back-check valve that restricts upward flow of fluid from the tubing back into the IV bag.
7. Additive port or distal Y-site: located near the needle adapter. This port provides a site through which medications can be directly infused into the vein. It contains a rubber diaphragm that can be punctured by a needle.

Manual setups of IV fluids using administration sets alone rely on gravity for infusing solutions and medications into the patient. Rates of infusion can be determined by observing the drip chamber and then adjusting the clamp to increase or decrease the rate. Infusion rate is also a factor of the tubing diameter. Macrodrip sets are wider and deliver 10, 15, or 20 gtt/mL, whereas microdrip sets are narrower and deliver 60 gtt/mL.

Administration sets are prone to contamination, so their intermittent replacement is required to prevent growth of microbes that might otherwise result in catheter-related bloodstream infections (CRBSIs). Data from studies reveal that replacing IV administration sets no more frequently than 72–96 hours following initial use is considered both safe and cost effective.[12] More recent studies suggest that administration sets may not require replacement for as long as 7 days if they are used with antiseptic catheters or if fluids that enhance microbial growth, such as parenteral nutrition or blood, have not been infused through the set.[12] Fluids that potentiate microbial growth, such as fat emulsions and blood, require more frequent changes of administration sets because they have been identified as risk factors for CRBSIs.[12] The Centers for Disease Control and Prevention (CDC) has issued recommendations regarding the frequency of replacing infusion sets, which are summarized in **Table 2-5**.

Secondary Sets

Additional tubing can be attached to a primary infusion set to infuse a secondary IV medication, or an IV piggyback (IVPB). The addition of a secondary set will interrupt the primary infusion to allow for the second medication to be infused. **Figure 2-16** depicts a secondary infusion set attached to a primary infusion set. To piggyback a medication, a secondary set is attached to the proximal Y-site of the primary infusion set. This allows for the primary solution, such as NS for fluid replacement, and another medication, such as an antibiotic, to be infused without the need to remove the primary infusion tubing. A back-check valve located on the primary infusion set prevents backflow of the second medication up through the primary IV tubing. Along with the back-check valve, hanging the secondary medication higher than the primary medication will cause its flow rate to overcome

Table 2-5   CDC Recommendations on Changing Infusion Set Tubing

Type of Product Infused	Frequency of Tubing Change
Any product in which the administration set is continuously used, including secondary sets and add-on devices Exceptions: • Blood • Blood products • Fat emulsions	No more frequently than 96-hour intervals, but at least every 7 days
Tubing used to administer the following products when combined with amino acids and glucose or when infused alone: • Blood • Blood products • Fat emulsions	Within 24 hours of initiating infusion
Propofol infusions	Every 6 or 12 hours, when the vial is changed, per the manufacturer recommendation
Intermittently used administration sets	No recommendation can be made

Source: Adapted from Centers for Disease Control and Prevention. Guidelines for the prevention of intravascular catheter-related infections. 2011. http://www.cdc.gov /hicpac/pdf/guidelines/bsi-guidelines-2011.pdf. Accessed November 25, 2012.

the flow rate of the primary infusion, thereby preventing mixing of the secondary solution into the primary solution.

IN-LINE FILTERS

Various studies have demonstrated the presence of particulate matter in solutions infused into patients, such as glass fragments from ampules, rubber pieces from coring, and particulate matter resulting from incompatibilities of parenteral nutrition additives or inherent within drug formulations.[13] Infusion of such particles can cause serious patient harm and potentially death as a result of blocked vessels from occlusive microemboli. Use of in-line filtration has been demonstrated to almost completely prevent

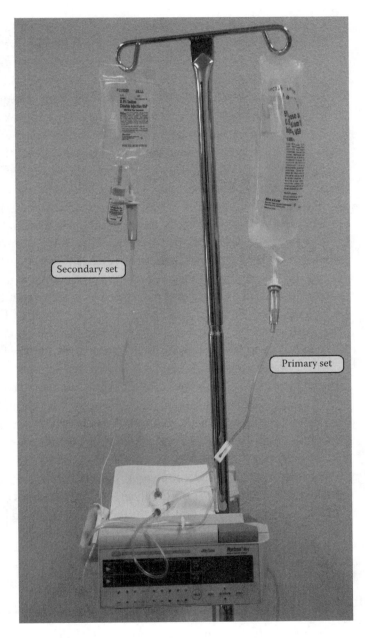

Figure 2-16 Primary and Secondary Infusion Sets

particulate matter from being infused.[13] In-line filters, available
as 0.22-micron and 1.2-micron filter sizes, are integrated in the
IV tubing of the administration set or as an add-on to existing
tubing. The 0.22-micron filters are used for crystalloid solutions
and carry a positive charge. Their use has been demonstrated
to retain particles, air, microorganisms, and endotoxins.[13] The
1.2-micron filter allows larger particles to be infused and should
be used when infusing medications consisting of larger particles,
such as lipids. When lipids are added as a secondary infusion,
it is important that the lipids be infused downstream from the
0.22-micron filter that is in the primary infusion set. If this setup
is not utilized, and the lipids are infused through the 0.22-micron
filter, the needed lipids will be filtered out. A 1.2-micron filter
should be used with liposomal medications, such as the liposomal
formulation of amphotericin B, so as to prevent the medication
from being filtered out prior to it reaching the patient. Certain
types of medications should always be infused with a filter, such
as total parenteral nutrition and mannitol. Mannitol crystallizes
readily, even at room temperature, and use of a filter will prevent
such crystals from being infused. Total parenteral nutrition has a
high propensity for incompatibilities resulting in particulate matter, so a filter should always be used when it is administered. It
is important to check the manufacturer's recommendations for
specific instructions regarding use of a filter, as several medications require their use.

Add-on filters that remove air are available to attach to IV
tubing. Because of the potentially grave consequences of air infusion, as described in literature, in-line air filters should be used in
patients at high risk of air embolisms, such as those with right-to-
left cardiac shunts and neonates.[14]

Infusion Pumps

External infusion pumps are utilized to safely and accurately
deliver fluids and medications to patients in controlled amounts.
Infusion sets are used in conjunction with infusion pumps by
threading the tubing through the pump so that flow rates can

be regulated electronically. Because of the personnel attention required for manual adjustment of flow rates and decreased accuracy with gravity infusions, electronic infusion pumps have mostly replaced manual setups in healthcare settings. Three types of infusion devices are used: large-volume pumps, syringe pumps, and pumps for patient-controlled analgesia (**Figure 2-17**).

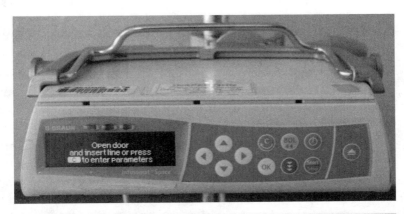

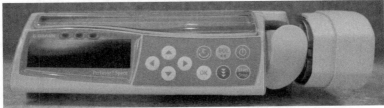

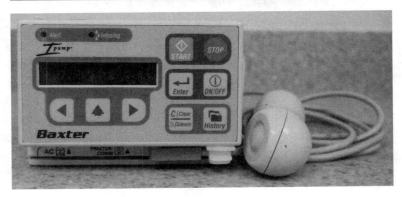

Figure 2-17   Infusion Pumps (Large Volume Pump, Syringe Pump, and Patient Controlled Analgesia Pump: in Order from Top to Bottom)

LARGE-VOLUME PUMPS

Rather than depending on gravity, large-volume pumps utilize pressure under resistance to force fluid into the vein. Because it is electronic, the nurse can program the pump to specify the rate at which the solution should be infused in milliliters per hour (mL/hr). Multiple solutions can be infused concurrently with infusion pumps, although compatibility between solutions should be ensured prior to infusion.

The most recent advancement in large-volume pumps is the advent of the smart pump. These software-driven pumps can be preprogrammed with drug libraries, which are databases that specify the exact rate that a specific solution should be infused. These sophisticated pumps can accommodate complex infusion regimens, assisting healthcare providers in calculating dose and delivery rates. This is beneficial for tapering or titrating medications or when it is necessary to deliver insulin or nutrition to coincide with meals. The internal alarm system alerts nurses when there is an error in the infusion rate, dose, or route of administration. Smart pump technology can be integrated into barcode scanning systems, computerized order-entry systems, and electronic medication administration records. The literature substantiates that, when used properly, the features available on smart pumps help prevent IV medication errors and reduce patient harm.[15]

SYRINGE PUMPS

Syringe pumps deliver small amounts of fluid at slow rates from medication-filled syringes. The syringe is placed in the pump chamber and the plunger is gradually depressed, delivering medications at a rate that has been programmed into the pump. Because syringe pumps are able to infuse small volumes, they are commonly used in pediatric settings or for fluid-restricted patients in whom small doses or volumes are typically administered. These pumps are also electronic, offering the advantage of programmable rates and alarm sensors.

PUMPS FOR PATIENT-CONTROLLED ANALGESIA

These pumps are similar to other electronic infusion pumps and use syringes filled with medications specific for patient-controlled analgesia (PCA). The technology within PCA pumps enables the patient to self-administer medication by pressing a control button attached to the IV pump. When the button is pressed, the patient will receive a prescribed amount of medication but cannot exceed a "lockout," or maximum allowed dose. For example, PCA pumps can be programmed to deliver loading doses, maximum doses per patient attempt, and maximum doses per hour. The pump can be set to deliver a basal rate of analgesia while allowing the patient to provide the bolus dose when the button is pushed.

BURETROLS

Buretrol, also known as Volutrol or burette, systems looks similar to a drip chamber with graduated marks on the outside of the chamber. The chamber sits between the patient's IV catheter and the bag of fluids, with a capacity ranging from 100 to 120 mL. The buretrol can be filled to a specific level based on the prescribed volume of solution or medication. It is used in conjunction with an infusion pump as a safety mechanism. In the event that the infusion pump malfunctions, the pump will administer only the volume that is present in the buretrol. This system is especially useful in pediatric and neonatal patients, although its use is decreasing as the use of syringe pumps and smart pumps increases.

Conclusion

This chapter reviewed fundamental supplies used in the preparation and administration of parenteral CSPs. Subsequent chapters will include additional supplies that are more specific and applicable to the topics covered. Having an overall understanding of available supplies and their role in the preparation and administration processes is essential for compounding sterile preparations in an efficient, effective, and safe manner. Knowledge on the types of supplies available can assist the operator when selecting the best container and diluents based on medication and patient-specific factors. Advancements made in the type and availability of supplies can improve workflow and patient safety, while reducing errors and drug wastage. Understanding administration of

CSPs is an important component in the overall concept of parenteral preparations.

Review Questions

1. Describe the influence of syringe size on accuracy.
2. Differentiate between single-dose and multidose solutions.
3. Describe the influence of open and closed systems on contamination
4. Which types of additives and diluents discussed in this chapter can result in patient death if directly infused?
5. When should products containing preservatives be avoided?
6. Which type of container should never be used in an emergent situation per FDA recommendations?
7. When should an in-line filter be utilized?
8. How often should infusion set tubing be changed when used to administer blood, blood products, or fat emulsions?
9. What are some benefits of smart pumps?

CASE STUDIES *Case 1*

You are a pharmacist working in the sterile compounding room when you are asked to verify a compounded sterile preparation that was prepared for a pediatric patient; the order requires a medication dose of 6.36 mL further diluted in a 50-mL bag. You notice that the technician has the dose drawn up in a 10-mL syringe.

1. Which error has the technician made?
2. How can this error be corrected?

Case 2

An order is received in your hospital for 10 units of insulin in 10 mL 0.9% NaCl. Insulin is provided as 100 units per 1 mL. You will be preparing this admixture for a pediatric patient. Describe the supplies and equipment that will be necessary for this admixture.

References

1. Pöll JS. The story of the gauge. *Anaesthesia.* 1999;54(6):575–581.
2. Iserson KV. The origins of the gauge system for medical equipment. *J Emerg Med.* 1987;5(1):45–48.
3. Erstad AJ, Erstad BL, Nix DE. Accuracy and reproducibility of small-volume injections from various-sized syringes. *Am J Health Syst Pharm.* 2006;63(8):748–750.
4. ISMP medication safety alert: a crucial and economical risk reduction strategy that has not been fully utilized. http://www.ismp.org/newsletters/acutecare/articles/20091022.asp. Accessed November 24, 2012.
5. Makwana S, Basu B, Makasana Y, Dharamsi A. Prefilled syringes: an innovation in parenteral packaging. *Int J Pharm Investig.* 2011;1(4):200–206.
6. Needleless prefilled glass syringes: stakeholder advisory—compatibility problems with needleless intravenous access systems: reports received on adenosine and amiodarone products. http://www.fda.gov/Safety/MedWatch/SafetyInformation/SafetyAlertsforHumanMedicalProducts/ucm234219.htm. Accessed November 20, 2012.
7. Rosenstock L. Department of Health and Human Services: statement for the record on needlestick injuries. 2000; updated May 27, 2009. http://www.hhs.gov/asl/testify/t000622a.html. Accessed November 25, 2012.
8. Fanikos J. Premixed products improve safe medication practices: recent innovations in amiodarone IV. *Pharmacy Pract News.* November 2011;56–57.
9. Ansel, Allen, Popovich. *Pharmaceutical dosage forms and drug delivery systems.* 7th ed. Lippincott Williams & Williams; 1999.
10. ISMP medication alert: water, water, everywhere, but please don't give IV. http://www.ismp.org/newsletters/acutecare/articles/20030123.asp. Accessed November 24, 2012.
11. U.S. Pharmacopeial Convention. Chapter <797>: pharmaceutical compounding-sterile preparations. In: *United States Pharmacopeia 36/National Formulary 31.* Rockville, MD: U.S. Pharmacopeial Convention; 2013.
12. Centers for Disease Control and Prevention. Guidelines for the prevention of intravascular catheter-related infections. 2011.

http://www.cdc.gov/hicpac/pdf/guidelines/bsi-guidelines-2011.pdf. Accessed November 25, 2012.

13. Jack T, Boehne M, Brent BE, et al. In-line filtration reduces severe complications and length of stay on pediatric intensive care unit: a prospective, randomized, controlled trial. *Intens Care Med.* 2012;38(6):1008–1016.

14. Wilkins RG, Unverdorben M. Accidental intravenous infusion of air: a concise review. *J Infus Nurs.* 2012;35(6):404–408.

15. Wilson K, Sullivan M. Preventing medication errors with smart infusion technology. *Am J Health Syst Pharm.* 2004;61(2):177–183.

CHAPTER 3

Calculations for Parenteral Compounding

José A. Vega and Pamella S. Ochoa

Chapter Objectives

1. Convert ratios and proportions to concentrations and percent strengths.
2. Calculate the amount of diluent needed for reconstitution of medications with displacement volumes.
3. Determine the volume of two products that must be added together to obtain a desired concentration using alligation.
4. Determine the volume of isotonic solution needed to render a final solution isotonic.
5. Calculate the osmolarity of solutions.
6. Calculate syringe and needle priming volumes.

Key Terminology

Reconstitute
Powder volume
Normal saline (NS)
Displacement volume

Alligation
Solution
Diluent
w/w
w/v
v/v
Percentage strength
Tonicity
Isotonic
Hypotonic
Hypertonic
Osmole (Osm)
Osmolarity

Overview

Calculations are routinely performed when compounding sterile preparations. Knowledge of basic algebra, at a minimum, is necessary to complete these calculations. Because the final preparation administered to the patient relies on the accuracy of the person doing these calculations, it is essential that personnel compounding parenteral preparations are knowledgeable on the types of calculations that are used and able to perform them with accuracy. It is important to understand that errors in calculations related to compounded sterile preparations (CSPs) can have significant ramifications, such as patient harm or death. Complete understanding of parenteral preparations is necessary for personnel involved in determining the volume and drug doses contained in CSPs. This chapter reviews several types of calculations, graduating in complexity, that accompany the compounding and use of common parenteral preparations.

Ratios and Proportions

Understanding ratios and proportions is fundamental to be able to perform higher-skill calculations related to parenteral preparations. A ratio, by definition, is the relationship in quantity, amount, or size between two or more things.[1] A proportion is a statement of equality between two ratios in which the first of the four terms divided by the second equals the third divided by the fourth.[2] The difference between ratios and proportions is that a ratio compares two numbers in relation to each other, while proportions are two ratios separated by an equal sign.

ALERT: *Always use a leading zero with decimal points (i.e., use "0.7" rather than ".7"). Never use a trailing zero with whole integers (i.e., use "20" rather than "20.0").*

For example:

- Ratio: 2/3 or 2:3
- Proportion: 4/6 = 2/3 or 4:6::2:3

In this example, the 4 and the 3 are referred to as the extremes, as they are on the extreme portion of the equal sign when set up as 4:6::2:3. Likewise, the 6 and 2 are referred to as the means.

Proportions are used frequently to "set up" calculations when needing to calculate an unknown. For example:

$$4/6 = X/3$$

The unknown, X, can be solved for by following these steps.

STEPS TO CALCULATE PROPORTIONS: METHOD 1

1. Multiply the means.
2. Multiply the extremes.
3. Place X on the left of an equal sign with the number being multiplied.
4. Place the product of the other two numbers on the right of the equal sign.
5. Solve for X.

For the example shown, here are the steps:

1. $6 \times X = 6X$
2. $4 \times 3 = 12$

3&4. $6X = 12$

5. $X = 12/6 = 2$

A second method can be used with the proportion set up as $4/6 = X/3$.

STEPS TO CALCULATE PROPORTION: METHOD 2

1. Cross-multiply on both sides of the equal sign.
2. Place the product of each multiplication on either side of the equal sign.
3. Solve for X.

Using these steps, we solve for X:

1. $\dfrac{4}{6} \diagup\!\!\!\!\diagdown \dfrac{X}{3}$
2. $6X = 12$
3. $X = 12/6 = 2$

Dosage Calculations

Performing dosage calculations for parenteral preparations is exceptionally important secondary to the patient harm that may occur if such calculations are not performed correctly. Even an error as small as one decimal place could result in serious patient harm. Common dosage calculations for parenteral preparations will involve ratios and proportions. A variety of equations may be used to arrive at doses for pediatric patients and patients receiving chemotherapy. For example, doses for pediatric patients are based on weight, in milligrams per kilogram body weight, and are based on body surface area (BSA) for chemotherapy. Using these dosing strategies in these patient populations provides more specific dosing that caters to the types of medication used and the size of the patient. Calculating the amount of medication that should be added to a solution can be accomplished by using equations based on either weight or concentration, depending on the type of information needed. Use the following steps to calculate doses.

STEPS TO CALCULATE DOSES BASED ON WEIGHT
1. Convert weight to kilograms (kg).
2. Set up a proportion equation. Use the prescribed dose of medication on one side of the equal sign and the unknown on the other side of the equal sign. Be sure units are balanced on either side of the equal sign.
3. Solve for X

EXAMPLE CALCULATION

A dose of vancomycin 20 mg/kg is ordered as a one-time dose for a patient who weighs 174 pounds. What is the dose that should be administered?

1. Convert weight to kilograms (kg).
   174 lb/2.2 = 79.1 kg

2. Set up a proportion equation.

$$\frac{20 \text{ mg}}{1 \text{ kg}} = \frac{X}{79.1 \text{ kg}}$$

3. Solve for X.
   $X = 20 \times 79.1 = 1582$ mg

Answer: 1582 mg of vancomycin is the equivalent dose of 20 mg/kg for this patient.

STEPS TO CALCULATE DOSAGES BASED ON CONCENTRATION
1. Determine the concentration of the available medication. This information will be found on the label of the drug or may be calculated.
2. Set up a proportion equation. Use the concentration of available medication on one side of the equal sign and the

desired dose on the other side of the equal sign. Be sure units are balanced on either side of the equal sign.
3. Solve for X.

EXAMPLE CALCULATION

The following order is received:

Gentamicin 320 mg IV Q8 hours

The following vial is stocked:

> 2 mL Single-dose
> **Gentamicin**
> Sulfate Injection, USP
> **80 mg/2 mL**
> (40 mg/mL as Gentamicin)

How many milliliters (mL) are needed? How many vials are needed?

1. Determine the concentration of the available medication. 80 mg/2 mL is the available concentration.

2. Set up a proportion equation.

$$\frac{80 \text{ mg}}{2 \text{ mL}} \underset{=}{\bowtie} \frac{320 \text{ mg}}{X \text{ mL}}$$

3. Solve for X.
$80X = 640$
$X = 640/80 = 8 \text{ mL}$

Answer: 8 mL (4 vials) of gentamicin 80 mg/2 mL is needed to achieve a dose of 320 mg.

Body Surface Area

Body surface area (BSA) is used for dosing of drugs, most commonly with chemotherapy. Various equations exist for calculating BSA, which can induce wide variances in total drug doses based on BSA calculations. The Mosteller and the DuBois and DuBois formulas are the most commonly used. The DuBois and DuBois formula was developed many years ago and was derived from studies of nine subjects.[4] The Mosteller formula provides a simple mathematical equation. Newer three-dimensional derived equations were developed and published in the literature around 2003.[4] In the event that large variances are noted when calculating doses using the different BSA equations, such as with chemotherapy, then institutional standards or manufacturer recommendations should be followed. BSA equations used for adults are provided here as examples:

Mosteller:
$$\text{BSA (m}^2) = \sqrt{([\text{height (inches)} \times \text{weight (lb)}]/3131)}$$
$$\text{BSA (m}^2) = \sqrt{([\text{height (cm)} \times \text{weight (kg)}]/3600)}$$

DuBois and DuBois:
$$\text{BSA (m}^2) = 0.007184 \times \text{height (cm)}^{0.725} \times \text{weight (kg)}^{0.425}$$

Boyd:
$$\text{BSA (m}^2) = 0.0003207 \times \text{height (cm)}^{0.5}$$
$$\times \text{weight (g)}^{0.7285 - (0.0188 \times \log\,(\text{weight (g)}))}$$

Gehan and George:
$$\text{BSA (m}^2) = 0.0235 \times \text{height (cm)}^{0.42246} \times \text{weight (kg)}^{0.51456}$$

Haycock:
$$\text{BSA (m}^2) = 0.024265 \times \text{height (cm)}^{0.3966} \times \text{weight (kg)}^{0.5378}$$

Although BSA equations vary, the calculated result should make logical sense. Thinking of the calculated result in the context of the adult average BSA, which is 1.72 m², serves to ensure that the calculated BSA is correct. For example, if the BSA was calculated for a patient who is of average weight and height and the BSA is 4, an error should be suspected. It is important to note that variances in estimation of BSA, compared to true BSA, become more significant in overweight and obese patients. In these patients, selection of the equations that perform best in this patient population should be used.

EXAMPLE

A patient is 71 inches tall and weighs 190 lb. The oncologist has ordered a dose of taxotere 75 mg per m². Calculate BSA using the Mosteller equation and determine the dose of taxotere to be administered.

$\sqrt{(71 \text{ inches} \times 190 \text{ lb})/3131} = 2.08$

BSA is 2.08 m².

75 mg/ m² × 2.08 m² = 156 mg of taxotere

Concentration Calculations

Determining the final concentration of a solution is often a required calculation when compounding sterile preparations. For example, some large-volume parenterals (LVPs) are available in premixed concentrations. At times, a different concentration that is not available directly from the manufacturer may be needed. Concentration calculations assist in determining the amount of additive needed to achieve the final prescribed concentration.

Calculation concentrations are also beneficial when working with different formulations of medications such as liquids and solids together. An important tip when performing these calculations is to ensure that the same units are being used when setting up proportion equations.

Certain patients may benefit from either a more concentrated or a more dilute preparation. For example, pediatric patients and fluid-restricted patients may benefit from smaller total volumes. In these situations, it may be appropriate to use higher concentrations, as long as the final concentration does not exceed the recommended maximum allowable concentration for both infusion and compatibility. In contrast, use of more dilute concentrations may be suitable for patients experiencing phlebitis with infusion of certain medications. Dilutions should also be considered when preparing medications for injections, as a minimum volume of 0.5 mL is needed, yet the volume cannot be more than 3 mL for intramuscular (IM) administration for adults. IM injection volumes for pediatric patients should not exceed 2 mL in older children, 1 mL in smaller children and older infants, and 0.5 mL in small infants.

> **TIP:** *Double-check units when setting up proportion equations to ensure they are balanced on either side of the equal sign.*

DILUTION CALCULATIONS

Accuracy with dilution is a consequence of both measurement and calculations. Dilution results from the addition of a solution, most commonly sterile water and normal saline (NS), to another solution or powder for reconstitution. While many medications require reconstitution with sterile water for injection, it is important not to confuse this additive with bacteriostatic water for injection. Bacteriostatic water for injection contains preservatives and is not interchangeable with sterile water for injection.

> **ALERT:** *Sterile water for injection and bacteriostatic water for injection cannot be interchanged.*

The volume of diluent added to a medication, as with reconstitution, will determine the final concentration of the solution. For example, assuming no displacement of volume, if a 1-g vial of ceftazidime is reconstituted with 20 mL, then the final concentration will be 1000 mg/20 mL or 50 mg/mL. Using 10 mL to reconstitute the medication will result in a final concentration of 1000 mg/10 mL or 100 mg/mL, which is twice as concentrated as the previous example. The volume to be withdrawn depends on the final concentration. To obtain a dose of 500 mg, as with the previous example, 10 mL should be withdrawn if the concentration is 50 mg/mL. A total of 5 mL should be withdrawn if the concentration is 100 mg/mL.

To calculate final concentrations, in which no volume displacement occurs, use a ratio equation according to the following steps.

Steps to Calculate Final Concentrations

1. Use the total amount of active ingredient as the numerator.
2. Use the total volume as the denominator.
3. Reduce the proportion, if needed, to obtain a denominator of 1.

EXAMPLE CALCULATION

The following inpatient order is received:

Vancomycin 1500 mg IV BID

A vial containing 10 g of vancomycin powder is available; 200 mL of sterile water for injection is added to the vial for reconstitution. Assuming no volume expansion of the powder, calculate the volume to be withdrawn to obtain a dose of 1500 mg.

1. Total amount of the active ingredient, vancomycin, is 10 g.
2. Total volume is 200 mL.
3. 10 g/200 mL can be reduced to 1 g/ 20 mL, which is the same as 50 mg/1 mL.

To calculate the volume to be withdrawn, use the steps for calculating unknowns in a proportion.

1. Cross-multiply on both sides of the equal sign.

$$\frac{50 \text{ mg}}{1 \text{ mL}} = \frac{1500 \text{ mg}}{X \text{ mL}}$$

2. Place the product of each multiplication on either side of the equal sign.
   $50X = 1500$

3. Solve for X.
   $X = 1500/50 = 30$ mL

Answer: 30 mL should be withdrawn from the vial, which is the equivalent of 1500 mg.

When two volumes and one concentration of a product are known or when two concentrations and one volume of a product are known, the following formula may be useful.

STEPS TO CALCULATE CONCENTRATIONS AND VOLUMES

1. Multiply the concentrations (C) and volumes (V) of known values.

$$C_1V_1 = C_2V_2$$

2. Multiply either the known volume or concentration by X.
3. Solve for X.

EXAMPLE CALCULATION

A medication is available as a 5% concentration. Calculate the volume of this medication required to achieve a desired volume of 10 mL of solution with a concentration of 2%.

1. Multiply the concentration and volume of known values.

> **TIP:** *Do not convert the percentages to decimal form when using the $C_1V_1 = C_2V_2$ equation.*

$$C_1V_1 = C_2V_2$$
$$(2\%)(10 \text{ mL}) = C_2V_2$$

2. Multiply either the known volume or concentration by X.
$$(2\%)(10 \text{ mL}) = (5\%)(X)$$

3. Solve for X.
$$X = 4 \text{ mL}$$

Answer: 4 mL of the 5% medication should be added to 6 mL of diluent to obtain a 2% solution with a final volume of 10 mL.

PERCENT STRENGTH

Percent strength calculations are used to determine the final concentration of a preparation. Percent strength and concentration are used interchangeably. Three different percent strength equations may be used depending on the type of formulation involved.

Percent Weight in Weight

Weight in weight, expressed as w/w, is used in percent strength calculations when all products involved in the calculation are in solid form. Weight in weight is used in mixtures of solids with other solids or semisolids and with mixtures of solids and liquids.

The w/w value represents the number of grams in a total of 100 g, or X g/100 g. Notice that both units are in grams, an expression of weight. For example, a 1% hydrocortisone ointment is 1 g hydrocortisone in 100 g ointment, numerically expressed as 1 g/100 g.

EXAMPLE CALCULATION

A prescription is received for a 2% zinc oxide diaper ointment with a dispensing size of 20 g. How many grams of zinc oxide should be used to make a 2% zinc oxide ointment?

We have 2% zinc oxide = 2 g/100 g
We are solving for X/20 g.

1. Cross-multiply on both sides of the equal sign.

$$\frac{2\text{ g}}{100\text{ g}} = \frac{X\text{ g}}{20\text{ g}}$$

2. Place the product of each multiplication on either side of the equal sign.
$100X = 40$

3. Solve for X.
$X = 40/100 = 0.4$ g

Answer: 0.4 g of zinc oxide should be added to 19.6 g of ointment for a resultant 2% zinc oxide ointment with a final size of 20 g.

Percent Weight in Volume

Expressed as w/v, weight in volume refers to the percent strength of preparations of solids in liquids. These calculations are similar to the w/w calculations, but the units will not be the same. D_5W, for example, contains 5% dextrose, or 5 g of dextrose in every 100 mL of solution.

EXAMPLE CALCULATION

Calculate the number of grams of sodium chloride (NaCl) in 1 L of ½NS (0.45% NS).

1. Cross-multiply on both sides of the equal sign.

$$\frac{0.45 \text{ g}}{100 \text{ mL}} \diagdown\!\!\!\!\!\diagup= \frac{X \text{ g}}{1000 \text{ mL}}$$

2. Place the product of each multiplication on either side of the equal sign.

$100X = 450$

3. Solve for X.

$X = 450/100 = 4.5$ g

Answer: One liter of ½NS contains 4.5 g of sodium chloride.

Percent Volume in Volume

Volume in volume, expressed as v/v, refers to the percent strength of liquid in liquid. For example, a 3% hydrogen peroxide solution contains 3 mL of hydrogen peroxide per 100 mL of solution. Notice that the units are the same for these calculations.

EXAMPLE CALCULATION

Rubbing alcohol contains 70% isopropyl alcohol. What volume of isopropyl alcohol is contained in 50 mL of rubbing alcohol?

1. Cross-multiply on both sides of the equal sign.

$$\frac{70 \text{ mL}}{100 \text{ mL}} \diagdown\!\!\!\!\!\diagup= \frac{X}{50 \text{ mL}}$$

2. Place the product of each multiplication on either side of the equal sign.

$100X = 3500$

3. Solve for X.

$X = 3500/100 = 35$ mL

Answer: 50 mL of rubbing alcohol contains 35 mL of isopropyl alcohol.

Ratio Strengths

Ratio strength is used when solutions are very dilute and is another way to express the concentration (percentage) of solutions. For example, epinephrine has a ratio strength of 1:1000 or 0.1%. Percentage strengths can be easily converted to ratio strengths, and vice versa.

EXAMPLE CALCULATION 1

Convert 1:5000 to percentage strength.

> **TIP:** *1:5000 is the same as 1/5000. Percentage strength is always "out of 100," or X/100.*

1. Cross-multiply on both sides of the equal sign.

$$\frac{1}{5000} = \frac{X}{100}$$

2. Place the product of each multiplication on either side of the equal sign.
   $5000X = 100$

3. Solve for X.
   $X = 100/5000 = 0.02$

Answer: The percentage strength of 1:5000 is 0.02%.

EXAMPLE CALCULATION 2

What is the ratio strength of 0.0001%?

> **TIP:** *Set up equations with percent strength expressed as "out of 100." Set up ratio strength with a numerator of 1, which is the same as 1:X.*

1. Cross-multiply on both sides of the equal sign.

   $$\frac{0.0001}{100} \diagtimes \frac{1}{X}$$

2. Place the product of each multiplication on either side of the equal sign.

   $0.0001X = 100$

3. Solve for X.

   $X = 100/0.0001 = 1{,}000{,}000$

Answer: The ratio strength of 0.0001% is 1:1,000,000.

Displacement Volume

Many drugs are manufactured as powders for reconstitution. Often, when reconstituted into solution, the powder displaces volume—which in turn creates additional volume compared to the volume that was added for reconstitution. The additional volume is referred to as displacement volume or powder volume. The total volume added is a factor in determining the final concentration, as numerically represented in the denominator of concentration ratios. Additional volume from displacement will affect the total volume, resulting in a more dilute concentration. Because of the potential error from displacement volume, the total volume of diluent needed to achieve the desired concentration should be calculated prior to reconstitution.

Calculation of displacement volume is particularly important with pediatric doses, which are smaller and are subject to errors with small changes in volume. To illustrate this effect, consider the following example using the following steps.

STEPS TO CALCULATE DISPLACEMENT VOLUMES

1. Calculate the powder volume.
2. Calculate the volume of diluent needed for the new concentration.
3. Subtract the powder volume (from Step 1) from the volume needed (from Step 2) to determine the final amount that should be added.

EXAMPLE CALCULATION

A medication order for a 6.6-kg pediatric patient with a respiratory infection is received, reading:

Ampicillin 250 mg (200 mg/mL) IM Q6 hours until IV access is established

Ampicillin for Injection, USP **1 gram per vial**	This vial contains ampicillin sodium equivalent to 1 gram ampicillin. Add 3.5 mL diluent. Resulting solution contains 250 mg ampicillin per mL.

Based on the label instructions, adding 3.5 mL of diluent to the vial containing 1000 mg will result in a concentration of 250 mg/mL.

1. Calculate the power volume for 250 mg/mL concentration.

> **TIP:** *250 mg/mL concentration is provided on the label instructions from the manufacturer.*

$$\frac{250 \text{ mg}}{1 \text{ mL}} \diagup\!\!\!\diagdown \frac{1000 \text{ mg}}{X \text{ mL}}$$

$$250X = 1000$$
$$X = 4 \text{ mL}$$

This answer represents the volume that would be added to the vial to achieve 250 mg/mL if no volume displacement occurs. Subtract the calculated volume from the diluent volume to determine powder volume:

> **TIP:** *3.5 mL diluent volume is provided on the label instructions from the manufacturer.*

$$4 \text{ mL} - 3.5 \text{ mL} = 0.5 \text{ mL}$$

The powder volume is 0.5 mL.

2. Calculate the volume of diluent to add for new concentration of 200 mg/mL.

> **TIP:** *The new concentration of 200 mg/mL is provided in the medication order.*

$$\frac{200 \text{ mg}}{1 \text{ mL}} \bowtie \frac{1000 \text{ mg}}{X \text{ mL}}$$

$200X = 1000$
$X = 5 \text{ mL}$

3. Subtract the powder volume from the new calculated volume to determine the volume of diluent to add for the new concentration.
   $5 \text{ mL} - 0.5 \text{ mL} = 4.5 \text{ mL}$

The diluent volume needed for a final concentration of 200 mg/mL is 4.5 mL.

To obtain a dose of 250 mg from a concentration of 200 mg/mL, the following calculations are performed:

1. Cross-multiply on both sides of the equal sign.

$$\frac{200 \text{ mg}}{1 \text{ mL}} \bowtie \frac{250 \text{ mg}}{X \text{ mL}}$$

2. Place the product of each multiplication on either side of the equal sign.
   $200X = 250$

3. Solve for X.
   $X = 250/200 = 1.25 \text{ mL}$

A total of 1.25 mL of a 200 mg/mL concentration would result in a dose of 250 mg for this pediatric patient.

In the event that the volume displacement of 0.5 mL went unaccounted for and the assumption was made that reconstituting with 5 mL would result in 1 g in 5 mL, then the following calculations illustrate the under-dosing that would occur:

$$\frac{1000 \text{ mg}}{5.5 \text{ mL}} \bowtie \frac{X \text{ mg}}{1.25 \text{ mL}}$$

$1250 = 5.5X$
$X = 1250/5.5 = 227 \text{ mg}$

If powder volume is not considered, the final concentration would be 1000 mg in 5.5 mL. This 1.25 mL dose would result in an actual dose of 227 mg, underdosing the patient by 23 mg per dose. This example outlines the importance of calculating powder volume prior to reconstitution.

Some drugs will not displace volume following reconstitution. For example, if 2 g of drug is in the vial and 20 mL is added, then the final concentration will be 2 g/20 mL or 0.1 g/mL. The package insert, or vial label, should be referenced to determine whether displacement will occur.

Flow Rates

When intravenous medications and solutions are infused, they should be administered at a specific flow rate that is neither too fast nor too slow. The appropriate rate of infusion, or flow rate, is determined by the following factors:

- Manufacturer recommendations
- Institutional standardized rates
- Per the prescriber

Patients experiencing complications with an infusion may require slower flow rates. For example, vancomycin infusion-related adverse effects are both concentration and rate dependent. A maximum rate of 1000 mg/hr (16.7 mg/min) is recommended for this medication. When vancomycin is infused faster than this recommended rate, it increases the risk of phlebitis and Stevens-Johnson syndrome (SJS).[3] If a patient develops these types of infusion-related events, the flow rate can be decreased and the adverse events often will subside. Conversely, some medications require quicker flow rates, either in emergent situations, due to a low adverse-event profile with quick infusions, or for some concentration-dependent medications.

Flow rates may also be calculated based on drop factors for the administration set tubing. The drop factor with gravity flow administration of solutions varies with the administration set tubing—for example, with microdrip versus macrodrip tubing. When calculating the flow rate, the drop factor must be known, because the flow rate is expressed in drops per minute (gtt/min). When an electronic infusion device, or infusion pump, is utilized, the rate needs to be programmed, in milliliters per hour (mL/hr), so that the device can regulate the flow to the desired rate. Smart pumps are often preprogrammed with maximum infusion rates and will alert nurses (via an alarm) when the infusion rate exceeds these parameters.

To calculate flow rates, the following steps should be used when given the total volume and time for infusion.

STEPS FOR CALCULATING FLOW RATES

1. Set up dimensional analysis using the information provided, ensuring that all units in the numerator and the denominator cancel so that the final units are in mL/hr or gtt/min or the desired rate units.
2. Multiply all numerators.
3. Multiply all denominators.
4. Divide the answer from Step 2 by the answer from Step 3, ensuring that all units in the numerator and the denominator have cancelled so that the final units are in mL/hr or gtt/min.

EXAMPLE CALCULATION

The following order is received:

Vancomycin 1500 mg in 500 mL NS to be infused over 90 minutes

The nurse calls the pharmacy and asks, "At what rate do I run the vancomycin?" The nurse states that an infusion pump is being used. Calculate the flow rate in mL/hr for programming the pump.

1. Set up dimensional analysis using the information provided, ensuring that all units in the numerator and the denominator cancel so that the final units are in mL/hr or gtt/min or the desired rate units.

$$\frac{500 \, \text{(mL)}}{90 \, \text{min}} \times \frac{60 \, \text{min}}{1 \, \text{(hr)}} = X \text{ mL/hr}$$

2. Multiply all numerators.
   $500 \times 60 = 30{,}000$

3. Multiply all denominators.
   $90 \times 1 = 90$

4. Divide the answer from Step 2 by the answer from Step 3, ensuring that all units in the numerator and the denominator have cancelled so that the final units are in mL/hr or gtt/min.
   $30{,}000/90 = 333.3$ mL/hr

Answer: The pump should be programmed to run the vancomycin at 333.3 mL/hr.

Now the nurse calls back stating that the pump is malfunctioning and the vancomycin will be administered by gravity flow. The administration set available delivers 20 drops per mL. Calculate the drip rate in drops/min.

1. Set up dimensional analysis using the information provided, ensuring that all units in the numerator and the denominator cancel so that the final units are in mL/hr or gtt/min or the desired rate units.

$$\frac{500 \, \text{mL}}{90 \, \text{(min)}} \times \frac{20 \, \text{(gtt)}}{1 \, \text{mL}} = X \text{ gtt/min}$$

2. Multiply all numerators.
   $500 \times 20 = 10{,}000$

3. Multiply all denominators.
   $90 \times 1 = 90$

4. Divide the answer from Step 2 by the answer from Step 3.
   $10{,}000/90 = 111.1$ gtt/min or 111 gtt/min

> **TIP:** *Because a fraction of a drop cannot be feasibly measured, calculated answers in gtt/min should be rounded to the nearest whole integer.*

Alligations

Alligation is a method used to calculate the final concentration of a solution when two solutions of different concentrations, but containing the same active ingredient, are mixed together. The final concentration of the CSP will numerically be between the two concentrations of the original products. For example, 7% hypertonic saline is used for inhalation in patients with cystic fibrosis to improve mucociliary clearance and to provide potential anti-inflammatory and antimicrobial benefits.[5] This percent strength of saline is not readily available and may need to be prepared using commercially available 3% and 10% hypertonic saline solutions. Alligations can be calculated to determine the volumes of both 3% and 10% to achieve a final percent strength of 7%.

Two different methods for calculating alligations can be used. Both methods are presented here, and the choice should be at the discretion of the individual performing the calculation.

TIP: *Sterile water for injection is considered to have a percent strength of zero when calculating alligations.*

STEPS FOR CALCULATING ALLIGATIONS: METHOD 1

This method is used when quantities and concentrations are known for the original products and the final concentration of a mixture is to be determined.

1. Drop the percent sign from the percent strengths for both original products.
2. Multiply each number from Step 1 by its respective volume for each original product.
3. Add the two numbers obtained in Step 2.
4. Add the volumes of the original products.
5. Divide the total volume of original products (from Step 4) by the sum obtained in Step 3 (i.e., Step 4/Step 3). The result is a percentage.

EXAMPLE CALCULATION

Calculate the final percent strength when 1500 mL of a 30% solution is mixed with 1100 mL of a 40% solution.

1. Drop the percent sign from the percent strengths for both original products.
   30% → 30 and 40% → 40

2. Multiply each number from Step 1 by its respective volume for each original product.
   $30 \times 1500 = 45{,}000$
   $40 \times 1100 = 44{,}000$

3. Add the two numbers obtained in Step 2.
   $45{,}000 + 44{,}000 = 89{,}000$

4. Add the volumes of the original products.
   $1500 + 1100 = 2600$

5. Divide the sum of the products (from Step 3) by the total volumes of both solutions obtained in Step 4 (i.e., Step 3/Step 4). The result is a percentage.
   $89{,}000/2600 = 34$

Answer: The final percent strength of the solution is 34%.

Percent strength may also be calculated by using decimal numbers instead of percentages; note that the final answer will need to be converted from a decimal number to a percentage.

$$\frac{(1500 \text{ mL})(0.30) + (1100 \text{ mL})(0.04)}{1500 \text{ mL} + 1100 \text{ mL}} = 0.34 \text{ or } 34\%$$

> **TIP:** *Double-check your answer. The number obtained for the final strength of the mixed preparation should be between the two strengths of the original products.*

STEPS FOR CALCULATING ALLIGATIONS: METHOD 2

This method is used when a desired concentration and quantity are known and at least two products, of greater and of lesser concentrations than the desired concentration, are being added together. It allows calculation of the number of parts of each original product that is needed to obtain the final preparation at the desired concentration and quantity. The following steps can be used:

1. Set up a grid using known concentrations. These numbers should be placed on the left of the grid, with the more concentrated value on the top and the less concentrated value on the bottom. Place the desired concentration in the middle.

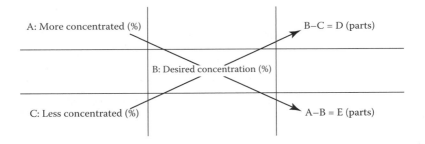

2. Subtract diagonally. Subtract in a manner that will result in a positive integer (B − C and A − B). The result will be the parts of each product (D is the number of parts needed for product A; E is the number of parts needed for product C).
3. Add, vertically, all the values from Step 2. The result is the total number of parts.
4. For each product, set up the following proportion:

Parts Needed
───────────
Total Parts

5. Multiply the desired quantity by the proportion for each product to obtain the quantity of each product to be used.

EXAMPLE CALCULATION

The following order is received:

7% hypertonic saline inhalation 5 mL via nebulizer QID for 14 days

The pharmacy does not stock this percent strength of saline, so it needs to be prepared. In stock are a 10% hypertonic saline solution and a 3% hypertonic saline solution. Calculate the volumes of these two solutions that should be added together to obtain a 7% hypertonic solution.

More concentrated = 10%
Less concentrated = 3%
Desired concentration = 7%
Desired quantity = 5 mL

1. Set up a grid using the known concentrations.

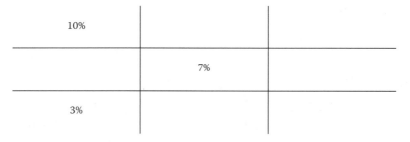

2. Subtract diagonally.
   10 − 7 = 3 and 7 − 3 = 4

3. Add, vertically, all the values from Step 2.
   4 + 3 = 7

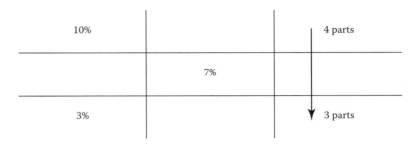

4. For each product, set up the following proportion:
   Parts needed
   ──────────────
   Total parts

   10% hypertonic saline: $\dfrac{4}{7}$

   3% hypertonic saline: $\dfrac{3}{7}$

5. Multiply the desired quantity by the proportion for each product.

   10% hypertonic saline: $\dfrac{4 \times 5 \text{ mL}}{7} = 2.9 \text{ mL}$

   3% hypertonic saline: $\dfrac{3 \times 5 \text{ mL}}{7} = 2.1 \text{ mL}$

Answer: 2.9 mL of 10% hypertonic saline should be added to 2.1 mL of 3% hypertonic saline to obtain 5 mL of 7% hypertonic saline.

> **TIP:** *When calculating alligations, double-check your answer by adding up the volumes for each product to see if the sum matches the total volume needed.*

The preceding example illustrates the case in which two products with different concentrations are used to obtain a different desired concentration. The same steps would be followed when using three or four different concentrations. For three products, two grids should be drawn with the lowest concentration used on the bottom of both grids. For example, if 5%, 30%, and 60%

concentrations are used to obtain a desired concentration of 15%, the grids should be set up as follows:

30%		
	15%	
5%		
60%		
	15%	
5%		

When performing calculations involving four products, two grids should also be drawn with all four numbers in two grids, with the lowest concentrations on the bottom. For example, if concentrations of 5%, 10%, 60%, and 70% are used to obtain a desired concentration of 30%, the grids should be set up as follows:

70%		
	30%	
5%		
60%		
	30%	
10%		

The parts of all products will need to be calculated and the total number of parts determined for all products. Similar to the examples with only two products, proportions for each product should be used to identify the quantities of each product that should be added to create the desired concentration.

Tonicity

Tonicity is a value that is expressed in relation to biological fluids, such as blood or tears. Solutions can be classified as isotonic, hypertonic, or hypotonic. Isotonic solutions are those that have the same tonicity as blood, tears, and normal saline. Tonicity is relative to the number of particles in a solution. Hypertonic solutions contain a higher concentration of solute particles per unit volume compared to isotonic solutions. Conversely, hypotonic solutions contain a lower concentration of solute particles per unit volume, comparatively speaking. Secondary to osmosis, intracellular and extracellular fluid, both interstitial and intravascular, is affected when hypotonic or hypertonic solutions are administered. The effect of tonicity on movement of water across cell membranes is the basis for understanding the effects experienced by blood cells in isotonic, hypotonic, and hypertonic environments.

- A solution is considered isotonic if there is no change in a cell's size when it is placed in a solution at equilibrium.
- A solution is considered hypotonic if, at equilibrium, there is an increase in the size of the cell.
- A hypertonic solution will result in shrinkage of the cell when at equilibrium.

Figure 3-1 illustrates the effects of tonicity on water osmosis. **Table 3-1** provides information on IV solutions commonly used for infusion and their tonicity.

Infusion rates of hypotonic and hypertonic solutions should be carefully chosen, and the solutions should be infused within the recommended rates for their respective concentrations. Too-rapid infusions of hypertonic solutions, such as with administration of

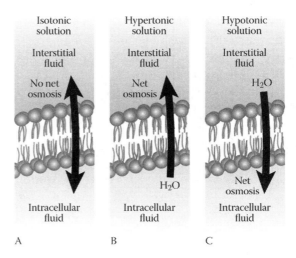

Figure 3-1 (A)   No concentration gradients are created with isotonic infusions causing no net effect in water exchange across cell membranes. **(B)** Hypertonic infusions result in more solutes in the intravascular space causing osmosis of water from the intracellular space into the intravascular space resulting in a decrease of the intracellular volume. **(C)** Hypotonic infusions result in fewer solutes in the intravascular space, which will result in osmosis of water into the intracellular space and expansion of the intracellular volume

Table 3-1   Tonicity of Common IV Solutions

IV Solution	Tonicity
0.45% sodium chloride (½NS)	Hypotonic
Dextrose 5% in water (D_5W)	Isotonic
Sodium chloride 0.9% (NS)	Isotonic
Lactated Ringer's (LR)	Isotonic
Dextrose 5% in 0.225% sodium chloride (D_5 ¼NS)	Isotonic
Dextrose 10% (D_{10})	Hypertonic
Dextrose 5% in lactated Ringer's (D_5LR)	Hypertonic
Dextrose 5% in 0.9% sodium chloride (D_5NS)	Hypertonic

3% hypertonic saline for correction of hyponatremia, can result in osmotic demyelination syndrome.[6] Hypotonic solutions that are infused too quickly can cause rapid movement of water into the cells, resulting in detrimental effects to the patient, such a hemolysis, hyponatremia, and hypotension.

> **ALERT:** *Infusion rates of hypotonic and hypertonic solutions should be carefully chosen and regulated to avoid too rapid infusion, which may result in patient harm.*

A solution that is not isotonic can be altered to achieve isotonicity through the addition of either sodium chloride or dextrose, allowing it to be infused without adverse consequences on cellular volumes. To do so, use the following steps.

STEPS FOR MAKING ISOTONIC PREPARATIONS

1. Calculate the amount of sodium chloride (NaCl) represented by each ingredient.

   Milligrams of ingredients × NaCl equivalents

2. Determine how much NaCl would be in the total volume to make the solution 0.9% (equivalent to 900 mg/100 mL).

   Volume (mL) × 900 mg/100 mL

3. Subtract the amount from Step 1 from the amount from Step 2.
4. If using something other than NaCl to make the solution isotonic, divide the amount from Step 3 by the NaCl equivalent (E).

> **TIP:** *E is the amount of sodium chloride that has the same osmotic effect as 1 g of the drug.*

EXAMPLE CALCULATION

How many milligrams of NaCl are needed to make 1:1000 epinephrine HCl isotonic in 50 mL of sterile water? Epinephrine: $E = 0.18$.

1. Calculate the amount of sodium chloride (NaCl) represented by each ingredient.
   Milligrams of ingredients × NaCl equivalents

> **TIP:** *Determine the milligrams of epinephrine in 50 mL by first converting 1:1000 to milligrams. 1:1000 is the same as 1/1000.*

$$\frac{1\ \text{g}}{1000\ \text{mL}} = \frac{X\ \text{g}}{50\ \text{mL}} \qquad X = 0.05\ \text{g} = 50\ \text{mg}$$

NaCl equivalent = 50 mg (0.18) = 9 mg NaCl
There are 9 mg of sodium chloride equivalents in 50 mL of 1:1000 epinephrine.

2. Determine how much NaCl would be in the total volume to make the solution have a concentration of 0.9% (equivalent to 900 mg/100 mL).
Volume (mL) × 900 mg/100 mL

$$\frac{900\ \text{mg}}{100\ \text{mL}} \times 50\ \text{mL} = 450\ \text{mg}$$

For the 1:1000 solution of epinephrine to be isotonic, it would need to contain 450 mg of sodium chloride in 50 mL.

3. Subtract the amount from Step 1 from the amount from Step 2.
450 mg – 9 mg = 441 mg NaCl

Answer: 441 mg of NaCl is needed to make the solution isotonic.

Osmolarity

Tonicity and *osmolarity* are terms that are routinely used interchangeably, but they do have subtle differences. Tonicity refers to the concentration of nonpermeable solute particles inside a cell versus the concentration outside the cell. Osmolarity is the measure of both the permeable and nonpermeable solute particle concentrations. Tonicity is used when referring to solutions, whereas osmolarity is typically used when referencing blood. Because tonicity has no unit of measure, it is used for comparative purposes. In addition to being distinguished based on their tonicity, solutions can be classified as isosmotic, hypo-osmotic, and hyperosmotic.

- Osmolarity of 280–310 mOsm/L: isotonic
- Osmolarity < 280 mOsm/L: hypotonic
- Osmolarity > 310 mOsm/L: hypertonic

Osmolality and osmolarity are often confused. Osmolality describes solute concentration in milliosmoles per kilogram of solution (mOsm/kg), referencing bodily fluid in a fluid-to-weight ratio. Osmolarity, in contrast, references solute concentration in a fluid-to-fluid ratio of milliosmoles per liter (mOsm/L). Recalling that 1 L of water weighs 1 kg, it becomes clear that mOsm/L equals mOsm/kg; these two terms may be used interchangeably. Osmolarity is more readily utilized for parenteral administration.

TIP: *Reference ranges for osmolality and osmolarity are the same.*

CALCULATING MOLES

Understanding calculations involving osmolality and osmolarity begins first with understanding moles. A mole (mol) is the amount of a substance equal to the molecular weight (MW) in grams. Millimoles (mmol) are more frequently used and represent the amount of substance equal to the MW in milligrams.

For example:

- MW NaCl = 58.5
- 1 mol NaCl = 58.5 g
- 1 mmol NaCl = 58.5 mg

When calculating moles of a solution with a known volume, use the following equation:

$$\text{moles} = \frac{\text{moles of substance (g)}}{\text{MW (g/mol)}}$$

EXAMPLE CALCULATION

Calculate mole and millimole equivalency for 100 g of sodium chloride.
MW NaCl = 58.5

$$\text{Moles} = \frac{100\text{ g}}{58.5\text{ g/mol}} = 1.709\text{ mol} = 1709\text{ mmol}$$

CALCULATING OSMOLES

The process of osmosis involves movements of active particles and/or molecules in a solution. These active particles result from some molecules dissociating into ions when dissolved in a solution. Osmoles are calculated as the number of moles multiplied by the number of particles present when dissolved in water. Osmolarity represents the number of osmotically active particles that are present in 1 L of solution.

EXAMPLE CALCULATION 1

Calculate the number of osmoles in 1 mole of dextrose.

> **TIP:** *Dextrose does not dissociate in a solution, so it is equal to 1 molecule.*

1 mol of dextrose × 1 = 1 Osm

EXAMPLE CALCULATION 2

Calculate the number of osmoles in 1 mole of KCl.

> **TIP:** *A potassium chloride molecule will dissociate into two ions when in solution.*

1 mol of KCl × 2 = 2 Osm

The concentration of many electrolytes (K, Na, Ca) is expressed in milliequivalents (mEq), from which osmoles can be calculated using the molecular weight and valence of the electrolyte.

Steps to Calculate mOsm from mEq

1. Calculate mOsm for each ion.

    For a univalent ion: mEq = mOsm
    For a divalent ion: mEq/valence = mOsm

2. Add the mOsm for all ions to obtain the total mOsm.

EXAMPLE CALCULATION

Calculate the mOsm in 20 mEq of KCl.

1. Calculate mOsm for each ion or molecule (for univalent ions: mEq = mOsm).

    > **TIP:** *Dissociation of potassium chloride results in two univalent ions.*

    20 mEq K = 20 mOsm Na
    20 mEq Cl = 20 mOsm Cl

3. Add the mOsm for all ions and molecules to obtain the total mOsm.
    20 mEq KCl = 20 mOsm K + 20 mOsm Cl = 40 mOsm

Answer: The total mOsm in 20 mEq of KCl is 40 mOsm.

Calculating Osmolarity

Osmolarity will need to be calculated to determine if a final solution is isosmotic for patient administration. This calculation is particularly useful when preparing parenteral nutrition to determine the influence of multiple additives on total osmolarity. Osmolarity dictates the type of access line through which solutions can be administered. Administration through a peripheral line can accommodate only solutions with an osmolarity of less than 900 mOsm/L, while central lines can tolerate infusions of more than 900 mOsm/L.

ALERT: *Osmolarity of solutions must be calculated to determine if the solution should be administered through a central or peripheral line.*

The following steps provide a guide to calculating osmolarity.

STEPS TO CALCULATE OSMOLARITY

1. Calculate the mOsm for the base solution.

$$\text{Osmolarity} = \frac{[\text{weight of substance (g/L)}](\text{number of species})(1000)}{\text{molecular weight}}$$

2. Calculate the mOsm for each additive (reference the section on calculating mOsm).
3. Calculate the total mOsm by adding all parts—both the base solution and all additives.

$$\frac{(\text{Osmolarity of A})(\text{volume A}) + (\text{Osmolarity of B})(\text{Volume B})}{\text{Total volume}}$$

EXAMPLE CALCULATION

Calculate the osmolarity of 500 mL of NS with 20 mEq of KCl (2 mEq/mL) and 10 mL of calcium gluconate (0.465 mEq/mL).

MW KCl = 74.5 g
MW NaCl = 58.5 g
MW calcium gluconate = 430.4 g

1. Calculate the mOsm for the base solution.

> **TIP:** *The base solution is NS, or 0.9% NaCl, resulting in a weight of 0.9 g/100 mL or 9 g/L.*

$(9 \text{ g/L})(2)(1000)/58.5 = 308 \text{ mOsm/L}$

2. Calculate the mOsm for each additive (reference the section on calculating mOsm).

> **TIP:** *KCl dissociates into univalent ions.*

20 mEq KCl = 20 mOsm K + 20 mOsm Cl = 40 mOsm
$(0.465 \text{ mEq/mL})(10 \text{ mL}) = 4.65 \text{ mEq calcium gluconate}$
$(4.65 \text{ mOsm/2}) \text{ Ca} + 4.65 \text{ mOsm gluconate} = 7.0 \text{ mOsm}$

3. Calculate total mOsm by adding all parts—both base solution and all additives.

> **TIP:** *The total volume to be used is the sum of the solution volume and all additives (10 mL of KCl and 10 mL calcium gluconate).*

$$\frac{308 \text{ mOsm/L } (0.5\text{L})}{0.52 \text{ L}} + \frac{40 \text{ mOsm}}{0.52 \text{ L}} + \frac{7 \text{ mOsm}}{0.52 \text{ L}}$$

Answer: The total osmolarity is 386.5 mOsm/L.

Syringe and Needle Priming Volume

Syringe and needle dead space is the space in a syringe and needle where solution is retained after the syringe plunger has been depressed completely. Dead space is also referred to as the syringe and needle priming volume. Typically, the solution retained in this space is not of concern—but on some occasions, it must be taken into account, such as with pediatric preparations. Other situations in which dead space becomes a factor are when mixing two drugs in a single syringe and when diluting a drug in a single syringe. With both of these situations, the significance of the dead space volume is increased when the medication volume is less than 1 mL. Dead space volume may also be of concern when the medication is relatively expensive or difficult to acquire. Avoiding mixing and diluting of drugs in a single syringe is ideal, but sometimes this approach is deemed necessary. Not accounting for syringe and needle dead space when mixing and diluting drugs in a single syringe may result in overdosing of the first medication and underdosing the second medication. The syringe and needle dead space volume varies by syringe manufacturer, the length of the needle, and gauge of the needle. Syringe dead space volume is approximately 0.04 mL, whereas needle dead space volume may vary from 0.01 mL to 0.06 mL. Exact syringe and needle dead space volumes may be obtained from the specific manufacturer or may be directly measured.

The following steps provide a guide to calculating the priming volume for two medications mixed in a single syringe.

Steps to Calculate Priming Volume

1. Calculate the proportion of the priming volume for Drug A.

$$\text{Priming volume} \times \frac{\text{Drug A volume}}{\text{Drug A volume} + \text{Drug B volume}}$$

2. Add the Drug A volume to the calculated priming volume for Drug A.

$$\text{Drug A volume} + \text{Drug A priming volume}$$

3. Calculate the proportion of the priming volume for Drug B.

$$\text{Priming volume} \times \frac{\text{Drug B volume}}{\text{Drug A volume} + \text{Drug B volume}}$$

4. Add the Drug B volume to the calculated priming volume for Drug B.

Drug B volume + Drug B priming volume

EXAMPLE CALCULATION

Syringe and needle system priming volume of 0.1 mL is known.

Drug A dosing volume = 0.2 mL
Drug B dosing volume = 0.5 mL

1. Calculate the proportion of the priming volume for Drug A.

$$0.1 \text{ mL} \times \frac{0.2 \text{ mL}}{0.2 \text{ mL} + 0.5 \text{ mL}} = 0.03 \text{ mL}$$

2. Add the Drug A volume to the calculated priming volume for Drug A.
   0.2 mL + 0.03 mL = 0.23 mL total for Drug A

3. Calculate the proportion of the priming volume for Drug B.

$$0.1 \text{ mL} \times \frac{0.5 \text{ mL}}{0.2 \text{ mL} + 0.5 \text{ mL}} = 0.07 \text{ mL}$$

4. Add the Drug B volume to the calculated priming volume for Drug B.
   0.5 mL + 0.07 mL = 0.57 mL total for Drug B

In addition to calculating the priming volume, unique compounding procedures requiring the utilization of three syringes must be followed to effectively accommodate the syringe and needle priming volume when mixing or diluting two drugs in separate syringes in a third syringe. The first syringe is used for measuring the Drug A dose volume and Drug A priming volume. A second syringe is used for measuring the Drug B dose volume and Drug B priming volume. The total volumes of Drug A and Drug B are then transferred into the third syringe. Transferring into the third syringe is accomplished using a special connector that attaches two syringe tips, allowing solutions to be transferred from one syringe to another. It is critical that the plunger of the third syringe be pulled back to a volume that exceeds the total volumes of both drugs to ensure that the solution does not overflow from the syringe tip. This air space also allows for the syringe to be agitated to ensure both drugs are properly mixed. Finally, the third syringe should be capped, visually inspected, and properly labeled for distribution.

Product Overfill Volume

Sterile products supplied from the manufacture typically contain a small amount overfill volume, above that of the labeled volume. The volume of overfill varies between manufacturers as well as between products and their various sizes. In most situations, overfill does not need to be addressed; however, in certain situations when the CSP is concentration dependent, the overfill volume may need to be accounted for or removed. The product manufacturer can provide the exact volume of overfill or it can be directly measured. Overfill volume may be accounted for by removing the overfill volume from the product prior to adding drug.

> **TIP:** *Overfill volumes may need to be considered when working with concentration dependent CSPs. In addition to the overfill volume, the volume of drug being added may also need to be removed from the product before the active drug is added.*

Conclusion

Patients and healthcare workers entrust the accuracy and sterility of parenteral CSPs to those who prepare them. Calculations are a fundamental step in preparing such preparations and require great accuracy. In a study evaluating the accuracy of dilutions of intravitreal antibiotics by pharmacists, ophthalmologists, and ophthalmic assistants, researchers found the least variability in accuracy among pharmacy personnel.[7] Pharmacists should be knowledgeable and capable of performing calculations accurately and employing self-check methods to verify their results. Electronic calculators should be utilized, when available, to decrease the potential for medications errors—a procedure that has been demonstrated to be effective with complex calculations involved in parenteral nutrition.[8] Online calculators are available for many calculations involved in compounding parenteral preparations, such as osmolarity and parenteral nutrition, and can be useful for pharmacists and other healthcare workers.

Review Questions

1. What is the percent weight in volume for 750 mg of levofloxacin in 150 mL of D_5W?
2. Convert 1:15,000 to a percent strength.
3. What is the final percentage when 800 mL of 90% isopropyl alcohol and 1500 mL of 50% isopropyl alcohol are mixed?
4. The following order is received:

Ceftriaxone 1 g IM one-time dose (in 3 mL)

Ceftriaxone for Injection, USP **2 gram per vial**	**For I.V. Administration:** Reconstitute with 19.2 mL of an I.V. diluent. Each 1 mL of solution contains approximately 100 mg equivalent of ceftriaxone.

How many milliliters of sterile water must be added to reconstitute the 2-g vial?

5. How many parts of 75%, 55%, 10% and 20% solution are needed to prepare a 35% solution?
6. How many milligrams of dextrose are needed to make 1% of cocaine HCl isotonic in 30 mL of sterile water?

Dextrose: $E = 0.16$
Cocaine HCl: $E = 0.16$

7. Calculate the mOsm in 20 mEq of CaCl.
8. Calculate the osmolarity of 500 mL D_5W ½NS and 40 mEq KCl. The concentration of the KCl solution is 2 mEq/mL.

MW dextrose = 180 g
MW NaCl = 58.5 g
MW KCl = 74.5 g

CASE STUDIES *Case 1*

A patient with lung cancer arrives in the oncology infusion clinic for her routine dose of Taxol (paclitaxel). You are the pharmacist who works in the infusion clinic and will be calculating the dose of chemotherapy for this patient. The order written by the oncologist reads: Taxol 200 mg/m². The patient weighs 125 pounds and is 5 feet 8 inches tall. What volume of Taxol should be removed from the vial and placed in the bag of diluent? How many vials will be needed?

Case 2

A patient in the hospital is found to be hypokalemic. The physician calls the main pharmacy and says she will be writing an order for intravenous potassium chloride shortly. The patient needs this treatment as quickly as possible. List all of the information you will need to gather prior to preparing the potassium chloride for both preparation of the intravenous admixture as well as for administration.

References

1. Ratio. 2011. Available at: http://www.merriam-webster.com /dictionary/ratio. Accessed November 20, 2012.
2. Proportion. 2011. Available at: http://www.merriam-webster .com/dictionary/proportion. Accessed November 20, 2012.
3. Vancomycin. In: *DRUGDEX® evaluations* [Internet database]. Greenwood Village, CO: Thomson Healthcare; August 30 2013.
4. Verbraecken J, Van de Heyning P, De Backer W, Van Gaal L. Body surface area in normal-weight, overweight, and obese adults: a comparison study. *Metabolism.* 2006;55(4):515–524.
5. Reeves EP, Molloy K, Pohl K, McElvaney NG. Hypertonic saline in treatment of pulmonary disease in cystic fibrosis. *Sci World J.* 2012;2012:465230. Epub May 3, 2012.
6. Vaidya C, Ho W, Freda BJ. Management of hyponatremia: providing treatment and avoiding harm. *Cleve Clin J Med.* 2010;77(10):715–726.
7. Narvaez J, Wessels IF, Mattheis JK, Beierle F. Intravitreal antibiotics: accuracy of dilution by pharmacists, ophthalmologists, and ophthalmic assistants, using three protocols. *Ophthalmic Surg.* 1992;23(4):265–268.
8. Lehmann CU, Conner KG, Cox JM. Preventing provider errors: online total parenteral nutrition calculator. *Pediatrics.* 2004;113(4):748–753.
9. Wilroy LJ, Garcia DE, Parks NP. *Pharmacy sterile products in-house training manual.* Houston, TX: Pharmacy Education Resources; 2009.
10. Potassium. In: *DRUGDEX® evaluations* [Internet database]. Greenwood Village, CO: Thomson Reuters Healthcare; August 20, 2013.
11. Potassium chloride. In: *Lexi-Drugs™* [Internet database]. Lexi-Comp. Accessed September 14, 2013.

CHAPTER 4

Microbiological Considerations in Parenteral Compounding

Pamella S. Ochoa and José A. Vega

Chapter Objectives

1. Summarize the implications of pyrogenicity and sterility in compounding sterile preparations.
2. Classify sterile preparations as low-, medium-, or high-risk preparations.
3. Describe the role of particulate matter in contamination.
4. Categorize sterile preparations based on their ISO class.
5. List influences on the sterility of compounded sterile preparations.
6. State the preferred disinfecting and antiseptic agents used for compounding environments and personnel.
7. Explain the responsibilities of personnel in preventing microbiological contamination.

Key Terminology

Sterility
Pyrogen
Pyrogenicity

Depyrogenation
Endotoxin
Primary engineering control
Aseptic technique
Beyond-use date
Pathogen
Particulate matter
ISO classification
Personal protective equipment
Risk levels
Fomite

Overview

Healthcare-associated infections (HAIs) have significant patient and economic consequences, with 1 out of 20 hospitalized patients experiencing a HAI in the United States. The burden of HAIs is estimated to exceed $33 billion in medical costs every year. Specifically, a central line bloodstream infection (CLBSI), a type of HAI, can add $16,550 in excess medical costs.[1] More astounding is that even though HAIs are preventable, the unfortunate loss of life secondary to HAIs is estimated at approximately 100,000 deaths each year.[2] While numerous efforts to reduce the rate of HAIs have been undertaken, much more work in this area is still needed.

Some HAIs result from contamination of parenteral preparations. Microbiological contamination can be introduced into parenteral preparations by several different modes. The most likely source of contamination is the operator involved in the preparation process. Different types of contamination can be introduced into the final preparation based on the original source of the bacteria. Because administration of parenteral preparations occurs through routes that readily introduce drugs into the body, such as the intravenous route, a contaminated preparation will result in direct introduction of the microbe into the patient. The types and amounts of bacteria that are introduced into the patient via parenteral contamination, as well as the level of immune function of the patient, influence the consequences to the patient. Further, specific types of microbes exist in institutional settings that can result in more significant consequences, such as infection with antibiotic-resistant bacteria, making it even more important to institute practices to prevent contamination. Historical examples of contamination of parenteral preparations are, unfortunately, abundant. Pharmacists and others involved in the preparation process should be knowledgeable as to the origin of contamination, the types of contamination, and measures that should be taken to prevent contamination.

Sterility

Sterility is defined as being free from viable microorganisms and is considered an absolute term, meaning that a preparation can be considered only either sterile or not sterile—there is no "in between" state. If not sterile, the preparation is considered contaminated. All parenteral preparations should be free from contamination. Preparing a sterile preparation takes understanding of the contamination process as well as utilization of methods and processes to prevent it.

The operator has an important role in ensuring sterility of parenteral preparations. This includes using specific preparation techniques, referred to as aseptic technique, consistently and appropriately. It also involves the attentive use of sterile equipment and supplies. Although care may be taken during the preparation process to prevent contamination by environmental control and use of proper preparation techniques, other risks to the sterility of the preparation exist. Further, nurses and other healthcare providers may be involved in preparing, withdrawing, or administering parenteral preparations or products. These processes may take place in areas that are not controlled, aseptic environments. Sterility can be compromised if proper techniques and environment are not carefully accounted for in these circumstances.

For low-risk preparations, the sterility of the preparation strongly depends on maintaining a proper compounding environment, ensuring operator competency and use of proper preparation techniques, and controlling for other influences that might potentially compromise sterility. High-risk preparations require sterilization of the final preparation, known as terminal sterilization, which can be achieved either physically or chemically. Physical sterilization involves the use of filtration, saturated steam, or dry heat. Chemical sterilization uses ethylene oxide gas or chemical liquids. Sterilization by filtration is the most common method of sterilization and is used for high-risk compounding.

High-risk preparations can be tested for sterility by ascertaining the probability of a microorganism existing in the final preparation following sterilization, also known as the sterility assurance level (SAL). Testing is an important step in quality assurance and control of parenteral preparations and is further discussed in the *Quality Assurance and Quality Control for Sterile Compounding* chapter.

Endotoxins and Pyrogens

Endotoxins are toxic, heat-stable lipopolysaccharide substances contained within the cell wall of gram-negative bacteria, including noninfectious gram-negative bacteria. Bacteria undergo cell lysis following ingestion by macrophages. When bacteria disintegrate, the toxins within them are released and recognized by the human immune system, resulting in immunogenic and toxic effects (**Figure 4-1**). The ensuing systemic reaction causes fever, diarrhea, and other inflammatory responses. Parenteral preparations are at risk of being contaminated with these types of endotoxins; consequently, USP Chapter <797> requires that specific types of parenteral preparations be tested to ensure that excessive bacterial endotoxins are not present.

Pyrogens include any substance that is foreign to the body and elicits a febrile response upon injection or infection.[3, p.462] A preparation can be considered sterile, but may still contain pyrogens. The most potent type of pyrogen is an endotoxin. Apyrogenicity refers to the absence of pyrogens. Pyrogens are produced by many microbes, including bacteria, yeasts, and molds, but the most

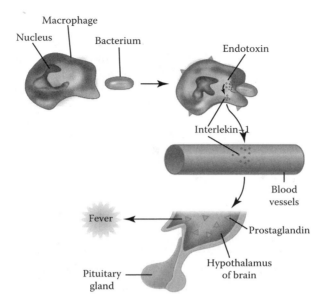

Figure 4-1 Release of Endotoxins

concerning types are those released from gram-negative bacteria. If large amounts of pyrogens are administered to a patient, they can lead to septic shock, organ failure, and ultimately death. In smaller amounts, pyrogens elicit biological effects including fever, pain, lethargy, and irritation and erythema at the injection site. Pyrogens are resilient substances that may become a source of contamination of parenteral preparations from equipment, containers, closures, chemical solutes, human touch, and aqueous vehicles such as water. Mostly found in moist environments, they can exist for long periods of time—up to years—in aqueous solutions or dried form.[4, p.27] Common sterilization processes are inadequate at eradicating pyrogens, so special sterilization processes should be employed for depyrogenation. Knowing that pyrogens are difficult to destroy helps us to understand the importance of preventing pyrogens from entering the human body. Thus the focus should be on preventing pyrogenic contamination by ensuring that the environment and all materials used in the preparation process are apyrogenic.

Testing of solutions for endotoxins and pyrogens is necessary for quality assurance to ensure patient safety. For further discussion of bacterial endotoxin and pyrogen testing, refer to the *Quality Assurance and Quality Control for Sterile Compounding* chapter.

Infection and Contamination

The difference between infection and contamination lies in the concentration of the microbiological source. For example, an infected wound is expected to have a larger concentration of bacteria compared to a contaminated wound. Contamination, however, can lead to an infection, just as a contaminated parenteral preparation can result in an infection if that preparation is administered to a patient. It is important to remember that microbes exist everywhere, including on people, objects, surfaces, water, food, soil, bodily excretions, and more. Many bacteria and viruses can survive for days or even weeks on surfaces, providing a persistent source of contamination. Healthcare workers are a source of contamination, as they often are colonized with bacteria that are unique to healthcare settings and can easily transmit such bacteria to patients, even if the workers themselves are not infected. Understanding the origin of infections and the method by which parenteral preparations become microbiologically contaminated serves as the foundational concept in ensuring a sterile preparation.

Infectious agents are transported from a reservoir through a portal of exit, are conveyed by a mode of transmission through an entry portal, and then infect a susceptible host (**Figure 4-2**). The reservoir from which the pathogen originates can be a human, animal, or environmental reservoir. The various modes of transmission, direct and indirect, are defined by the Centers for Disease Control and Prevention (CDC) as follows:[5]

- Direct: pathogens are transmitted directly from the reservoir to the host
    - Direct contact: pathogens are transmitted through direct skin-to-skin contact

- Droplet spread: sprays from coughing, sneezing, talking, and chewing gum
■ Indirect: pathogens are transmitted from the reservoir to the host by air particles, inanimate objects (vehicle), or animate intermediaries (vectors)
  - Airborne: transmission occurs when pathogens are carried on dust or droplets that are suspended or resuspended in air
  - Vector-borne: vectors such as mosquitos or ticks can transmit infections to a host by either direct carrier means or through changing the pathogen
  - Vehicle-borne: food, water, blood and other biological sources, and fomites can be a source of contamination

Parenteral preparations may be contaminated from droplet spread, such as when personnel engage in coughing, sneezing,

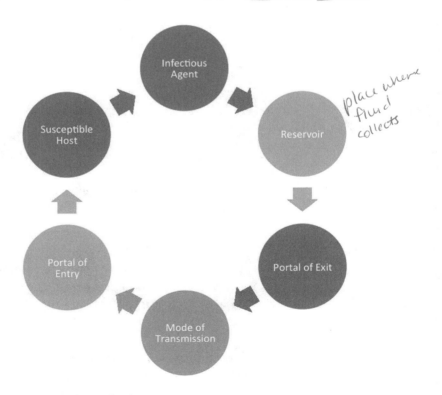

place where fluid collects

Figure 4-2 Chain of Infection

talking, or chewing gum when compounding the preparation. Touch contamination, by way of vehicle-borne transmission of pathogens, is considered the most common source of contamination for parenteral preparations. Contamination by touch occurs when an operator touches critical parts, known as critical sites, of the container, syringe, or needle that are associated with an increased likelihood of contamination of the final preparation when touched. Airborne transmission of pathogens is a concern because particles introduced during the preparation process may potentially lead to contamination of the admixture. In all of these cases, either the operator or the environment serves as a reservoir, while the parenteral preparation serves as the mode of transmission. The pathogen then is administered to the patient along with the parenteral preparation, at which point the patient becomes the host. Considering that the evolution of this cycle begins with a reservoir, every effort should be taken to control these factors. If the operator consistently and properly applies aseptic compounding technique during the preparation process and the environment is strictly controlled, such efforts will minimize the potential for contamination.

ALERT: *Touch contamination is the most common source of contamination of parenteral preparations.*

Various forms of contamination exist. USP Chapter <797> classifies contamination into three different categories: microbial, chemical, and physical.

MICROBIAL CONTAMINATION

Microbial contamination relates to the presence of microbes or pathogens. When introduced into parenteral preparations, and subsequently to a patient, microbial contamination results in bloodstream infections or other infections based on the location of administration.

The literature describes many incidents of adverse patient outcomes secondary to microbial contamination. Most recently, a 2012 outbreak of fungal meningitis—a rare type of meningitis that usually occurs in immunocompromised patients—resulted from contamination of compounded preservative-free intrathecal methylprednisolone used for spinal injections. This devastating outbreak affected more than 700 patients and resulted in hospitalization of numerous patients experiencing meningitis, vertebral osteomyelitis, epidural abscesses, systemic infections, and stroke; it also led to the deaths of more than 50 patients.[6] Upon observation during an investigation, one fourth of the steroid vials had a "greenish black foreign matter" visible to the naked eye.[6] Testing revealed different types of fungi as the source of microbial contamination, including fungal species such as *Aspergillus tubingensis*, *Aspergillus fumigatus*, *Cladosporium* species, and *Penicillium* species.[7]

In 2011, the U.S. Food and Drug Administration (FDA) received reports of an outbreak of *Serratia marcescens* infection leading to bacteremia in patients, many of whom died.[8,9] During an investigation by the CDC, *Serratia marcescens* was isolated from a tap water faucet in the pharmacy. A container and stirrer that were used during reconstitution of powder amino acids for total parenteral nutrition admixtures were rinsed in tap water from the contaminated faucet.[9]

CHEMICAL CONTAMINATION

[handwritten margin note: causes discomfort to death]

Endotoxins are not bacteria themselves, but rather chemicals released from bacteria that can cause contamination of parenteral preparations. Chemical contamination with endotoxins can lead to serious patient outcomes if a contaminated preparation is administered.

Aluminum is another example of chemical contamination. The products and supplies used in preparing parenteral nutrition (PN) may be contaminated with aluminum, making PN a potential source of high aluminum exposure. Raw materials and by-products alike may be contaminated with aluminum from the manufacturing process, such as with calcium gluconate and phosphate salts.[10] Recent focus has centered on the adverse effects of aluminum accumulation in neonatal and pediatric patients receiving PN. While the FDA has set maximum daily exposure limits for cumulative aluminum exposure at 5 mcg/kg/day, these limits are easily exceeded with normal preparations of PN for smaller patients.

PHYSICAL CONTAMINATION

Physical contamination of parenteral preparations can result from sources such as objects, personnel, solid or liquid matter, supplies, equipment, and the environment. Coring, for example, is a common source of physical contamination. It results from improper entry of a needle through the rubber closure of a vial, such that a piece of rubber is bored from the closure and remains in the shaft of the needle. When the solution is expelled from the syringe and into the final preparation, the piece of rubber closure is simultaneously ejected into the final preparation.

Glass ampules also pose a high risk of physical contamination. When opening a glass ampule, glass shards may enter the ampule and consequently be ejected into the final preparation if a filter needle is not used.

Particles resulting from ingredients not fully solubilized into solution or from incompatibilities are other sources of physical contamination.

Administration of preparations that are contaminated physically can lead to severe complications in patients, such as occlusion of vessels, damage to organs from thrombus formation, phlebitis, and possibly death.

Influences on Contamination

ENVIRONMENT

Compounding in conditions in which air quality does not meet specific requirements may influence the likelihood of microbial contamination, both in direct compounding areas and in areas nearby. Parenteral medications are often prepared in patient care areas, rather than in controlled aseptic environments. For example, in the event of an emergency, admixtures are often prepared at the patient bedside. Other places where medications are prepared in a hospital include the operating room, recovery units, radiology, and emergency departments.

The influence of the environment on the sterility of parenteral preparations was evidenced in a study in which syringes were prepared using standard procedures in the intensive care unit (ICU) and compared to syringes prepared by pharmacy technicians in standard aseptic conditions of the pharmacy compounding room. The syringes were prepared from either vials or ampules, the difference being an open system or a closed system. The rate of contamination in the syringes was significantly higher in those prepared in the ICU, outside of the aseptic conditions.[11]

Further discussion of environmental conditions for compounding can be found in the *Primary and Secondary Engineering Controls* chapter.

OPERATOR

While the environmental air quality and cleanliness in which compounding occurs influence the sterility of a preparation, compounding in a controlled environment alone will not result in a sterile preparation. Personnel involved in the preparation process have the most influence on the sterility of the final preparation, as touch contamination is considered the most common source of contamination. Proper hand washing, along with wearing proper personal protective equipment (PPE), using aseptic technique, using adequate and proper disinfecting agents, and ensuring supplies and equipment are sterile, can prevent contamination of the preparation. Additionally, no talking, sneezing, coughing, smoking, eating, drinking, or chewing of gum should be done when compounding parenteral preparations; these activities are known to introduce droplets into the compounding environment and may also result in fluctuations in air currents.

Healthcare workers pose a special risk of microbial contamination because of the amounts and types of microorganisms that they carry. For example, antibiotic-resistant bacteria can be found on the hands of healthcare workers; their presence is minimized with hand washing but is not fully eliminated with this measure. Healthcare workers also introduce a significant amount of particles into the environment.

ALERT: *No sneezing, coughing, talking, smoking, eating, drinking, or chewing gum when compounding sterile preparations.*

ALERT: *Operator transfer of microbes through direct contact is the most common cause of contamination in compounded preparations.*

Nails

It is important to realize that debris, whether visible or invisible to the naked eye, harbors bacteria. Despite proper hand cleansing procedures, including removal of debris from under fingernails using a nail cleanser or use of surgical scrubs, a substantial number of pathogens will remain in the nail spaces.[12] Recognizing that hands come in intimate contact with the preparation and that touch contamination is the most frequent source of contamination, the importance of keeping the nails trimmed and clean becomes obvious. If fingernails are long, not only does the increased length provide more area for bacterial or fungal growth, but it also increases the likelihood of tearing of gloves during preparation. The CDC recommends a maximum nail length of 0.25 inch; however, recent studies indicate that a shorter length may further minimize risk of contamination, with an association being found between nail lengths greater than 2 mm and increased carriage rate of *Staphylococcus aureus*.[12,13]

Artificial nails have been implicated as a source of infection and have been linked with serious patient consequences, such as with hemodialysis-related bacteremia and an outbreak of extended-spectrum beta-lactamase–producing *Klebsiella pneumoniae* in a neonatal intensive care unit.[14,15] Although using proper hand cleansing procedures may reduce bacterial load associated with artificial nails, a higher number of pathogens will remain on the hands following cleaning with either antimicrobial soap or alcohol-based gel for those persons with artificial acrylic nails compared to those persons without such artificial nails.[16] Furthermore, healthcare workers with artificial nails are more prone to harbor gram-negative bacteria on their fingertips, both before and after hand washing.[12] Like longer nails, artificial nails also introduce the risk of breaking or tearing through gloves, often going unnoticed during the preparation process. USP Chapter <797> states that "the wearing of artificial nails or extenders is prohibited while working in the sterile compounding environment."[17]

Cosmetics and Jewelry

All cosmetics are known to shed, although such shedding is not always visible to the naked eye. This effect contributes to the overall particulate count in compounding environments, as cosmetics can flake off and land on supplies, equipment, hands, or preparations. Besides physical contamination, cosmetic flaking or shedding may contribute to microbial contamination. For similar reasons, nail polish should not be worn. Per USP Chapter <797>, cosmetics should not be worn by those personnel involved in compounding sterile preparations. Cosmetics to avoid when compounding sterile preparations include face or eye makeup (mascara, false eyelashes, lipstick, eye shadow, eyebrow pencil or powder, eye liner), hair products (hair spray, mousse), perfumes, aerosols, and aftershave.

Jewelry or piercings that interfere with the effectiveness of proper PPE should not be worn.[17] Essentially, this includes all types of jewelry, such as rings, earrings, watches, and other types of jewelry. The importance of this recommendation is substantiated by reports in the literature, in which the effects of jewelry and hand lotion on hand microbiology were demonstrated. For example, researchers found enhanced bacterial counts on the hands of healthcare workers who wore watches compared to those who did not.[13] Similar results were found among healthcare workers who wore finger rings as well as among those who recently applied hand lotion.[13] Thus no jewelry should be worn by personnel involved in compounding sterile preparations. Approved skin lotion can be considered to reduce skin flaking.

ALERT: *No jewelry, makeup, or artificial nails should be worn while involved in compounding parenteral preparations. Unapproved hand lotion should be avoided and nails should be no longer than 2 mm.*

Illnesses and Wounds

If the operator is experiencing any type of illness that is of microbiological origin, he or she should not be involved in compounding. There is an increased likelihood of an ill operator contaminating both the area of compounding and the final preparation. Considering the acuity of patients in the hospital and other settings in which compounded sterile preparations (CSPs) are administered, this can wager high risks for patients, especially those who may be immunocompromised. Thus it is imperative that no one with a suspected communicative illness, such as conjunctivitis or respiratory infection, be allowed to compound parenteral preparations.

Wounds are also of concern, as they can transmit bacteria if infected. Further, some types of wounds, such as sunburns, can result in shedding of particles at an increased rate. Personnel with rashes, sunburns, open wounds, or weeping sores should not compound parenteral preparations. Minor wounds that are not open (i.e., in which the skin is intact) should be completely covered with appropriate nonshedding bandages and then covered with the usual PPE, such as gloves.

Any compounding personnel with illnesses or wounds should not compound preparations and should not enter ISO Class 5 or ISO Class 7 environments.[17]

ALERT: *Personnel with any suspected illness of microbiological origin must not be involved in preparing CSPs and must not enter controlled compounding environments.*

Multidose Vials

While all types of vials have been implicated in cases of contamination, multidose vials (MDVs) can pose an increased risk secondary to being entered multiple times as well as being stored in between uses. MDVs provide the convenience and cost-effectiveness of being able to remove small portions of solutions on multiple occasions. They differ from single-dose vials, which are for one-time use only, in that MDVs usually contain antimicrobial preservatives. This does not, however, exempt the preparation from risk of contamination if proper procedures are not followed concerning their storage and beyond-use dating. There also exists an increased risk of contamination in MDVs that do not contain preservatives. If a MDV is not opened or accessed, its expiration date reverts to that assigned by the manufacturer. If it is opened or accessed, however, the vial should be discarded 28 days after its opening or accessing.[17] Thus it is important that the vial be marked with the date and time that it was opened or accessed. When the vial is not in use, it should be sealed with a sterile seal and placed in an environment that will prevent its contamination (**Figure 4-3**).

Because of the risk of both direct and indirect contamination, MDVs that enter an immediate patient treatment area, such as a patient room or operating room, should be dedicated to a singular patient and discarded after use. Additionally, vials should be disinfected prior to each entry and only clean, sterile needles and syringes should be used with each preparation.

Reports of adverse patient outcomes secondary to improper use of MDVs have been described in the literature. For example, an outbreak of acute hepatitis C infections was found to result from improper use of MDVs. In this incident, 12 patients were infected with acute hepatitis C after being treated in an outpatient gastroenterology center. Following an investigation, it was determined that multidose anesthetic vials, intended for single-patient use, were used on multiple patients during operations. Further, new needles were not used upon reentering the vial when more medication was needed. These practices were believed to be the cause of transmission of hepatitis C between patients, which could have been prevented with proper use of MDVs.[18]

TIP: *The time and date that a multidose vial is accessed or opened should be clearly and consistently recorded.*

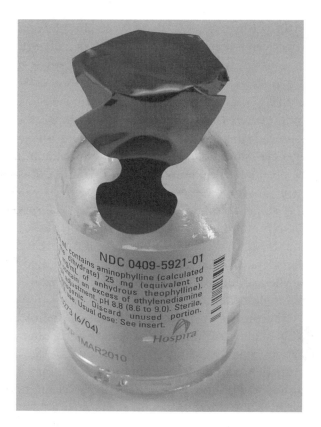

Figure 4-3 Vial Seal

OPEN AND CLOSED SYSTEMS

Open systems, as discussed in the *Supplies and Equipment for Compounding and Administering Sterile Preparations* chapter, allow the exchange of free air into and out of the container. An open ampule is an example of an open system. In contrast, closed systems do not accommodate free air exchange, as with vials with rubber closures. Open systems are much more vulnerable to contamination, compared to closed systems, because contact with air increases the likelihood that particulates and microbes will enter the container. Preparations that have been compounded from ampules, for example, have been shown to have greater rates of contamination as those prepared from vials.[11]

Chemical and Environmental Characteristics

Certain conditions are more conducive to microbial growth and can result in extended colonization of bacteria in a solution. For example, pH, temperature, and exposure to oxygen can either favor or not favor microbial growth. Solutions with a neutral pH are more likely to provide the environment necessary to promote growth of bacteria following contamination. The presence of oxygen, or lack thereof, also influences the growth of aerobic and anaerobic bacteria. Temperatures at or near room or body temperature are conducive for the proliferation of most microorganisms, which explains why many preparations are refrigerated or frozen to extend their beyond-use date. Additionally, storage conditions may influence bacterial contamination of parenteral preparations. Longer storage times result in increased risk of microbial growth.

Discussion of the influence of chemical and environmental conditions on stability of CSPs can be found in the *Principles of Compatibility and Stability* chapter. Compounding processes that involve multiple transfers and/or increased amount of time for the completion of the compounding also put the final preparation at risk of contamination.

Types of Preparations

The types of drugs used in CSPs influence the likelihood of microbial contamination. In particular, the use of sterile versus non-sterile components of a preparation will affect the risk of contamination. Additionally, some ingredients provide a more robust environment that promotes the growth and proliferation of certain types of bacteria. For example, propofol and insulin have been shown to have higher rates of contamination in syringes prepared by nurses in the ICU.[19] Microbes require nutrients to proliferate, such as carbohydrates, fats, proteins, and vitamins. Parenteral nutrition (PN) contains many of these ingredients and is known to have high risk of microbial growth, especially if administered over a long period of time. PN has been implicated in several incidents of microbial contamination, as these preparations contain ingredients that readily foster microbial growth.

Particulate Matter

USP Chapter <788> defines particulate matter as "mobile, randomly-sourced, extraneous substances, other than gas bubbles, that cannot be quantified by chemical analysis due to the small amount of material that it represents and to its heterogeneous composition."[20] Particulate matter consists of minute liquid or solid particles and may include dust, lint, paper, cellulose and cotton fibers, glass, rubber, metals, undissolved chemicals, dandruff, and more. Particulates may originate from a variety of sources, such as the environment, equipment, personnel, containers, closures, vehicles, and solutes. The CDC defines droplet nuclei, a type of particulate, as "dried residue of less than 5 microns in size."[5] These nuclei can remain suspended for a long time in the air. They also have the ability to be blown over a significant distance, especially in the presence of air currents.

Particulate matter, such as dust and droplets, influences air quality as well. Consequently, its minimization is important in both compounding areas and adjacent areas. Particles that are suspended in the air may include airborne particles that have settled and then become resuspended by air currents. One can easily visualize the presence and number of dust particles suspended in the air by opening window blinds on a bright, sunny day and allowing sunlight inside, thereby illuminating the many particles suspended in the air that might otherwise go unseen. Environments in which parenteral compounding is undertaken are not exempt from this same potential for particulate matter, especially if the air quality is not sufficiently controlled.

In a compounding area, particles generated from personnel are a significant contributor to the overall particulate load. It has been demonstrated that a human will shed approximately 1 billion skin cells every day and approximately 100,000 skin particles per minute when sitting.[21,22] By increasing activity level to walking at a leisurely 1.9 miles per hour, the number of skin particles shed becomes 5 million per minute.[22] Not only do skin cells significantly contribute to the particle level indoors, but it is also believed that bacteria are associated with such skin cells.[21] For instance, each square centimeter of skin on the human hand will have a concentration of 10^2 to 10^7 bacteria.[23] Skin cells may become deposited onto floors and surfaces from which they can later become resuspended in the air.[24] Resuspension of skin cells and other particles is highly influenced by air currents, which are mostly attributable to traffic in compounding areas. For this reason, along with the increase in skin particles shed with increased activity levels, the number of personnel and amount of traffic in compounding areas should be minimized.

The size of particles is an important consideration in controlling environmental conditions and contamination risk. Particles smaller than 40 microns cannot be seen with the naked eye.[22] To put this into perspective, the flu virus is 0.07 micron, bacteria are 1 to 10 microns, dust particles can be 0.1 to 100 microns, and hair ranges in size from 50 to 150 microns.[22] Particulate matter injected into the human body that is larger than the size of an arteriole or a capillary, which can be 20–50 microns and 8 microns, respectively, can block downstream blood flow.[25] The clinical consequences of injecting or infusing particulate matter into a patient include phlebitis, inflammation, occlusion of veins or capillaries, formation of thrombi or microthrombi, immunogenic reactions, or even death.

Particles can be classified as viable or nonviable. Viable particles are those that contain one or more living microorganisms. These types of particles can contaminate surfaces or other objects, leading to subsequent contamination of final preparations. Viable particles usually range from about 0.2 to 30 microns in size. Airborne microorganisms do not float freely, but rather associate with, or are transported on, larger particles such as those of size 10 to 20 microns.[26] Nonviable particles do not contain living microorganisms; instead, they serve as transporters for viable particles. While a direct correlation between particles and microbiological contamination has not been confirmed, dependence between the two has been established.[3, p.621] Furthermore, it is generally accepted that controlling the airborne microorganisms in the environment will influence the quality and sterility of inter-mediate or final preparations.[26]

Because of the numerous adverse patient outcomes that can result if particulate matter is injected, USP Chapter <788> provides limits for the maximum number of particulates that can be present in a preparation—specifically, 600 particulates of size 25 microns for small-volume injections, and 3 particulates of no more than 25 microns per 1 mL.[20] Additionally, because of the interdependence between microbial contamination and particulate matter, it is important to control both the number and the size of particles, both in direct compounding areas and in nearby areas. There are three methods by which particulates in the environment can be controlled:[22]

- Eliminating existing particles in the room air
- Preventing new particles from being imported into the environment
- Preventing new particles from being generated in the environment

ISO Classification of Particulate Matter — measuring particulates

The environment in which parenteral preparations are compounded should be controlled because of the increased likelihood of contamination when increased numbers of viable and nonviable particulate matter are present. The number of particles in a given space should be measured to evaluate air quality. For example, preparations that have a high likelihood of contamination should be prepared in an environment that has very low particulate count.

Environments in which direct compounding takes place, as well as adjacent environments, can be categorized according to air quality. These categories, referred to as ISO classifications, are summarized in **Table 4-1**. ISO classification is used to determine the necessary air quality for given environments. Formerly, classifications were measured as particulate count per cubic feet and were referred to differently (i.e., Class 1000). Today, all

Table 4-1 ISO Classification of Particulate Matter in Air

Class Name		Particle Count	
ISO Class	Former Class	ISO (per m³)	Particulate Count (per ft³)
3	Class 1	35.2	1
4	Class 10	352	10
5 *hood*	Class 100	3520	100
6	Class 1000	35,200	1000
7 *buffer area*	Class 10,000	352,000	10,000
8 *anteroom*	Class 100,000	3,520,000	100,000

Source: Modified from U.S. Pharmacopeial Convention. Chapter <1072>: disinfectants and antiseptics. In: *United States Pharmacopeia 36/National Formulary 31*. Rockville, MD: U.S. Pharmacopeial Convention; 2013.

classifications should be referred to by their ISO class and measured as particulate count per cubic meter. For example, direct compounding areas should be an ISO Class 5 environment. The particle limits for the various ISO classes refer to the number of particles that are 0.5 micron and larger found per cubic meter of air. For example, an ISO Class 5 environment (formerly referred to as a Class 100 environment) should not have any more than 3520 particles that are 0.5 micron or larger in each cubic meter of air. Air quality evaluation, in which total particle counts are measured, should be performed no less often than every 6 months and whenever primary engineering controls are relocated or the structure of the compounding rooms and surrounding areas is altered.[17]

> **TIP:** *Use the ISO class and particulate count per cubic meter when referencing ISO classifications.*

Microbial Contamination Risk Levels

USP Chapter <797> provides guidance as to classification of compounded sterile preparations CSPs based on risk of contamination. These risk levels—low, medium, or high—are assigned based on the preparation's propensity for microbial, chemical, and physical contamination. Risk levels indicate the potential for microbial contamination during compounding for low- and medium-risk preparations, or the risk of inadequate sterilization for high-risk preparations.[17] These risk levels should be determined immediately after compounding. If sterilization is required, then the risk level should be determined after final sterilization is performed. For preparations to be classified as low, medium, or high risk, the conditions shown in **Figure 4-4** should be met, as taken from USP Chapter <797>.[17]

An example of a low-risk preparation would be one that involves a single transfer of a drug from a vial into a bag. A "banana bag," which is administered intravenously to alcoholic patients, includes the addition of folic acid, thiamine, and multivitamins into a liter of normal saline. This type of preparation cannot be classified as low risk because it contains four ingredients (the diluent counts as one of the maximum of three products allowed in a single preparation). In this example, the banana bag would be classified as medium risk. PN preparations are also examples of a medium-risk preparation. An example of a high-risk preparation is one that is made from a non-sterile bulk drug, which then requires terminal sterilization. Amino acid powders, for example, are available in bulk and need to be dissolved to form a solution that can then be used to prepare PN.

Most parenteral compounding in healthcare settings is low or medium risk. Determining the risk levels of preparations that will be compounded is important, as storage and quality assurance requirements differ for each level. Consideration of these requirements should guide pharmacies to evaluate the risk level that would best accommodate their compounding needs.

Immediate-Use Sterile Preparations

In many urgent patient circumstances, parenteral preparations are compounded in environments that are not controlled, referred to as unclassified space. These types of occurrences usually involve an immediate need for a CSP for which compounding and transporting of the parenteral preparation would be too

Low-Risk Level

- Compounding is performed in an ISO class 5 or better environment
- Only sterile ingredients, products, components, and devices should be used
- Only standard aseptic manipulations involving transferring, measuring, and mixing should be used
- No more than 3 commercially manufactured packages of sterile products should be used
- No more than two entries into any single sterile container or package of sterile product or administration container/device for preparation
- Manipulations are limited to aseptically opening ampules, penetrating disinfected stoppers on vials with sterile needles and syringes, and transferring sterile liquids in sterile syringes to sterile administration devices, package containers of other sterile products, and containers for storage and dispensing

≤ 12 hour BUD under certain circumstances

BUD can't exceed 48h CRT, 14 days cold, 45 days frozen

Medium-Risk Level *Class 5*

- Multiple individual or small doses of sterile products are combined to compound a preparation that will be administered to multiple patients or to one patient on multiple occasions
- Compounding process involves complex aseptic manipulations other than the single-volume transfer
- Compounding process requires usually long duration (dissolution of homogenous mixing)

High-Risk Level *Known contamination*

- Nonsterile ingredients, including manufactured products not intended for sterile routes of administration
- Nonsterile device is employed before terminal sterilizations
- Any of the following are exposed to air quality worse than ISO Class 5 for more than 1 hour:
  - Sterile contents of commercially manufactured products
  - Preparations that lack effective antimicrobial preservatives
  - Sterile surfaces of devices and containers for the preparation, transfer, sterilization, and packaging of preparations
- Compounding personnel are improperly garbed and gloved
- Nonsterile water-containing preparations are stored for more than 6 hours before being sterilized
- It is assumed that the chemical purity and content strength of ingredients meet their original or compendial specifications in unopened or in opened packages of bulk ingredients

Figure 4-4   Risk Levels

time consuming and would compromise patient care. In these situations, other healthcare providers typically will compound the preparation at the patient bedside or on the nursing unit. Examples include medications involved in cardiopulmonary resuscitation, treatments in the emergency department, and other critical therapies. Preparations compounded for immediate use also include those utilized as diagnostic agents.

USP Chapter <797> provides specific guidelines regarding the use and classification of immediate-use preparations. High- and medium-risk sterile preparations cannot be compounded as immediate-use preparations. Thus all immediate-use preparations should meet the criteria for the low risk level. Such preparations should not be stored. If the following criteria, defined in USP Chapter <797>, are met, then the preparation can be exempt from low-risk criteria:

- Only simple transfers are conducted of no more than three commercial sterile products or diagnostic radiopharmaceutical products. These transfers must originate from the original containers, and no more than two entries are allowed into any single container or package of sterile solutions or administration container/device.
- Compounding is a continuous process and does not last more than 1 hour, unless required for the specific preparation.
- Administration begins within 1 hour from the time the compounding begins.
- Aseptic technique is followed. If the preparation is administered immediately, then the preparation should be under continuous supervision to ensure it does not come in contact with non-sterile surfaces, particulate matter, or biological fluids, as well as to ensure that the preparation does not get mixed up with other preparations.
- In the event that the preparation is not administered completely and immediately following preparation, a label should be placed on the preparation with the following information:
  - Patient identifying information
  - Names of all ingredients
  - Amounts of all ingredients
  - Name or initials of the preparer
  - Beyond-use date and time (1 hour from the start of the preparation process)
- If administration of the compounded preparation is not initiated within one hour following the start of the

compounding process, the preparation should be promptly, properly, and safely discarded.

Disinfectants and Antiseptics

Disinfectants are used on surfaces for the following purposes:[3, p.249]

- Destroy or remove microorganisms
- Prevent entry of microorganisms into compounding areas
- Prevent dissemination of microorganisms throughout compounding areas
- Eliminate and prevent accumulation of pyrogens

Proper and consistent disinfecting is an important step to prevent the transmission of pathogens to patients. Not all equipment and supplies require sterilization, but may require disinfecting. Proper disinfection should eliminate many or all pathogenic microorganisms.

Although many types of disinfectants are available, the most commonly used disinfecting agents include alcohol, phenolics, quaternary ammonium compounds, aldehydes, chlorine compounds, hydrogen peroxide, and peracetic acid.[3, p.250] Disinfecting agents available today offer the benefit of having a broad spectrum of activity. When selecting the type of disinfectant, the following factors should be considered:[17]

- Microbicidal activity
- Inactivation by organic matter
- Residue
- Shelf-life

Ethyl and isopropyl alcohols are the type of disinfecting agent most commonly used for processes involving parenteral preparation, such as cleaning work surfaces and equipment, disinfecting gloves, and disinfecting rubber vial closures, ampule necks, and container ports. Methyl alcohol has lower bactericidal activity compared to ethyl and isopropyl alcohol, which has led to recommendations against its use. Alcohols exhibit bactericidal characteristics at concentrations of 60% to 70%, with higher concentrations being less effective.[3, p.236] USP Chapter <797> recommends the use of residue-free sterile 70% isopropyl alcohol (IPA).

IPA works by inducing denaturation of proteins found in living cells. Because of this mechanism of action, sufficient contact time with surfaces should be allowed. If supplies, equipment, or gloves are not allowed to dry for an adequate amount of time, disinfection becomes less effective. USP Chapter <797> recommends allowing alcohol to remain on a surface for at least 30 seconds prior to using the surface. Sterile, residue-free, 70% IPA swabs should be used to disinfect vial closures and ampule necks. These surfaces should remain wet for at least 10 seconds and then allowed to dry before use.[17] Often, surfaces become soiled with organic matter, which decreases the efficacy of alcohols.[3, p.236] If organic matter is present on surfaces, a cleaning step should be included. This step involves cleaning the surface with an agent that will solubilize the matter, such as sterile water. After complete removal of the matter, a disinfecting agent should be applied to the surface and allowed to dry completely. The cleaning step removes organic matter so that the alcohol can effectively disinfect the surface.

Bacterial spores are difficult to eradicate, as they are not inactivated by many conventional disinfectants and require physical removal or use of disinfecting agents with sporicidal activity.[27] Agents with sporicidal activity include chlorine compounds, hydrogen peroxide, peracetic acid, and iodine compounds.[3, p.247] Some alcohols are not sporicidal and may, in themselves, contain spores. Sterile 70% IPA has been filter sterilized to remove spores from its formulation. For this reason, sterile 70% IPA—rather than non-sterile 70% IPA—should be used for disinfecting purposes, particularly for critical sites. In addition to daily use of disinfectants, sporicidal agents can be used on a daily, weekly or monthly basis. Because these agents tend to corrode equipment and create potential safety issues with chronic operator exposure, it is generally not recommended to use sporicidal agents on a daily basis.[28] The type of sporicidal agent and frequency of its use should be determined by each facility.

Table 4-2 Antiseptic Agents for Hand Hygiene

Alcohols
Chlorhexidine
Chloroxylenol
Hexachlorophene
Iodine and iodophors
Quaternary ammonium compounds
Triclosan

Source: Data from U.S. Pharmacopeial Convention. Chapter
<1072>: disinfectants and antiseptics. In: *United States
Pharmacopeia 36/National Formulary 31*. Rockville, MD: U.S.
Pharmacopeial Convention; 2013.

Antiseptics are used to inhibit or destroy microorganisms
on living tissue, such as for purposes of hand hygiene, and are
not as potent as disinfectants. **Table 4-2** lists various antiseptics.
The most commonly used antiseptics include 4% chlorhexidine,
10% povidone–iodine, 3% hexachlorophene, 70% isopropyl alcohol, and 0.5% chlorhexidine in 95% alcohol.[28] If hands are visibly
soiled, they should be washed with either a non-antimicrobial
or antimicrobial soap, followed by use of antiseptic hand scrub.
In the absence of visible soiling, antiseptic hand scrub should be
used routinely. Utilization of antiseptics for hand hygiene has
been demonstrated to be more effective than soap and water in
reducing bacterial load on skin. Repeated use of antiseptics will
reduce bacterial load further, although some types of antiseptics
may cause irritation with frequent use.[28] Per USP Chapter <797>,
waterless, alcohol-based antiseptic hand scrub with persistent
activity should be used. Use of scrub brushes during hand washing is not recommended secondary to causing irritation and skin
damage, leading to skin fissuring or areas of open skin.[17]

Recent increases in rates of *Clostridium difficile* in institutional settings in the United States, along with concerns of *Bacillus anthracis* infections associated with contaminated items sent
through the postal system, have resulted in evaluation of hand
hygiene related to spore-forming bacteria. Antiseptic hand wash
and hand-rub preparations do not provide reliable sporicidal

activity against *Clostridium* or *Bacillus* species.[12] Spores must be physically removed using hand washing with either antimicrobial or non-antimicrobial soap.

Preventing Contamination

Prevention of contamination results from implementing fundamentals of compounding as part of everyday practices (**Figure 4-5**). All personnel involved in compounding parenteral preparations have an ultimate responsibility to protect patients from harm ensuing from contamination of CSPs. While there are various methods of doing so, examples of methods to prevent contamination include the following:

- Use consistent and proper aseptic technique.
- Use recommended PPE and environmental controls.
- Disinfect vial and ampule closures with each access using sterile 70% alcohol, including disinfecting rubber closures of MDVs with each access.
- Store and discard sterile products and preparations properly in accordance with manufacturer recommendations.
- Consider risk level and ISO classifications when compounding.
- Maintain vials in ISO Class 5 environments and use sterile seals when needed.

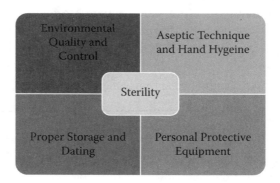

Figure 4-5   Contributing Factors for Sterility

- Use single-dose vials and prefilled syringes when possible.
- Do not administer drugs from a single-dose vial to multiple patients.
- Do not combine residual solutions from different vials or syringes for future use.
- Assign conservative beyond-use dates based on reliable references.
- Change administration tubing for PN, lipids, and propofol often and limit hang time for these drugs.
- Discard single-use vials after one use.

- consider risk lvl + Iso classifications when cmpding

Conclusion

There exist an unfortunate abundance of cases in which adverse patient outcomes resulted from contamination of parenteral preparations. It is important that there is no misconception that the controlled environment and use of primary engineering controls guarantees a sterile preparation. This assumption can lead to lackadaisical practices that can result in contamination of parenteral preparations. All individuals involved in sterile compounding are accountable for protecting patients from preparations that are contaminated. While recommendations, such as those from the Healthcare Infection Control Practices Advisory Committee of the CDC as well as the United States Pharmacopeia, can guide us in preventing contamination, the implementation of such recommendations becomes the responsibility of compounding personnel.

Review Questions

1. Which of the following is a clinical manifestation of injection or infusion of an admixture contaminated with pyrogens?
   a. Transient ischemic attack
   b. Myocardial infarction
   c. Immunogenic response
   d. Pneumonia

2. A compounding pharmacy is outsourced to compound sterile preparations involving non-sterile components. Which risk level are these preparations?
   a. High risk
   b. Medium risk
   c. Low risk
   d. Intermediate risk

3. Which of the following statements is false?
   a. Particles contribute to the overall air quality, with increased particles causing poorer air quality.
   b. Nonviable particles do not cause contamination.
   c. People are a significant source of particles.
   d. Touch is the most common source of contamination.

4. True or False: An ISO Class 7 environment should have no more than 352,000 particles of size 1 micron or larger per cubic meter of air.

5. List factors that influence the sterility of parenteral preparations.

6. Which disinfecting agents should be used for critical sites?

7. How long should alcohol remain on surfaces before beginning compounding?

8. Explain the responsibilities for personnel in preventing microbiological contamination.

9. Which of the following is a true statement regarding hand antisepsis?
   a. Spores are most effectively eliminated with antiseptics containing triclosan.
   b. Spores are most effectively removed with hand washing.
   c. Frequent hand washing is preferred over frequent use of antiseptics.
   d. USP Chapter <797> recommends the use of a water-less, hydrogen peroxide–based hand antiseptic.

10. In the event that a surface is visibly soiled, describe the steps that should be taken to disinfect the surface.

CASE STUDY

You are a third-year pharmacy intern shadowing a hospital pharmacist on your introductory pharmacy practice experience (IPPE). While at the hospital, you attend a pharmacy departmental meeting in which it is announced that there is a medication shortage for a particular IV medication. The IV room pharmacist later shares with you that, because of the shortage, he needs to use a multidose vial of the medication to prepare all four daily doses for a patient. He explains that because the preparation involves a single multidose vial, he is able to categorize it as a low-risk compound. Please present your concern to the pharmacist regarding his risk level classification.

After preparing all four daily doses for the patient, the multidose vial contains four more doses of medication. Because of the shortage, the IV pharmacist would like to save it for use tomorrow. Can the vial be stored for future use? Which type of labeling would be required?

References

1. Centers for Disease Control and Prevention policy toolkit. Available at:http://www.cdc.gov/hai/pdfs/toolkits/toolkit-HAI-POLICY-FINAL_01-2012.pdf
2. Reed D, Kemmerly SA. Infection control prevention: a review of hospital-acquired infections and the economic implications. *Ochsner J.* 2009;9(1):27–31.
3. Williams KL, Swarbrick J, eds. *Microbial contamination control in parenteral manufacturing.* New York, NY: Marcel Dekker; 2004:621.
4. Buchanan EC, Schneider PJ. *Compounding sterile preparations.* Bethesda, MD: American Society of Health-System Pharmacists; 2009:27.
5. Centers for Disease Control and Prevention. Principles of epidemiology in public health practice, 3rd edition: introduction to epidemiology. Available at: http://www.cdc.gov/osels/scientific_edu/ss1978/lesson1/Section10.html. Accessed May 3, 2013.
6. Arnold C. Fungal meningitis outbreak affects over 700. *Lancet Neurol.* 2013;12(5):429–430.

7. Centers for Disease Control and Prevention. Medication safety programs recalls: information about additional medical products from New England Compounding Center. Available at: http://www.cdc.gov/medicationsafety/recalls/necc/. Accessed May 12, 2013.

8. U.S. Food and Drug Administration. CDC and ADPH investigate outbreak at Alabama hospital, products recalled. Available at: http://www.fda.gov/Safety/Recalls/ucm249068.htm. Accessed May 20, 2013.

9. Sacks GS. Microbial contamination of parenteral nutrition: how could it happen? *J Parenter Enteral Nutr.* 2011;35(4):432.

10. Poole RL, Pieroni KP, Gaskari S, et al. Aluminum exposure in neonatal patients using the least contaminated parenteral nutrition solution products. *Nutrients.* 2012;4(11):1566–1574.

11. van Grafthorst JP, Norbert F, Nooteboom, F, et al. Unexpected high risk of contamination with staphylococci species attributable to standard preparation of syringes for continuous intravenous drug administration in a simulation model in intensive care units. *Crit Care Med.* 2002;30(4): 833–836.

12. Centers for Disease Control and Prevention. Guideline for hand hygiene in health-care settings. *MMWR.* Available at: http://www.cdc.gov/handhygiene/Guidelines.html. Accessed May 10, 2013.

13. Fagernes M, Lingaas E. Factors interfering with the microflora on hands: a regression analysis of samples from 465 healthcare workers. *J Adv Nurs.* 2011;67(2):297–307.

14. Gordin FM, Schultz ME, Huber R, et al. A cluster of hemodialysis-related bacteremia linked to artificial fingernails. *Infect Control Hosp Epidemiol.* 2007;28(6):743–744.

15. Gupta A, Della-Latta P, Todd B, et al. Outbreak of extended-spectrum beta-lactamase–producing *Klebsiella pneumonia* in a neonatal intensive care unit linked to artificial nails. *Infect Control Hosp Epidemiol.* 2004;25(3):210–215.

16. McNeil SA, Foster CL, Hedderwick SA, Kauffman CA. Effect of hand cleansing with antimicrobial soap or alcohol-based gel on microbial colonization of artificial fingernails worn by health care workers. *Clin Infect Dis.* 2001;32(3):367–372.

17. U.S. Pharmacopeial Convention. Chapter <797>: pharmaceutical compounding: sterile preparations. In: *United States*

Pharmacopeia 36/National Formulary 31. Rockville, MD: U.S. Pharmacopeial Convention; 2013.

18. Branch-Elliman W, Weiss D, Balter S, et al. Hepatitis C transmission due to contamination of multidose medication vials: summary of an outbreak and a call to action. *Am J Infect Control.* 2013;41(1):92–94.

19. Kerenyi M, Borza Z, Csontos C, et al. Impact of medications on bacterial growth in syringes. *J Hosp Infect.* 2011;79(3):265–266.

20. U.S. Pharmacopeial Convention. Chapter <788>: particulate matter in injections. In: *United States Pharmacopeia 36/National Formulary 31.* Rockville, MD: U.S. Pharmacopeial Convention; 2013.

21. Milstone LM. Epidermal desquamation. *J Dermatol Sci.* 2004; 36:131–140.

22. *Basic guide to particle counters and particle counting.* Boulder, CO: Particle Measuring Systems; 2011:6–8. Available at: http://www.pmeasuring.com/wrap/filesApp/BasicGuide/file_1/ver_1317144880/basicguide.pdf. Accessed May 25, 2013.

23. Leyden JJ, McGinley KJ, Nordstrom KM, Webster GF. Skin microflora. *J Invest Dermatol.* 1987;88:65s–72s.

24. Hospodsky D, Qian J, Nazaroff WW, et al. Human occupancy as a source of indoor airborne bacteria. *PLoS One.* 2012;7(4): e34867.

25. Stranz M. *When is solution filtration necessary?* Paper presented at AVA 18th Annual Conference, Vancouver, British Columbia, September 2004.

26. U.S. Pharmacopeial Convention. Chapter <1116>: microbiological control and monitoring of aseptic processing environments. In: *United States Pharmacopeia 36/National Formulary 31.* Rockville, MD: U.S. Pharmacopeial Convention; 2013.

27. Rutala WA, Weber DJ. Centers for Disease Control: guideline for disinfection and sterilization in healthcare facilities, 2008. Available at: http://www.cdc.gov/hicpac/pdf/guidelines/Disinfection_Nov_2008.pdf. Accessed May 27, 2013.

28. U.S. Pharmacopeial Convention. Chapter <1072>: disinfectants and antiseptics. In: *United States Pharmacopeia 36/National Formulary 31.* Rockville, MD: U.S. Pharmacopeial Convention; 2013.

CHAPTER 5

Primary and Secondary Engineering Controls

Pamella S. Ochoa and José A. Vega

 Where this icon appears, visit http://go.jblearning.com /OchoaCWS to view the corresponding video.

Chapter Objectives

1. Differentiate between primary engineering controls and secondary engineering controls.
2. Describe airflow patterns of primary engineering controls.
3. Describe the cleaning methods for primary engineering controls.
3. Describe the construction and characteristics of secondary engineering controls.
4. Explain the role of primary and secondary controls in compounding sterile preparations.

Key Terminology

Workbench
Work surface
First air
Zones of turbulence
Clean zone

Buffer area

Ante-area

Direct compounding area

Clean room

Closed-system vial-transfer devices (CSTDs)

Flow control

Dilution control

Overview

Primary engineering controls (PECs) and secondary engineering controls are utilized to maintain environmental quality in areas in which compounded sterile preparations (CSPs) are processed. Regulations and quality assurance standards provide guidance as to the type and specifications of PECs to be used for sterile compounding. Secondary engineering controls work as adjuncts to PECs to control room air quality in both compounding areas and adjacent areas. Collectively, primary and secondary controls include constructions and characteristics that are used to improve air quality by decreasing particle counts within controlled zones. While the use of these controls alone does not ensure the sterility of CSPs, it does minimize the risk of airborne contamination.

Controls are utilized and maintained not only to protect the preparation from contamination, but also to protect the operator from exposure to hazardous agents in some circumstances. PECs include laminar airflow workbenches, biological safety cabinets, compounding aseptic isolators, and compounding aseptic containment isolators. All of these PECs are designed to maintain ISO Class 5 air quality within the work zone. To meet ISO Class 5 requirements, the air quality within the PEC must not contain more than 3520 particles sized 0.5 micron or larger in every cubic meter. Air quality sampling is performed for PECs and secondary engineering controls to ensure adequate air quality is maintained. Secondary engineering controls should provide air quality of ISO Class 7 and ISO Class 8, depending on their locations relative to direct compounding areas. Because the consequence of contamination to the patient is of great concern, it is important that products be prepared in a controlled environment, whenever possible.

Primary Engineering Controls (PEC)

LAMINAR AIRFLOW WORKBENCHES

Laminar airflow workbenches (LAFWs) are also referred to as laminar airflow hoods, laminar flow workbenches, horizontal or vertical hoods, or (more casually) "hoods" (**Figure 5-1**). LAFWs provide a controlled area for preparing compounded sterile preparations (CSPs). Any product at risk of contamination through environmental factors should be prepared in a LAFW.

Laminar airflow can be described as airflow that moves within a confined area in a unidirectional, linear manner. LAFWs produce unidirectional air at a fixed velocity moving along parallel

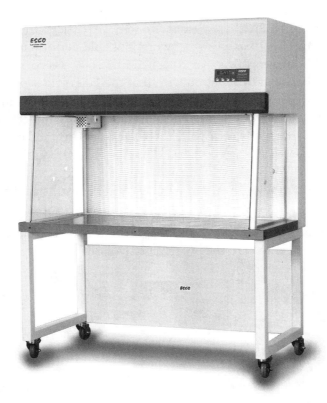

Figure 5-1   Laminar Airflow Workbench

ESCO Technologies Inc. Hospital Pharmacy Isolator Solutions for USP <797> Compliance from Esco. http://www.escoglobal.com/resources/pdf/HPI-consolidated-product .pdf. Accessed February 11, 2013. Reprinted by permission of ESCO Technologies, Inc.

HEPA air not sterile

lines in either a horizontal or vertical fashion. This air is referred to as "first air" or "clean air," because the cleanest air is that which exits the high-efficiency particulate absorption (HEPA) filter first. The role of the LAFW in sterile compounding is to create a controlled environment, or clean zone, within the LAFW by producing first air in the area in which sterile processing, including critical site exposure, occurs. The air is produced with a constant

90 ft/min ± 20%

and positive flow at a velocity that prevents room air from entering the clean zone. If the air outside the clean zone exceeds the velocity of the first air, room air will backwash into the clean zone. First air represents room air that has been extensively filtered. The filtering process will remove particles and microorganisms

99.97% removed

that are 0.3 micron or larger, preventing them from entering the clean zone.

HEPA doesn't filter gas

HEPA filters are rated to remove particles that are 0.3 micron or larger based on the worst possible performance of the filter; however, PECs are classified as ISO Class 5. The discrepancy between the environment that the HEPA filter provides and the ISO classification is based on principles of contamination related to the differences between viable particles and carriers for those particles. Because particles of size 0.5 micron and larger may transport viable particles, the air quality is based on this classification.

Horizontal Laminar Airflow Workbenches

Horizontal laminar airflow workbenches (HLFWs) produce first air in a horizontal manner directed from the back of the workbench toward the operator, or front of the bench.

> **ALERT:** *Because airflow is directed toward the operator, only nonhazardous products should be prepared in a HLFW.*

Parts of a HLFW

The main parts of a HLFW are illustrated in **Figure 5-2**. These parts include the following components:

- Pre-filter
- Exhaust blower

- Plenum
- HEPA filter
- Workbench surface

Pre-filter

The pre-filter is typically located at the base or top of a HLFW and is protected with an intake grille. The corrugated structure of the filter increases the surface area, allowing it to remove more particles. Room air is drawn through the pre-filter to remove large particles, such as lint and dust. Removal of large particulate matter will prevent clogging of the HEPA filter, through which air passes downstream from the pre-filter. Items that may carry contaminants, such as a trashcan, should not be placed near the pre-filter. The pre-filter should be inspected monthly and replaced per institutional policy.

[handwritten annotation: monthly replacement]

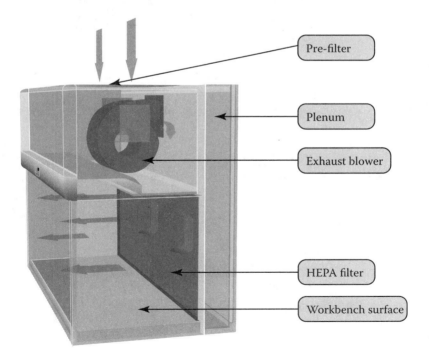

Figure 5-2 Main Parts and Airflow of a Horizontal Laminar Airflow Workbench

Reprinted by permission of ESCO Technologies, Inc.

Exhaust Blower

Air that has passed through the pre-filter for removal of large particulate matter will subsequently pass through the exhaust blower. The blower takes in filtered air and directs it toward the plenum. Blowers may be located below or above the work surface of a HLFW.

Plenum

The plenum is located between the HEPA filter and the exhaust blower. It receives air from the exhaust blower, accelerates it, and consistently distributes it to the HEPA filter.

HEPA Filter

The HEPA filter is located at the back of a HLFW, facing the opening of the workbench. It is typically covered by a protective screen with openings to allow sufficient airflow to pass. HEPA filters further remove particulate matter, including microorganisms. First air exits the HEPA filter, with 99.97% of particles that are 0.3 micron or larger being removed by the HEPA filter.[1] HEPA filters consist of pressed borosilicate fibers that are then made into flat sheets and treated with a water repellant binder.[1] These sheets are corrugated to increase the filter's overall surface area. Aluminum separators between each of the corrugated pleats provide stability and assist in directing airflow within the HEPA filter in an outward direction.

ALERT: *If turned off, laminar airflow workbenches should run for at least 30 minutes prior to their use.*

Workbench Surface

The surface of the workbench is a large, flat area that provides a clean zone for compounding sterile preparations. First air is directed into this clean zone, affecting the manner in which manipulations must be conducted.

Airflow in a HLFW

Airflow within a HLFW travels in a linear, horizontal fashion, exiting the HEPA filter and directed toward the opening of the

HLFW. An air velocity of 90 feet per minute ± 20% should be maintained.[1] This velocity of airflow is sufficient to blow particulate matter within the workbench outward. Airflow should be regularly tested to ensure adequate velocity is being maintained. **Figure 5-2** illustrates the airflow pattern in the HLFW. Movement within the workbench or the environment directly outside of the workbench can easily overcome the velocity of the outward flow of first air, allowing air from the room to enter the workbench, known as backwashing of air. Thus workbenches should be strategically placed in areas of low traffic. Additionally, there should be no talking, coughing, or sneezing in or near the workbench area, as these actions will create air velocities into the workbench that are greater than the outward velocity of the first air.

Airflow patterns can also be disrupted by the simple placement of hands or objects within the workbench. Zones of turbulence, similar to eddies in a river, can occur within the workbench. These zones are created when an object is placed in the workbench, disrupting the laminar flow of first air behind the object. Other objects placed either within these areas or directly downstream, as well as manipulations that occur within these zones, are at risk of contamination because first airflow is compromised. When turbulence occurs near the front of the workbench, it can potentially extend outside of the workbench, causing air from outside the workbench to enter. Air turbulence occurs three times the diameter of an object when that object is placed in an area in which first air is on all sides of the object, such as the central portion of the workbench surface. When an object is placed in an area in which first air passes on only one side of the object, such as along the side of the workbench surface, zones of turbulence will extend to six times the diameter of the object. For this reason, objects should be placed with careful consideration of airflow patterns, and all manipulations performed in the HLFW must be performed within the central-most portion of the workbench surface, which can be defined as follows:

- Six inches into the workbench area from the edge of the LAFW
- Three inches from the back of the LAFW (HEPA filter)
- Six inches from each side of the LAFW

ALERT: *In a HLFW, always perform manipulations 6 inches from the sides, 6 inches from the front, and 3 inches from the back of the workbench.*

ALERT: *Activities that result in velocities of air greater than that exiting the HEPA filter should be restricted. These actions include talking, sneezing, and coughing.*

Laminar airflow workbenches should not be turned off. Because of the extensive filtering of air that must take place, if the HLFW is turned off, the workbench should be turned back on and allowed to run for at least 30 minutes prior to use to allow purging of contaminants and full circulation of first air. This period should be followed by cleaning of the HLFW.

 ### Cleaning the HLFW

Cleaning the HLFW is an important step to ensure disinfection of the workbench. Utilization of a disinfectant that does not leave a residue, such as sterile 70% isopropyl alcohol (IPA), is preferred for general use in cleaning a HLFW, along with clean, lint-free wipes. Cleaning the HLFW is a process of moving particles and other contaminants from the area closest to the HEPA filter outward toward the operator, always moving in the direction of first air flow. The concept can be thought of as cleaning in the direction of the cleanest to the least clean. The top of the HLFW should always be cleaned first, because cleaning it can cause contaminants to fall downward to the work surface. Lint-free wipes should be used for cleaning. During cleaning, streaks of alcohol should be visible when wiping with a saturated cloth and should overlap to ensure that all areas are cleaned on every surface of the workbench.

Surfaces cleaned with IPA should dry for at least 30 seconds. Manipulations involving glass vials on a wet surface can introduce safety issues. For example, a wet surface can cause a glass vial to easily slip when the operator is entering it with a needle. Therefore, allowing the workbench surface to dry completely prior to beginning vial manipulations can circumvent mishaps from working on a wet surface.

To clean the HLFW, all of the steps in **Table 5-1** should be followed in the order listed.

Sterile water, more so than alcohol, easily dissolves residue and soiling resulting from spills during manipulations in a HLFW. Therefore, when the surface of the HLFW is visibly soiled, the workbench should be cleaned by applying sterile water to the soiled area, allowing it to stand, and then wiping with a lint-free wipe. After this procedure is complete, the usual disinfecting process should be employed using sterile 70% IPA.

Table 5-1   Steps for Cleaning the Horizontal Laminar Airflow Workbench

1. Stack a pile of clean, lint-free wipes (approximately one wipe per surface) on the work surface of the HLFW.
2. Saturate the pile with disinfecting agent, ensuring the bottom of the stack is adequately saturated.
3. Grab a lint-free wipe and use it to clean one surface of the HLFW at a time in the following order:

    - *Upper surface (top)*: The top of the HLFW should be cleaned using a side-to-side motion in a horizontal fashion from one side of the HLFW to the other.
    - *Pole and hooks*: The pole of the HLFW should be cleaned next. A wipe should be wrapped firmly around the circumference of the pole at one end of the pole. Using a straight continuous motion, the pole should be cleaned to the other side of the HLFW. Do not use a back-and-forth motion from one side of the HLFW to the other side of the HLFW.
    - *Sides*: Each side of the HLFW should be cleaned by starting in the upper corner closest to the HEPA filter. Cleaning should proceed from the top of the HLFW to the bottom in a vertical fashion, working from the back of the HLFW toward the front of the HLFW.
    - *Workbench*: The workbench should be cleaned last, as it is the most important surface to ensure disinfection. Cleaning should begin at the back corner closest to the HEPA filter and proceed from side to side in a horizontal fashion from the back of the HLFW to the front edge.

4. Allow all surfaces to completely dry for at least 30 seconds prior to compounding.

> **ALERT:** *Cleaning of surfaces in the PECs with an appropriate disinfectant agent (e.g., sterile 70% IPA) should occur at the beginning of each shift, prior to each batch preparation, after spills, and when contamination of the surface is known or suspected to have occurred. Otherwise, if preparations are ongoing, then no more than 30 minutes should pass between cleaning.*

It is preferable that alcohol be dispensed from the original container for cleaning the HLFW. Spray bottles should not be used within the workbench for various reasons. First, spray bottles brought into the workbench area can introduce contaminants. Second, sprays of liquid from the bottle could reach the HEPA filter. If the HEPA filter gets wet, small holes in the filter can result, thereby compromising its effectiveness. Sprayed droplets of IPA may suspend microorganisms that can settle on compounding surfaces. Finally, alcohol that is sprayed within the workbench area can reach the intake grille, resulting in possible circulation of alcohol vapors.

> **ALERT:** *Sterile 70% IPA should remain on surfaces for at least 30 seconds and be allowed to dry completely.*

The HEPA filter screen should not be cleaned as part of the routine cleaning of the workbench, as removal of the screen is necessary for proper cleaning. The protective screen should be removed and cleaned every 6 months.

VERTICAL LAMINAR AIRFLOW WORKBENCHES

Vertical laminar airflow workbenches (VLFWs) produce laminar airflow in a vertical fashion, from the top of the VLFW downward toward the workbench surface (**Figure 5-3**). Air intake is similar to that of a HLFW, but the HEPA filter is located on the ceiling of the VLFW, resulting in a downward exit of air from the HEPA filter. Air exits the workbench out toward the operator, as with the HLFW. Because of this airflow pattern, hazardous agents should

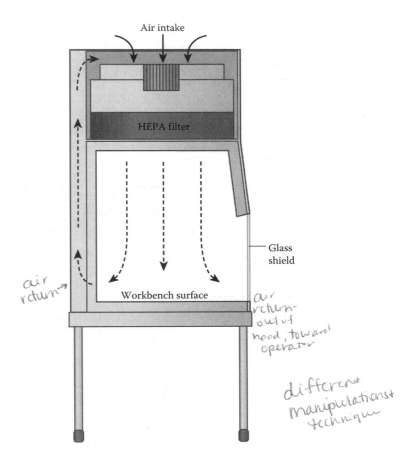

Air intake

HEPA filter

Glass shield

air return →

Workbench surface

air return - out of hood, toward operator

different manipulationst technique

Figure 5-3 Vertical Laminar Airflow Workbench

not be prepared in a VLFW, as it does not provide protection to the operator from fumes or aerosols.[1]

Manipulations within the VLFW and cleaning of the VLFW must be altered because first air is directed in a vertical—rather than horizontal—fashion. For personnel who frequently prepare products in both HLFWs and VLFWs, consistently accounting for changes in manipulations may prove challenging. More discussion on proper manipulation techniques for both types of workbenches is discussed in the *Aseptic Technique and Compounding Manipulations* chapter.

The parts of the VLFW are similar to those of a HLFW, but may also include a glass sash, or shield, at the front of the VLFW. While this addition offers better physical protection to the operator, airflow continues to be directed through an opening under the sash and toward the operator.

BIOLOGICAL SAFETY CABINETS

The principal functions of biological safety cabinets (BSCs) are to provide product, environmental, and personnel protection. Operator and environmental protection are accomplished by creating an inward flow of air at the front opening to protect the operator and exhausting air from the cabinet through a HEPA filter. BSCs are categorized based on their characteristics for providing product, environmental, or personnel protection (**Table 5-2**). Class II BSCs are the most commonly used and the type that the National Institute for Occupational Safety and Health (NIOSH) states should be used for aseptic processing. According to NIOSH, the B2 type of cabinet is preferred, as it is the only type of BSC that does not recirculate air internally.

Table 5-2 Categories of Biological Safety Cabinets Based on Level of Protection

Class of BSC	Protection Provided			Risk Level
	Personnel	Product	Environment	
I	Yes	No	Yes	Low- to moderate-risk biological agents (BSL 1–3)
II (A1, A2, B1, B2)	Yes	Yes	Yes	Low- to moderate-risk biological agents (BSL 1–3)
III; II when used in suit room with suit	Yes	Yes	Yes	High-risk biological agents (BSL 4)

Source: U.S. Department of Health and Human Services. Appendix A: primary containment for biohazards: selection, installation and use of biological safety cabinets. In: Chosewood LC, Wilson DE, eds. *U.S. biosafety in microbiological and biomedical laboratories.* 5th ed. Washington, DC: U.S. Department of Health and Human Services; 2009:311.

While BSCs and VLFWs both produce laminar air in a vertical fashion, they differ in terms of their utility. VLFWs provide product protection only and may be used to prepare nonhazardous IV preparations. Because the airflow is directed outward, under the sash, toward the operator, no operator protection is provided. BSCs are a type of VLFW, but a VLFW may not necessarily be a BSC.

Similar to HLFWs, BSCs utilize HEPA filtration to remove particles and microorganisms. Filtered air moves in a vertical and laminar fashion to provide first air to products being prepared in the cabinet, creating an environment conducive to aseptic processing. A protective sash is located at the front of the BSC to protect the operator from accidental sprays during manipulations. Additional operator protection results from an inward airflow through the front opening of the cabinet.

BSCs utilize special exhaust mechanisms, which is factored into their classification. For example, all Class II BSCs use HEPA filters not only at their air supply points, but also at their exhaust points. Air exiting the BSC is directed through a HEPA filter and out of the cabinet into a designated area using one of two different mechanisms. Class I BSCs exhaust air into existing exhaust systems through direct connection into the ductwork. A clearance of 12 to 14 inches above the cabinet may be required, depending on the manufacturer's recommendations, and should be considered for proper placement of a BSC.[1] This needed space is important to allow for sufficient air intake to maintain proper intake velocity of air into the workbench and to prevent backpressure on the exhaust filter. Adequate clearance is also required on all sides of the workbench to ensure that air from the cabinet that is recirculated to the clean room is not obstructed as well as for maintenance access.[1] The second, and most expensive, exhaust mechanism in BSCs directs air into a designated and separate exhaust system, which is then exhausted outside. If the separate exhaust system through which air is directed contains multiple ducts, the design must ensure that air exhausted from the BSC is not recirculated.[1]

Because HEPA filters are ineffective at filtering vapors or gases, both NIOSH and USP Chapter <797> require outside venting of any BSC used for chemicals that may volatilize, or vaporize, while being handled or after HEPA filtration. Class II Type B cabinets provide protection to the operator when working with vapors and gases that need to be processed in an aseptic environment. The B1 and B2 subtypes of Class II cabinets exhaust 70% and 100% of airflow, respectively, making them the preferred type of cabinets for working with hazardous vapors and gases. Although Class II Type A cabinets do not provide protection to the operator from gases and vapors, if only trace amounts of volatile chemicals are used, Class II Type A2 cabinets may suffice.

BSCs can be used for any type of aseptic process. However, because of the protective sash and inward airflow at the opening of the cabinet, they should be used when preparing hazardous agents, such as chemotherapies, that require additional personnel and environmental protection.

ALERT: *All hazardous agents should be prepared in a biological safety cabinet or compounding aseptic containment isolator.*

Parts of a BSC

A BSC is illustrated in **Figure 5-4**. The main parts of a BSC include the following:

- Sash
- Exhaust blower
- Air intake grilles
- HEPA filter
- Work zone (workbench surface)

Sash

The glass sash, also referred to as the shield, is located at the very front of the BSC. Its purpose is to protect the operator from exposure to hazardous agents, including accidental or unknown exposures. The sash contains an 8-inch opening along the bottom

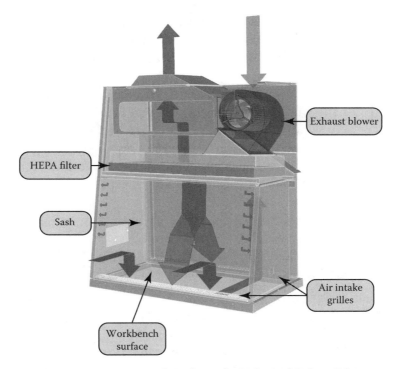

Figure 5-4 Main Parts and Airflow of a Biological Safety Cabinet
From http://www.escoglobal.com/products/download/1334038968.pdf, p. 2. Courtesy of ESCO Technologies, Inc.

side, where the hands of the operator enter the cabinet to perform manipulations. The entire sash can be lifted for cleaning, but
should remain in the down position during manipulations. The
opening at the bottom of the sash should never be blocked, as it
is needed for proper airflow through the cabinet.

Exhaust Blower
The exhaust blower facilitates the circulation of air back into the
cabinet for exhausting.

Air Intake Grilles
Air intake grilles are located at the front and, at times, the back
of the BSC. Negative pressure at the opening of the sash draws
vapors exiting the cabinet away from the operator. Air from the

intake grilles gets recirculated through the BSC and eventually exhausted. Some BSCs also have a rear air intake grille.

HEPA Filter

As in HLFWs, HEPA filters in BSCs remove particulate contaminants and microorganisms; however, BSCs contain two HEPA filters. The filter located at the top of the BSC sends first air downward toward the work surface. Another filter located within the exhaust mechanism allows air from the BSC to be filtered prior to being exhausted.

Work Zone

The surface of the cabinet is a large, flat area that provides a clean zone for sterile preparations. Laminar first air is directed into this work zone, affecting the manner in which manipulations must be conducted.

Airflow in a BSC

BSCs are able to provide operator protection by creating an inward airflow at the front opening of the cabinet. First air is derived from air taken in through the intake grille, recirculated within the BSC, and blown downward through a HEPA filter toward the work surface in a vertical laminar fashion. Figure 5-4 illustrates the airflow pattern in the BSC.

When the cabinet has both front and rear grilles, air moving downward from the HEPA filter "splits" prior to reaching the work surface. Part of the air is drawn up through the front grille, and the rest moves through the rear grille and is recirculated. In most cabinets, this split occurs halfway between the front and rear grilles and between 2 and 6 inches above the work surface.[1]

Airflow disruptions can also occur within a BSC. Because the direction of the airflow is downward, first air will not reach items that are located underneath items placed within the work zone. Therefore, care must be taken when placing objects within the cabinet. For example, if a bag of IV solution is hung from the pole inside the cabinet, any items placed under the bag will not be in the flow of the first air exiting the HEPA filter. Additionally, the quality of first air decreases at the sides of the work surface. Given these factors, the recommended work zone area for a BSC is defined as follows:

- Between the front and rear air intake grilles
- At least 4 inches in from the front grille
- Six inches from each side of the BSC

BSCs should run continuously to optimize their performance. If the BSC is turned off, the blowers should run continuously for at least 4 minutes to purge suspended particulates from the cabinet prior to performing any aseptic processes within the cabinet. This should be followed by cleaning of the BSC.

Cleaning the BSC

Cleaning of the BSC is similar to cleaning of the HLFW but differs in the direction and order of cleaning. Thinking back to the concept of cleaning from the cleanest area to the least clean area, the direction of cleaning will move from top to bottom in a BSC. Additionally, the sides of the cabinet should be cleaned in a horizontal side-to-side motion, which is the opposite direction when cleaning the HLFW. To remember the direction in which to clean, remember that cleaning should proceed in a direction opposite to the airflow direction. For example, horizontal strokes should be used to clean a vertical airflow workbench.

Cleaning of the BSC with an appropriate disinfectant agent (e.g., sterile 70% IPA) should occur at the beginning of each shift, prior to each batch preparation, after spills, and when contamination of the surface is known or suspected to have occurred. Otherwise, if preparations are ongoing, then no more than 30 minutes should pass between cleaning.[2] In addition to disinfecting the BSC, decontamination, such as with sodium hypochlorite, may be necessary when working with certain hazardous agents. Decontamination is further discussed in the *Preparation of Hazardous Drugs for Parenteral Use* chapter. Lint-free wipes

Table 5-3 Steps for Cleaning a Biological Safety Cabinet or Vertical Laminar Airflow Workbench

1. Stack a pile of clean, lint-free wipes (approximately one wipe per surface) on the work surface.
2. Saturate the pile with disinfecting agent, ensuring the bottom of the stack is adequately saturated.
3. Grab a lint-free wipe and use it to clean one surface of the BSC at a time in the following order:
   - *Pole and hooks*: The pole of the BSC should be cleaned first, and hooks if applicable. The wipe should be wrapped firmly around the circumference of the pole at one end of the pole. Using a straight continuous motion the pole should be cleaned to the other side of the BSC. Do not use a back-and-forth motion from one side of the BSC to the other side of the BSC.
   - *Back*: The back of the BSC should be cleaned next. Starting in an upper corner, use a horizontal side-to-side motion from the top of the BSC to the bottom, using overlapping strokes.
   - *Sides*: Each side of the BSC should be cleaned by starting in the upper corner closest to the HEPA filter at the top of the BSC. Cleaning should proceed from the top of the BSC to the bottom in a horizontal fashion.
   - *Sash*: The glass sash should be cleaned next, beginning in the upper corner near the HEPA filter. Overlapping strokes should be used in a side-to-side horizontal fashion, working from the top of the sash to the bottom.
   - *Workbench*: The workbench should be cleaned last, as it is the most important surface to ensure disinfection. Cleaning should begin at the back corner closest to the back side and proceed from side to side in a horizontal fashion from the back of the BSC to the front edge.
4. Allow all surfaces to completely dry for at least 30 seconds prior to preparing products.

are also recommended for cleaning the BSC. Similar to the case when cleaning a HLFW, sterile water may be used to clean the workbench when it is visibly soiled, followed by disinfection with an appropriate disinfectant agent (e.g., sterile 70% IPA). **Table 5-3** lists the steps for cleaning a vertical laminar airflow workbench or a BSC, as both of these controls produce air in a vertical manner.

TIP: *When cleaning laminar airflow workbenches, cleaning strokes should be in a direction perpendicular to that of the airflow.*

COMPOUNDING ISOLATORS

Compounding isolators, also known as "glove boxes," are used to compound sterile pharmaceutical preparations. These isolators allow the worker to prepare sterile compounds by inserting his or her hands into gloves that are attached and sealed to the box (**Figure 5-5**).

USP Chapter <797> adopted terminology for two types of compounding isolators: compounding aseptic isolator (CAI) and compounding aseptic containment isolator (CACI). As their names imply, these compounding isolators differ in their design and functionality for aseptic processing of sterile compounds.

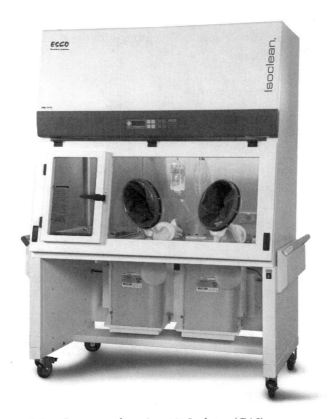

Figure 5-5 Compounding Aseptic Isolator (CAI)

ESCO Technologies Inc. Hospital Pharmacy Isolator Solutions for USP <797> Compliance from Esco. http://www.escoglobal.com/resources/pdf/HPI-consolidated-product
.pdf. Accessed February 11, 2013. Reprinted by permission of ESCO Technologies, Inc.

While both isolator types use HEPA-filtered air, CAIs are primarily used for nonhazardous preparations because they employ positive pressure within the isolator. CACIs, which use negative pressurized air and contain exhaust mechanisms, are used to prepare hazardous agents and provide better protection to the operator.

While isolators provide a closed and pressurized environment of ISO Class 5 quality, the enclosure of a glove box alone does not provide sterility to the aseptic process. Rather, it is the enclosure in addition to proper airflow that ensures the sterility of products prepared in the isolator.

Isolators offer several advantages over LAFWs, such as improved protection to the operator as well as decreased influence of room air on sterile preparation. Studies demonstrate improved protection to operators with the use of isolators, especially compared to BSCs.[3,4]

Parts of an Isolator

The main components of an isolator include the following elements:

- HEPA filters: HEPA filters provide first air to the work zone and are also used at exhaust points for exiting air.
- Gloves port: Gloves are attached to the enclosed isolator with an airtight seal.
- Exhaust: Exhaust systems must be in place to ensure that all exiting air is exhausted to the outside, rather than into the workroom. When working with hazardous drugs that may volatilize, air cannot be recirculated and must exit to the outside atmosphere.
- Work zone: Manipulations occur in this area.
- Transfer hatch: This "pass-through" is the part of an open-system isolator in which products are passed in and out through a door or opening. Closed-system isolators are connected to auxiliary equipment and transfer of the preparation is conducted aseptically.

■ Monitoring system: These systems include gauges that can be read to determine whether the isolator is operating within the design parameters. An alarm system provides an alert when the isolator does not meet the intended design parameters.

Airflow in Compounding Isolators

Airflow within an isolator is produced by either flow control or dilution control methods, depending on the type of isolator.[8] The flow control method eliminates particles from the work zone by utilizing HEPA-filtered unidirectional airflow to sweep particles away from the compounding area. A dilution control compounding isolator dilutes airborne contaminants with HEPA-filtered air—a process that results in a lower concentration of contaminants within the isolator. This type of airflow is referred to as turbulent airflow because contaminants remain suspended for a longer amount of time prior to being cycled out of the isolator, which depends on the volume of HEPA-filtered air used for dilution. Because unidirectional airflow sweeps HEPA-filtered air over the preparation areas and carries particulates to an air return, flow control isolators provide for a cleaner work zone environment. A study compared flow control and dilution control isolators, using unidirectional and turbulent airflow isolators, respectively. The investigators demonstrated that isolators using unidirectional flow met ISO Class 5 requirements in the work zone with an alcohol drying time of 16 seconds; by comparison, the turbulent airflow isolator did not meet the same standards and demonstrated a 6-minute alcohol drying time.[5]

Isolators utilize either positive or negative pressurized air. Open-system isolators use positive pressurized air to prevent backwash of air from the pass-through into the isolator. The pressure differential between the two spaces must be adequate to prevent contaminants from entering the isolator. Because HEPA filtration will remove particles and aerosols, but not fumes, air from the isolator must be exhausted to the outside if volatile substances are used within the isolator.

Cleaning Compounding Isolators

Considering that isolators are enclosed, less time is needed to purge them of contaminants if these controls are turned off. If the isolator has been turned off for less than 24 hours, it should run for 2 minutes prior to using it. If it has been turned off for more than 24 hours, the isolator should be sanitized and allowed to run for at least 10 minutes following disinfection.[8] Special isolator cleaning tools are useful in cleaning CAIs and CACIs. Most commonly, a small flat-surface mop, wipers, swabs, and detergents are used. The type of detergent selected should be based on which type of soil is to be removed and if decontamination is needed. **Table 5-4** outlines the steps for cleaning compounding isolators as described by manufacturers.[7]

Cleaning of isolators poses difficulty in accessing all surfaces due to the limited reach of gloves within the enclosed area. Because of this constraint, specialized cleaning tools can be used for cleaning, such as those with telescoping handles. Lint-free mops and wipers are used for cleaning surfaces and can be attached to cleaning tools. Appropriate detergents for cleaning

Table 5-4   Steps for Cleaning a Compounding Isolator

1. Clean
   - Clean all surfaces using quarter-folded wipers and linear overlapping strokes with an appropriate detergent
   - Clean in a pattern from areas most clean to those least clean
   - Use wipers for areas which can be reached with arms and cleaning tools with a telescopic handle for areas beyond the reach of the arm.
2. Rinse
   After cleaning, rinsing removes detergent residues. The purpose in rinsing is to provide a clean, bare surface for contact of a disinfecting agent.
   - Wet mop or wiper with residue-free disinfecting agent (e.g., sterile 70% IPA), or sterile deionized water and rinse in a similar pattern to cleaning.
3. Disinfect
   - Follow steps outlined in cleaning and rinsing using appropriate disinfecting agents.
4. Second Rinsing
   - Wet mop or wiper with residue-free disinfecting agent (e.g., sterile 70% IPA), or sterile deionized water and follow pattern used for cleaning.
5. Gaseous Sterilization

should be chosen based on the type of product prepared in the isolator. Detergents may include bleach, hydrogen peroxide, and ammonia compounds. Surfaces can be examined to ensure adequate cleaning and disinfection using surface sampling. Based on surface sampling results, only the disinfection, rinsing, and gaseous sterilization steps may be needed if the isolator has not been contaminated since the previous cleaning. A second rinsing similar to that following cleaning is performed to remove residue from disinfecting agents, which can result in buildup of residue and staining of work surfaces if not removed. Gaseous sterilization may be required if all surfaces of the isolator cannot be easily reached for physical disinfection. If required, the isolator can be sterilized as with vaporized hydrogen peroxide.

Cleaning and disinfection of the isolator should occur prior to each shift. Additionally, cleaning and disinfection of the isolator should be performed between preparations to avoid cross-contamination.

CERTIFICATION OF PRIMARY ENGINEERING CONTROLS

USP Chapter <797> outlines standards for expected quality control, such as air quality. The Controlled Environment Testing Association (CETA) provides recommendations to guide the certification process for compliance with USP Chapter <797>— namely, "Certification Guide for Sterile Compounding Facilities." These recommendations include "an industry-based minimum set of criteria appropriate for performance evaluation and certification of facility and environmental controls used for compounding sterile preparations."[9]

PECs should be certified upon initial installation to ensure proper functioning of the device. Additionally, PECs must be certified by a certified professional at the following times:[2]

- Device or room is moved: Moving a BSC can cause the seals around the HEPA filter to break. Additionally, the cabinet risks breaking if moved.
- Following a major repair: Recertification can verify that the cabinet is functioning appropriately following a repair, such as replacement of a HEPA filter or a motor.

- Major service to the facility: When construction or other major service to the facility is performed, it can compromise the air integrity during compounding practices. Recertification can ensure that air quality is maintained during construction.
- Every 6 months: Routine recertification is required.

During certification, air sampling within the PEC is conducted to ensure that an ISO Class 5 environment is maintained under dynamic operating conditions. For testing, an electronic discrete particle counter is used. The measurement needed for recertification should be no more than 3520 particles sized 0.5 micron and larger per cubic meter of air.[2,10] Additional testing is performed to evaluate air quality and patterning, such as airflow smoke pattern, HEPA filter leak, downflow velocity, negative pressure/ventilation rate, cabinet integrity, and face velocity. Tests are also conducted to certify that alarms and alerts are functioning properly, if applicable.

Secondary Engineering Controls

Direct compounding areas (DCAs) are critical areas that are directly exposed to first air, as within a PEC. While PECs maintain an ISO Class 5 environment, the surrounding areas also need to be controlled to prevent contamination of CSPs. Secondary engineering controls work as adjuncts to PECs to provide an environment that meets the requirements for air quality and to reduce the likelihood of contamination of final preparations. Secondary engineering controls include the environment leading to and in which the ISO Class 5 PECs are located. USP Chapter <797> provides specific criteria for air quality, design, and construction of secondary engineering devices.

A clean room, by USP Chapter <797> definition, is "a room in which the concentration of airborne particles is controlled to meet a specified airborne particulate cleanliness class."[2] Clean rooms should be supplied with HEPA-filtered air and restricted to personnel who are trained in compounding sterile preparations or those who require access for facility maintenance. The supply air in the clean room should be of sufficient volume and pressurization to ensure that introduction of airborne contaminants is controlled. Clean rooms may include buffer areas and ante-areas, both of which are considered secondary controls. **Figure 5-6** provides an example of a design for a clean room for nonhazardous sterile compounding.

ALERT: *Compounding facilities should be well lighted and maintain a temperature of 20°C or cooler to provide a comfortable environment for compounding personnel.*

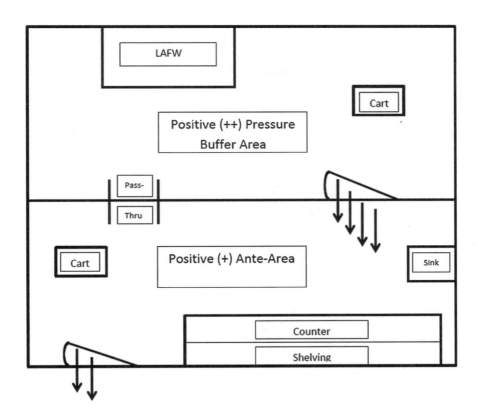

Figure 5-6   Example Clean Room Design

BUFFER AREA

Buffer areas are designed to maintain at least ISO Class 7 conditions for 0.5-micron particles under dynamic conditions. PECs should be located within this area, but should be situated so as to avoid conditions that might compromise their functioning. Traffic flow should not occur near the PEC, and room air supply should also be considered when selecting a place for the PEC. Activities that take place within the buffer area should be limited to only those that are necessary for working within a controlled environment, as with those directly involving aseptic processing. Hand washing should not occur in the buffer area; thus this area should not contain floor drains or sources of water, such as a sink. Items that are brought into the buffer area should be limited, and equipment and other items routinely used in the buffer area should not be removed except for maintenance and servicing. Items needing to be brought into the buffer area must first be cleaned and disinfected.

ALERT: *Supplies must be wiped down with an appropriate disinfecting agent prior to being introduced into the buffer area.*

TIP: *Traffic flow in and out of the buffer area should be minimized to minimize risk of contamination and compromise of air quality.*

Because sterile processing occurs in this area, air quality is of utmost importance. Thus HEPA-filtered air should supply the buffer area. USP Chapter <797> recommends that this air be supplied through vents in the ceiling, with return vents located low on the wall, thereby creating a top-down dilution of air. Buffer areas should be segregated from surrounding spaces that are not ISO classified to reduce influx of contaminants into the buffer area. USP Chapter <797> specifies that buffer areas with physical separation from the ante-areas should maintain a minimum

(handwritten margin notes: (normal conditions); no water – source of organisms, pyrogens)

of 0.02- to 0.05-inch water column positive pressure. Buffer areas not physically separated should use the principle of displacement airflow. This concept requires an air velocity of 40 feet per minute or greater across the line of demarcation from the buffer area to the ante-area. In general, during low- and medium-risk nonhazardous drug compounding, the buffer area and the ante-area can be in the same room, albeit separated by a line of demarcation. The buffer area must have positive pressure relative to the ante-area, and the ante-area must have negative pressure relative to the buffer area but positive pressure relative to the general pharmacy area. USP Chapter <797> provides further specifications for buffer rooms not preceded with an ante-room.

ALERT: *The principle of displacement airflow cannot be used for high-risk compounding. A wall with a door must separate the buffer area from the ante-area.*

ALERT: *USP Chapter <797> states that buffer areas should have at least 30 air changes per hour (ACPH) or as little as 15 ACPH if a LAFW provides 15 ACPH.*

SEGREGATED COMPOUNDING AREA

A segregated compounding area, by USP Chapter <797> definition, is "a designated space, either a demarcated area or room that is restricted to preparing low-risk level CSPs with 12-hour or less BUD."[2] A segregated compounding area will contain an ISO Class 5 PEC and should not contain devices that are extraneous to compounding. Furthermore, this area should not be located near unsealed windows or doors that have access to high-traffic areas or to the outside.

ALERT: *Sinks should not be located near the immediate area of the ISO Class 5 PEC.*

ALERT: *External cartons should not be taken into the buffer area or segregated compounding area.*

ALERT: *Outer garments, all visible jewelry or piercings, all cosmetics, and false nails should not be worn in the buffer area or segregated compounding area.*

ANTE-AREA

The ante-area should satisfy ISO Class 8 conditions for 0.5-micron and larger particles under dynamic conditions. The ante-area is located just outside the buffer area and is supplied with HEPA-filtered air. It is in this area that hand hygiene, garbing, staging, order entry, and labeling should take place. Any other activity that might potentially generate a high particulate count should be performed in the ante-area, rather than in other areas. Outer garments, cosmetics, and all jewelry should be removed in the ante-area, prior to entering the buffer area. Supplies that may be needed for compounding, such as needles, syringes, tubing, and other parenteral supplies, should be removed from their cartons and wiped down with an appropriate disinfectant in the ante-area.

ALERT: *All outer garments, cosmetics, and all jewelry should be removed prior to entering the buffer area.*

ALERT: *Artificial nails should not be worn in sterile compounding environments.*

ALERT: *Only nonshedding gowns that have not been soiled may be removed in the ante-area and redonned during the same shift.*

Ante-areas and buffer areas both require that a comfortable temperature be maintained at 20°C or cooler. Considering the required garb for those involved in compounding, these personnel should be able to perform flawlessly given the environmental conditions.

USP Chapter <797> provides standards on the surface characteristics for both ante-areas and buffer areas. For example, dust-collecting overhangs should be avoided, such as ceiling utility pipes, ledges, and windowsills. Additionally, carts used in these areas should be constructed of stainless steel wire, nonporous plastic, or sheet metal construction. Further, the casters of carts should of good quality and cleanable to promote good mobility.[2] More characteristics and construction requirements are illustrated in **Figure 5-7**.

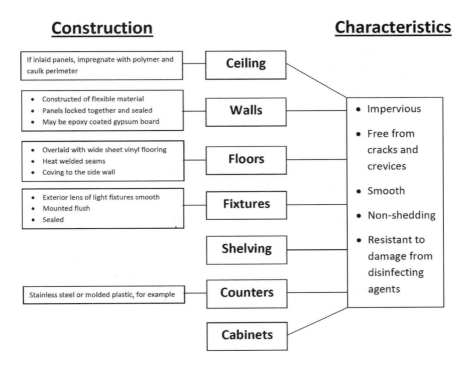

Construction

		Characteristics
If inlaid panels, impregnate with polymer and caulk perimeter	**Ceiling**	
• Constructed of flexible material • Panels locked together and sealed • May be epoxy coated gypsum board	**Walls**	• Impervious
• Overlaid with wide sheet vinyl flooring • Heat welded seams • Coving to the side wall	**Floors**	• Free from cracks and crevices
• Exterior lens of light fixtures smooth • Mounted flush • Sealed	**Fixtures**	• Smooth
	Shelving	• Non-shedding
		• Resistant to damage from disinfecting agents
Stainless steel or molded plastic, for example	**Counters**	
	Cabinets	

Figure 5-7 Characteristics and Construction Requirements for Secondary Engineering Controls

In going from the entry point of ante-areas to the direct compounding area, air quality improves. Environmental sampling for viable and nonviable testing must be performed to ensure that requirements for air quality are met. To help maintain these standards, the pressure differential between the buffer area and the ante-area requires monitoring, as does the differential between the ante-area and the general environment outside the compounding area. Results from the readings of a pressure gauge or velocity meter should be reviewed and documented at least every work shift or by a continuous recording device. USP Chapter <797> provides further specifications regarding pressure differentials.

To facilitate minimizing risk of contamination, floors and work surfaces of the ISO Class 7 buffer area and ISO Class 8 ante-area, as well as segregated compounding areas, need to be cleaned and disinfected daily. Walls, ceilings, and storage shelving need cleaning on a monthly basis.[2] Only nonshedding supplies should be used for cleaning. USP Chapter <797> provides further requirements for cleaning of the ante-areas and buffer areas in addition to the direct compounding areas.

BUFFER AREA AND ANTE-AREA FOR HAZARDOUS COMPOUNDING

When preparing hazardous preparations, the BSC or CACI must be located in an ISO Class 7 negative-pressure buffer area with no less than 0.01-inch water column negative pressure and separated from the other preparation areas. The buffer area must be adjacent to an ISO Class 7 positive-pressure ante-area. The ante-room must have positive pressure relative to both the buffer area and the general pharmacy area. The BSC and CACI should be 100% vented to the outside, with the air first passing through a HEPA filter prior to exiting to the outside. In situations where the CACI is utilized outside a buffer area (non-clean room), the compounding area must have a 0.01-inch water column negative pressure and a minimum of 12 ACPH. When utilizing closed-system vial-transfer devices in low-volume hazardous drug facilities, two tiers of containment should be used—for example, closed-system vial-transfer devices with a BSC or a CACI that is not located in a negative-pressure room.

ALERT: *Chewing gum, food, candy, and drinks cannot be taken into ante-areas, buffer areas, or segregated compounding areas. Materials exposed to patient care and treatment areas should never be introduced into areas where components and ingredients for sterile preparations are present.*

Conclusion

PECs and secondary engineering controls are essential for controlling overall contamination and maintaining an environment conducive for aseptic compounding. Primary engineering controls provide controlled environments in direct compounding areas where critical site exposure takes place. For secondary engineering controls, the air quality in direct compounding areas, buffer areas, and ante-areas influences the ability to maintain an acceptable environment for sterile processing. USP Chapter <797> provides guidance on requirements regarding both PECs and secondary engineering controls. These standards should be maintained at all times. Because of the impact of air quality and the importance of minimizing risk of contamination for compounding sterile preparations, focus should always remain on patient safety in adhering to all specifications provided. Maintaining a clean environment, in accordance with set standards, should be considered an adjunct to using aseptic technique to prepare CSPs that are safe for patient administration.

Review Questions

1. How often should the surface of the workbench be cleaned?
   a. Daily
   b. Every shift
   c. Every hour
   d. Prior to each manipulation

2. Which type of primary engineering control is most appropriate for use for preparation of nonhazardous products?
   a. Horizontal laminar airflow workbench
   b. Biological safety cabinet
   c. Compounding aseptic isolator
   d. Any of the above
3. Describe the differences and similarities between cleaning a horizontal laminar airflow workbench and a vertical laminar airflow workbench.
4. List the ISO classifications for the following environments:
   a. Direct compounding area
   b. Primary engineering control
   c. Buffer area
   d. Ante-area
5. How often should cleaning take place for primary and secondary engineering controls?

CASE STUDY

The University Hospital inpatient pharmacy is undergoing renovations to meet regulatory standards for its IV room. The pharmacy director is contemplating changes that need to be made to the IV room. The director has asked for pharmacist input regarding the arrangement of the rooms to meet current requirements. Using a schematic for illustration, provide an example of a room design that meets the requirements for secondary engineering controls in an IV room for compounding both hazardous and nonhazardous drugs. Indicate the pressure differences with arrows.

References

1. U.S. Department of Health and Human Services, Centers for Disease Control and Prevention. Appendix A: primary containment for biohazards: selection, installation and use of biological safety cabinets. In: Chosewood LC, Wilson DE, eds. *U.S. biosafety in microbiological and biomedical laboratories.* 5th ed. Washington, DC: U.S. Department of Health and Human Services; 2009:290–325.

2. U.S. Pharmacopeial Convention. Chapter <797>: pharmaceutical compounding: sterile preparations. *United States Pharmacopeia 36/National Formulary 31*. Rockville, MD: U.S. Pharmacopeial Convention; 2013.

3. Crauste-Manciet S, Sessink PJ, Ferrari S, et al. Environmental contamination with cytotoxic drugs in healthcare using positive air pressure isolators. *Ann Occup Hyg*. 2005;49(7):619–28.

4. Kopp B, Crauste-Manciet S, Guibert A, et al. Environmental and biological monitoring of platinum-containing drugs in two hospital pharmacies using positive air pressure isolators. *Ann Occup Hyg*. October 22, 2012 [Epub ahead of print]. Accessed February 9, 2013.

5. Peters GF, McKeon MR, Weiss WT. Potential for airborne contamination in turbulent- and unidirectional-airflow compounding aseptic isolators. *Am J Health Syst Pharm*. 2007;64(6):622–631.

6. Mason HJ, Blair S, Sams C, et al. Exposure to antineoplastic drugs in two UK hospital pharmacy units. *Ann Occup Hyg*. 2005; 49(7):603–610.

7. ESCO Technologies Inc. Hospital pharmacy isolator solutions for USP <797> compliance from Esco. Available at: http://www.escoglobal.com/resources/pdf/HPI-consolidated-product.pdf. Accessed February 11, 2013.

8. American Society of Health System Pharmacists Guidelines. Drug distribution and control: quality assurance for pharmacy-prepared sterile products. Available at: http://www.ashp.org/DocLibrary/BestPractices/PrepGdlQualAssurSterile.aspx. Accessed February 11, 2013.

9. Controlled Environment Testing Association. *CAG-003-2006-11: certification guide for sterile compounding facilities*. Raleigh, NC: Controlled Environment Testing Association; 2012:1–18.

10. ISO 14644-1. International Organization for Standardization. Geneveve 20, Switzerland. Case Postale 56. CH-1211.

11. A USP 797 compliant clean room. Hartley Medical Blog. Available at: http://hartleymedical.com/blog/a-usp-797-compliant-clean-room/. Accessed February 8, 2013.

CHAPTER **6**

Aseptic Technique and Compounding Manipulations

Pamella S. Ochoa and José A. Vega

 Where this icon appears, visit http://go.jblearning.com /OchoaCWS to view the corresponding video.

Chapter Objectives

1. List the proper steps for performing hand washing.
2. Properly sequence the donning of personal protective equipment.
3. Describe the relationship between aseptic technique and patient safety.
4. List critical sites of the vial, bag, needle, and syringe.
5. Describe techniques for withdrawing solutions from an ampule and a vial.
6. Summarize the process for reconstituting lyophilized products.
7. Explain manipulations for accommodating positive and negative pressure.
8. List core elements of a label for compounded sterile preparations.
9. Describe workflow processes for compounding sterile preparations.

Key Terminology

Personal protective equipment
Garb

Batch compounding
Buffer area
Ante-area
Coring
Filter needle
Milking
Critical sites
First air
Reconstitution
Auxiliary label

Overview

The presence of microorganisms, pyrogens, or particulate matter in parenteral preparations can have harmful consequences to patients. The manner in which these sterile preparations are compounded, the environment in which the preparation process takes place, and the utilization of methods to prevent contamination are important aspects of ensuring the sterility of preparations for patient administration. Utilizing the correct techniques with consistency is the foundation of compounding sterile preparations, which should be employed by all personnel involved in the compounding process. During initial training of such personnel, the focus should be on refining technique prior to addressing efficiency. To skillfully master a good technique for parenteral preparation requires much guided practice; however, once this skill is perfected, personnel can perform manipulations efficiently without compromising their technique.

Factors in Compounding a Sterile Preparation

A combination of factors related to the preparation process must be taken into account to prevent contamination and ensure the sterility of parenteral preparations:

- Environmental quality
- Proper hand washing and hand hygiene
- Personal protective equipment

- Primary and secondary engineering controls
- Maintenance of equipment and environment
- Aseptic technique

Each of these factors involves steps that can prevent contamination of the end preparation.

 ## HAND WASHING

Hand washing should be performed in the ante-area and is an essential and critical component of preventing contamination. The number of normal flora on hands can range from 10^2 cfu/cm^2 to 10^3 cfu/cm^2.[1] While the normal flora on the hands help to limit colonization of pathogenic microorganisms, healthcare workers, including pharmacy personnel, have been found to have both transient and resident bacterial flora that are associated with healthcare-acquired infections.[2,3] Additionally, healthcare workers can become persistently colonized with a variety of pathogenic flora. Hand washing can reduce levels of transient flora by ensuring their physical removal.[3] Specifically, spore-producing bacteria, such as *Clostridium difficile*, are best removed with hand washing. Hand washing also provides the benefit of removing particles that have accumulated on the hands, which risk being introduced onto objects in areas requiring limited particle exposure. Although gloves are worn during the manipulation process, it is important to remember that touch contamination can occur when donning gloves. Without proper hand washing, gloves can be contaminated and subsequently result in contamination of the end preparation.

The effect of time is an important factor in proper hand washing; that is, sufficient time spent on hand washing is necessary to achieve adequate microbial reduction. Washing hands with plain soap and water for 15 seconds has been shown to reduce bacterial counts by 0.6–1.1 $\log_{10}$, while washing for 30 seconds can reduce bacterial counts by 1.8–2.8 $\log_{10}$.[4] USP Chapter <797> recommends washing hands and forearms for at least 30 seconds. Hand washing should be used as an adjunct to use waterless alcohol-based surgical hand sanitizer for good hand hygiene in preparation for compounding sterile preparations (CSPs).

TIP: *Hands and forearms should be washed for at least 30 seconds.*

As noted earlier in this text, personnel preparing parenteral admixtures cannot wear artificial nails. Artificial nails have been shown to introduce bacteria and fungi and can pose a risk of contamination of the CSP to be administered to the patient. For similar reasons, nails should be kept short and trimmed. Like artificial nails, longer nails not only can harbor bacteria, but also can cause punctures or tears in gloves, sometimes unbeknownst to the operator. Thus nails should be kept as short as possible, but certainly no longer than 2 mm. For more information regarding the influence of nails on microbiologic contamination, refer to the *Microbiological Considerations in Parenteral Compounding* chapter.

When performing hand washing, imagine moving particles and debris from the area that should be the cleanest to that which is the dirtiest, such as from the fingertips to the elbow. All steps performed should focus on this aspect of cleaning by ensuring that once an area is cleaned or dried, the area is not touched again. For example, using an up-and-down motion along the entire forearm when drying will move particles from dirtier areas (i.e., the elbows) to cleaner areas (i.e., the wrists). Because manipulations will be performed with the hands and fingertips, it is important for these areas to be the cleanest. It is also important that no objects, such as the faucet, be touched immediately following the hand washing process and prior to gloving, in an effort to avoid contamination.

Steps for Hand Washing

The following steps should be followed by all personnel prior to performing parenteral preparations and when "scrubbing in" is warranted:

1. Gather supplies needed.
   a. Scrub brush (if warranted)
   b. Nail cleaner

      c. Hand cleanser (either antimicrobial or non-antimicrobial)

      d. Lint-free disposable towels (at least five)

      e. Access to warm water

2. Turn on the warm water.

      a. Water should be a temperature that is warm but not hot. Regular hand washing with hot water can cause irritation, drying, and possible cracking of skin, which can result in open skin exposure and introduce the potential for contamination of preparation.

3. Wet the hands and forearms.

4. Use nail cleaner to clean under all nails on each hand. Nails should be cleaned under warm running water.

5. Discard the nail cleaner into a waste container.

6. Wet the the foam side of the scrub brush and squeeze a few times to work up lather.

7. Use the scrub brush to gently clean all sides of each finger of both hands.

8. Scrub the palm of one hand, and then the palm of the other hand.

9. Scrub the backs of both hands to the wrist.

10. Beginning at the wrist, use small circular motions of the scrub brush to clean around the circumference of the wrist.

11. Move down, slightly overlapping with the area previously cleaned on the wrist, and continue to use small circular motions to clean around the circumference of the arm.

      a. Do not use an up-and-down motion to clean the forearm area.

12. Continue to move down slightly each time, repeating Step 11, until the elbow area is reached.

13. Rinse the scrub brush under running water and squeeze a few times to work up lather.

14. Beginning at the wrist of the opposite arm, repeat Steps 10 through 12.

15. Discard the scrub brush into a waste container.

16. Holding the arms in an upward manner, with the fingertips pointed up and the elbows down, rinse the hands so that the water runs from the fingertips downward toward the elbows.

  a. Keep the hands and arms in this position for the entire rinsing process and until the hands are completely dry.

  b. Prevent dripping of water toward the fingertips. Water dripping from the elbows will indicate that the proper position is being used.

17. Grab at least two disposable towels, select one hand to dry, and dry the fingertips first, followed by the palm and back of the hand.

  a. Ensure that wrist does not drop below elbow when grabbing the towels.

18. Dry the wrist next, going around the circumference of the wrist area.

19. Dry the forearm using the same manner used for cleaning, by going around the circumference of the arm in different levels downward until reaching the elbow.

  a. Do not use an up-and-down motion when drying the arm, as this will move particles up to areas that are already clean.

  b. Once an area is dry, do not return to this area, as doing so will recontaminate the area.

20. Discard the disposable towels used for drying into a waste container.

  a. Ensure that the wrist of wet hand does not drop below the elbow when disposing towels.

  b. If necessary, use the dry hand to grab the used towels (clean side of the towel touching wet hand) from the wet hand.

21. Grab two new disposable towels and repeat the same drying process on the opposite hand and arm.

22. Discard the used disposable towel in a waste container.

23. Grab a new disposable towel to turn off the water faucet, if needed.

24. Discard the disposable towel used to turn off the faucet.

  a. The faucet should not be turned off until the hands are completely dry and the hand washing process has been completed.

USP Chapter <797> recommends against the use of a scrub brush, as this can lead to irritation of skin and possible breaks in the skin. Many institutions still utilize scrub brushes for hand cleaning. The use of scrub brushes should be evaluated by institutions and strict discretion used when deciding on their continued use. If continued, use of scrub brushes should be significantly limited. For example, personnel may "scrub in" initially, such as at the beginning of a shift and when returning from a lunch break. Hand washing, not scrubbing in, should be performed often, such as when hands are known to be or are visibly soiled or contaminated, upon entering the buffer area (each time), and prior to gloving. The same steps listed previously should be followed for regular hand washing; however, rather than using a scrub brush, personnel should use their hands in the same manner that the scrub brush is manipulated.

Following hand washing, garbing should take place immediately, and only supplies used in the garbing process should be touched. No other objects should be touched, as this would risk recontamination of hands following cleaning.

PERSONAL PROTECTIVE EQUIPMENT

Personal protective equipment (PPE) consists of clothing and gear that is worn when compounding. The process of donning PPE is commonly referred to as "garbing." PPE is utilized for two main purposes: (1) to protect the preparation from the operator and (2) to protect the operator from the preparation. As described in the *Microbiological Considerations in Parenteral Compounding* chapter, the operator introduces a significant amount of particles into clean areas, as well as microorganisms. PPE keeps such particles and microorganisms contained and prevents them from contaminating the final preparation as well as assists in maintaining better environmental control. Moreover, PPE is made of materials that demonstrate low particle emission rates, thereby decreasing the number of particles released into the controlled environment. In cases in which chemotherapy or other hazardous agents are prepared, PPE can also protect the operator from sprays or spills. Often, sprays or fumes cannot be seen with the naked eye but still occur. PPE is essential in these types of situations to protect the operator from the preparation.

The requirements for the type of PPE donned vary depending on the type of product being prepared. Donning requirements for hazardous agents will be discussed later, as the type of PPE used when preparing hazardous agents is specific to such scenarios. For nonhazardous preparations, the following PPE should be worn:

- Shoe covers
- Beard cover
- Hair cover
- Face mask
- Jacket/gown
- Gloves

The sequence of garbing should be completed by donning garb from areas that are considered most dirty to areas considered cleanest. For the PPE described here, the operator should begin with shoe covers, as shoes are considered to be dirtiest, and move to gloves, as hands are considered and should be maintained as the cleanest. PPE should also be donned in specific areas and in a sequence relative to hand washing and sanitizing, as illustrated in **Figure 6-1**.

Shoe Covers

Shoe covers intended for use in sterile or controlled environments should be donned in the ante-area. Shoe covers are available in a range of sizes. Most commonly, one range accommodates most

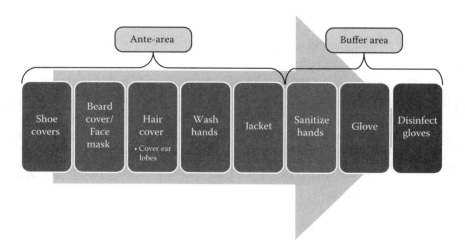

Figure 6-1 Sequence for Donning PPE

common shoe sizes, but larger sizes are also available. A fit that covers all or the majority of the shoe is most appropriate. Shoe covers should be replaced with new ones when reentering compounding areas.[5]

Beard Cover and Face Mask

Covers specifically made for beards are available as commercial products. Beard covers should be worn if the operator has facial hair, as facial hair can be a source of particle emission and contamination. All facial hair should be completely covered with the beard cover, and such a cover should be worn at all times when in the clean room. Face masks should be worn by all operators. The face mask should be placed such that the nose piece sits over the bridge of the nose. The operator may bend the nose piece for a better fit. A beard cover and face mask may be donned prior to the hair cover, as donning either of these requires the removal of the hair cover. If a hair cover is donned prior to the beard cover and face mask, the ear loops of the cover and face mask can be placed atop the hair cover. Donning a beard cover and mask prior to the hair cover is also more convenient for those personnel who wear eyeglasses. Operators with facial hair must don a beard cover first, then don a face mask over the beard cover. Beard covers and face masks should be donned in the ante area and replaced with a new ones when reentering compounding areas.[5]

Hair Cover

A significant number of particles are released from the hair. Hair covers assist in preventing these particles from entering the workbench and diminishing the cumulative particle count in the environment. Because hair emits so many particles, it is necessary to completely cover all hair to prevent particles from falling onto garb or CSPs. Hair covers should fit so that all the hair is covered.

Two types of hair covers are typically used: one that has an elastic band around the circumference of the edge and one that ties in the back of the head. Hair covers that contain an elastic band provide a secure fit around the perimeter of the hair cover so as to cover the hair in its entirety and hold hair within the cover. These types of hair covers are preferred because they do not leave any hair exposed. Hair covers that tie in the back of the head cover only a portion of the hair, which can introduce particles and the potential for contamination.

It is best practice to utilize hair covers that cover all hair for all personnel involved in compounding sterile preparations. Hair covers should be donned so that ear lobes are completely covered. Further, hair at the nape of the neck should be securely tucked under the hair cover. Hair covers should be donned in the ante area and replaced with a new hair cover when reentering compounding areas.[5]

Jacket/Gown

Low-particle-emitting jackets should be selected. Jackets that are waterproof are available, but are most appropriate when working with hazardous agents. Jackets should be at least knee length to ensure good coverage and protection. The sleeve cuffs should fit snug around the wrist to ensure gloves can be placed over the cuffs. All buttons should be buttoned, including the one nearest the collar. Jackets should be donned in the ante area.

Gloves

Sterile, powder-free gloves should be donned in the buffer area. Compounding of hazardous agents requires two sets of gloves, an inner pair and an outer pair, with the outer pair being gloves that meet specifications for use in chemotherapy preparations.

Gloves are available in a variety of sizes. When choosing an appropriate size, fit should be considered. Gloves that are too loose can prevent the operator from performing manipulations with ease. In contrast, gloves that are too tight become prone to ruptures or tears. A snug fit is considered most appropriate, and size should be selected based on this standard.

Sterile 70% IPA should be used for sanitizing gloves. Gloves should not be washed and reused. It is recommended to replace gloves when torn or compromised, or when gloves are known to be contaminated or are visibly soiled.

After proper hand washing, hands should be disinfected using alcohol based hand scrub. Gloves should then be donned once hands are completely dry. Subsequently, gloves should be

Table 6-1	Schedule for Disinfecting Gloves

Immediately after being donned

Prior to and after cleaning the laminar airflow workbench (LAFW)

Prior to each preparation

Prior to reentering an ISO Class 5 environment (e.g., LAFW, biological safety cabinet [BSC])

If suspected or known to be contaminated or if visibly soiled

Periodically during prolonged durations of compounding in the primary engineering control (PEC)

Source: U.S. Pharmacopeial Convention. Chapter <797>, Pharmaceutical compounding-sterile preparations. United States Pharmacopeia 36/National Formulary 31. Rockville, MD: U.S. Pharmacopeial Convention, Inc.; 2013.

disinfected with sterile 70% IPA when donned, prior to cleaning the workbench, upon reentering the workbench if taken out during product manipulation, during prolonged compounding, and prior to each product preparation (**Table 6-1**). Gloves should be changed every 30 minutes for extended manipulations, such as with batch compounding.[5]

Aseptic Technique

Aseptic technique comprises a series of techniques that are employed during the preparation of CSPs and that ensure a product free of microorganisms, pyrogens, and particular matter. It involves manipulation of syringes and vials, with consideration of airflow, to reduce the likelihood of contamination of the end preparation.

CRITICAL SITES AND AIRFLOW

Critical sites are areas on the syringe, vial, and needle that are at greatest risk of contamination (**Table 6-2**). Contamination of critical sites can occur through touch, moisture, or contact with unclean air. Touch contamination can occur through human touch or touching of the critical site to an unclean object, such as the laminar airflow workbench (LAFW). As the area of exposure increases, so does the risk of contamination. For example, an opened ampule, which is an open system and exposed to air, has

Table 6-2	Critical Sites

Needle

- Hub of the needle
- Tip of the needle
- Shaft of the needle

Syringe

- Tip of the syringe
- Ribs of the plunger

Vials and Ampules

- Rubber closure when penetrated
- Opening of an ampule

Additive Bags

- Additive/injection port

a greater risk of contamination than does a vial, which is a closed system, or than a needle tip, which has a smaller surface area. The type of critical site can influence the risk of contamination. For example, rough surfaces, surfaces with ridges, and porous surfaces are more difficult to disinfect and, therefore, carry a higher risk of contamination. Greater time of exposure of critical sites and greater number of manipulations performed can increase the risk of contamination as well. Thus it is important to be organized and work efficiently, yet accurately, and to disinfect gloves periodically during extended manipulations.

First air, also referred to as clean air, is air that has been processed through the primary engineering device and exits the high-efficiency particulate absorption (HEPA) filter into the LAFW surface. Because the risk of contamination of critical sites is significant, it is important that all critical sites are exposed to the path of first air from the HEPA filter—a practice that mitigates this risk. It is also important that critical sites are never touched or exposed to air outside of the LAFW during, or prior to, the preparation process. The direction of first air flow must be considered during manipulations. The operator must always be aware of airflow direction in regard to critical sites as well as for placement of objects within the LAFW.

Consistent airflow of first air from the HEPA filter to all critical sites during the compounding of sterile preparations is of utmost importance. Blocking of airflow to critical sites should never occur during compounding. Airflow to critical sites can be disrupted when passing a hand, or parts of the hand, between the HEPA filter and a critical site. Additionally, blocking the path of first air to critical sites will result from passing the critical site behind an object, such as a vial. Awareness of contamination risks is important so that consistent methods can be employed during the preparation process to avoid contamination of the CSP.

ALERT: *The path of first air to all critical sites must never be blocked during compounding.*

STEPS OF ASEPTIC TECHNIQUE

1. Gather Supplies

After following the steps described previously for cleaning the LAFW in the *Primary and Secondary Engineering Controls* chapter, all needed supplies should be collected to avoid the need to exit the LAFW once the preparation process has been initiated. Items needed include, but are not limited to, the following:

- Vial or ampule
- Needle of appropriate gauge
- Filter needle, if using an ampule
- Syringe of appropriate size
- Bag, vial, or solution to which additives will be added
- Diluent for reconstitution, if needed
- Sterile, lint-free, alcohol wipes
- Sterile 70% IPA
- Label and calculations available for reference during manipulation (should not be taken into the LAFW)

wipe down everything

ALERT: *Sterile supplies that are stored individually need to be wiped down with an appropriate disinfectant prior to being passed into the buffer area. Sterile supplies that are removed from sealed outer wrappers and immediately passed into the buffer area do not need to be wiped.*

2. Disinfect Vials, Ampules, and Injection Ports

The protective cap should be removed from the top of the vials being used for the preparation. Next, a sterile, unused, and lint-free alcohol wipe should be removed from the package and used to wipe the surface of the rubber closure three times in the direction of the operator, thereby disinfecting and removing any particles from the closure. Back-and-forth motions should be avoided. A clean alcohol wipe should be used each time a new vial is cleaned to avoid contamination and delivery of particles from one vial to the next. Ampules should be disinfected by using a new, sterile, and lint-free alcohol wipe, wrapping the wipe around the neck of the ampule, and using a twisting motion to ensure that all surfaces of the neck are cleaned. Surfaces should remain wet for at least 10 seconds.[5] After disinfecting either the vial or the ampule, the alcohol should be allowed to dry to aid in the disinfecting process. The additive port of the bag or container to which drugs are added should also be disinfected by wiping with a sterile, lint-free, alcohol wipe three times in the same direction and in a direction parallel to the airflow from the HEPA filter. Disinfecting vials, ampules, and injection ports at this point in the preparation process will allow sufficient time for drying prior to entry.

3. Prepare Syringe

Remove Syringe

The workflow process tends to be easiest if the syringe is opened from its package prior to removing the needle from the packaging. To do so, the unopened syringe should be placed at least 6 inches inside the LAFW. This will ensure that immediate exposure of the critical sites of the syringe occurs in a clean environment. To remove the syringe from the packaging, peel the plastic overwrap in the manner intended by the manufacturer. Once the syringe has been removed, it should be held with the tip facing the HEPA filter. It is important that critical sites of the syringe never come in contact with the workbench or be touched, as these actions can result in contamination. The tip of the syringe should remain in contact with first air during removal of the needle from its package as well as throughout the duration of the preparation process.

Remove Needle

Next, the needle should be removed from its packaging at least 6 inches inside the LAFW. This practice will ensure that immediate exposure of the critical sites of the needle occurs in a clean environment. When removing the needle, the plastic protective wrap should be peeled off as intended by the manufacturer. It is important that the needle is not removed by forced exit through the paper covering, such as by pushing the hub of the needle through the paper package, as this will introduce a large number of particles into the clean environment of the workbench. After its removal from the package, the hub of the needle should be faced toward the HEPA filter while preparing the syringe, as this positioning will allow good flow of first air to the hub of the needle. The needle should not be placed on the work surface of the workbench, as doing so would result in contamination of the hub, which is a critical site.

> **ALERT:** *Never push syringes or needles through their packaging when removing from their outer wrapper. Doing so will introduce significant particles into the ISO Class 5 environment of the LAFW.*

 Attach Needle to Syringe and Remove Cap of Needle

As discussed in the *Supplies and Equipment for Compounding and Administering Sterile Preparations* chapter, needles can have either a slip-tip or Luer Lock hub. If using a slip-tip needle, first ensure that the syringe tip can accommodate a slip-tip needle and is not a Luer Lock. The hub of the needle should be pushed onto the slip-tip syringe with a slight twist to ensure that the needle is firmly attached. If using a Luer Lock needle and syringe, screw the hub onto the syringe tip with slight tension. To remove the cap, a push–pull technique should be employed to prevent injury. To do so, use one continuous motion by first pushing the needle cap toward the hub of the needle, and then pulling the needle cap off (**Figure 6-2**). An alternate method can be used for safely

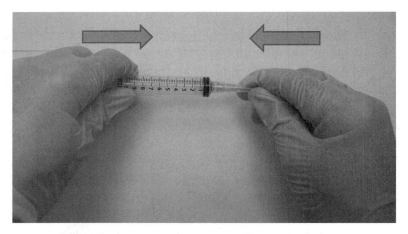

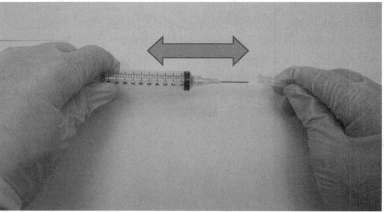

Figure 6-2 Push-Pull Technique

removing the needle cap: place wrists together—palms of hands facing each other—while holding the syringe in one hand and the cap in the other. Pull cap off while keeping wrists together. As a reminder, recapping of needles should be avoided. If necessary, the "scoop" method should be employed; it is discussed later in this chapter.

 4. Enter Vial

The manner in which the needle enters the vial is important, as coring can result from improper entry. Coring occurs when the needle bores a small hole through the rubber closure, with rubber becoming lodged within the needle shaft. When the contents of the vial are subsequently drawn into the syringe, the piece of rubber closure can ultimately end up in the final admixture, posing a significant risk to the patient if infused.

When entering the vial with a needle, the vial should be securely placed standing upright on the workbench surface. Entering the vial with a needle while the vial is in mid-air poses needle stick risks to the operator. Thus it is recommended that the vial be held with one hand, with the bottom surface of the vial resting on the workbench, and the other hand be used to manipulate the syringe.

The needle should be placed against the rubber closure with the bevel facing upward. The needle should be angled at 45 degrees while applying pressure downward and then pushed through the rubber closure. **Figure 6-3** illustrates the proper method for entering a vial with a needle. Once the bevel enters the vial, the needle can be positioned upright.

Using this technique will help prevent coring. Coring is also influenced by gauge size, with smaller gauges being more likely to result in this problem. The final admixture should always be

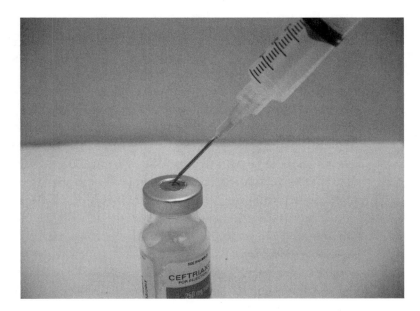

Figure 6-3   Entering a Vial

inspected for rubber particles resulting from potential coring prior to being dispensed.

 ### 5. Withdraw Contents

Withdrawing from a Vial

It is important to remember that the insides of most vials are at an equal pressure with the outside atmosphere. Because of this, an equal amount of air should be added to the vial as the volume to be withdrawn in an effort to maintain pressure equilibrium within the vial. To withdraw contents from a vial, the volume of solution to be removed from the vial should be determined. An equivalent volume of air should be drawn up into the syringe prior to entering the vial. Once the rubber closure has been punctured, the vial and attached syringe should be inverted so that the vial is above the syringe. The syringe, and attached vial, should be held directly upright in a completely vertical fashion to ensure that first air is able to reach all critical sites.

When inverting the vial and syringe, a horizontal "see-saw" motion should be used. To do so, place one hand on the bottom of the vial with the palm facing the HEPA filter, holding the vial between the thumb and forefinger. The other hand should grasp the syringe barrel closest to the flange, between the thumb and forefinger, with the palm of the hand facing the HEPA filter. The vial can then be rotated upward to a vertical position while allowing the syringe to rotate downward. Using this "see-saw" motion will prevent rotation of the vial toward the HEPA filter, which will block first air to the critical sites during inversion. **Figure 6-4** depicts the inversion of the vial and syringe in a manner to prevent blocking of first air to critical sites using a "see-saw" motion. Following inversion, the vial and syringe should appear vertically linear, which will provide flow of first air to all critical sites.

Once in position, a "milking" technique should be used by pushing and releasing the plunger of the syringe. Milking uses pressure to withdraw a solution from a vial and involves pushing some of the air within the syringe into the vial until slight resistance is felt. The plunger of the syringe should then be released to allow the added pressure in the vial to push the solution back into the syringe. This process should be repeated until all the air

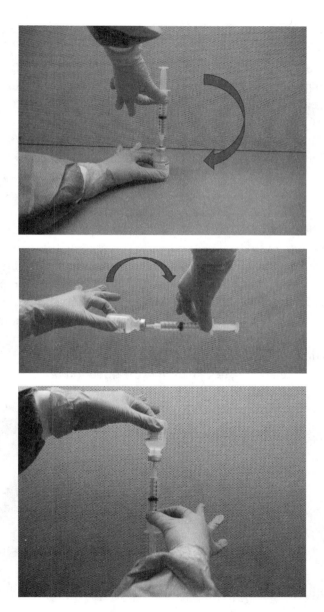

Figure 6-4 Inversion of Vial and Syringe

within the syringe is in the vial and the desired amount of solution is in the syringe. It is important to not push all air into the vial at once, especially when a large volume of air is involved. Doing so puts too much air into the vial, which can result in spraying of the solution out through the rubber closure and, although unlikely, bursting of the vial.

To avoid pressure issues related to withdrawing contents, a vented needle can be used. When using a vented needle, air does not need to be added to the syringe prior to withdrawing contents and "milking" is not necessary.

Manipulating the syringe, while inserted into the vial, is a skill that requires practice. The most important concepts during manipulations are twofold. First, it is important that no critical sites are touched. Second, the flow of first air to critical sites must be maintained at all times during manipulations.

When only one hand is used to manipulate the syringe, the method is referred to as a "one-handed technique" (**Figure 6-5A**). With this technique, one hand manipulates the syringe and the other holds the vial. The tip of one finger of the hand manipulating the syringe is placed on the flange of the plunger, in the space between two ribs, and is pushed downward when withdrawing solution. When expelling air or solution from the syringe, the fingertip is relocated to the opposite side—the outward side—of the flange and pushes in an upward direction. A one-handed

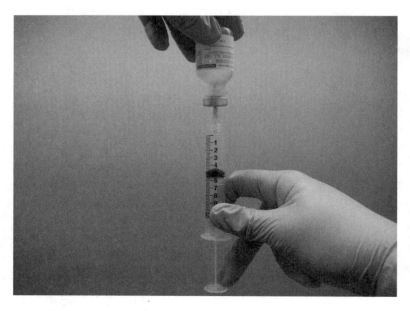

Figure 6-5A   One-handed Technique

technique is a useful skill to master, as it is less likely to result in disruption of first air to critical sites.

When two hands are used to manipulate the syringe, the method is referred to as a "two-handed technique." Many individuals are more comfortable with a two-handed technique compared to a one-handed technique. With this technique, one hand holds the syringe plunger while the other hand alternates between holding the vial and the syringe when withdrawing solution. While this method can feel more secure, it has a greater potential to block the syringe tip and rubber closure from first air as the hand moves up and down between the syringe and the vial. If a direct linear motion is used during this maneuver, the hand will come between first air and critical sites. Thus, when moving to and from the vial from the syringe, the hand should move in a horseshoe formation or similar to a C (not to be confused with the C-grasp). **Figure 6-5B** depicts a two-handed technique and the proper movement pattern when transitioning from the syringe to/from the vial.

Some personnel prefer to grasp the vial and the syringe concomitantly with one hand, referred to as the "C-grasp"

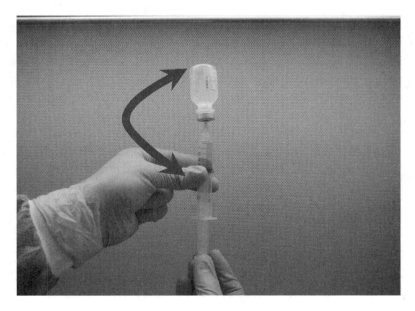

Figure 6-5B   Two-handed Technique

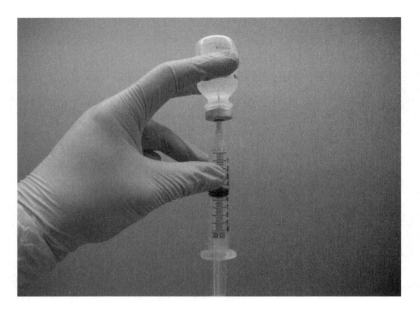

Figure 6-5C C-grasp

(**Figure 6-5C**). With this technique, the vial is secured between the forefinger and the middle finger. The syringe is grasped between the thumb and the ring finger of the same hand. Holding both the syringe and the vial with one hand frees up the second hand to pull the plunger of the syringe so as to withdraw the solution. When using this technique, it is important to consider how the position is initially obtained. For example, many individuals grasp the syringe first, then move their forefinger and middle fingers onto the vial. When doing so, the middle finger will pass between the HEPA filter and the rubber closure and syringe tip, blocking first air. To prevent this, the C-grasp should be formed away from the vial and syringe, followed by bringing the hand, already in position, onto the vial and syringe.

Regardless of which technique used, the vial should always be grasped toward the bottom, farthest away from the rubber closure. Lackadaisical technique often results in "cupping" the vial in one hand or allowing "free" fingers to fall downward, both of which cause fingers to block the path of first air to the rubber closure and syringe tip. Figure 6-4 serves as a good illustration of proper finger placement for "free" fingers, as well as indicates where the vial should be grasped. These positions should be maintained throughout the compounding process. In addition, when pulling the plunger during withdrawal of solution, it is important to avoid touching the ribs of the plunger.

> **TIP:** *First air should not be blocked when inverting the vial and syringe. Using a "see-saw" motion during inversions will ensure consistent flow of first air to critical sites.*

> **TIP:** *Use a "milking" technique when removing solution from a vial.*

 Removal of Air Bubbles

After the desired volume is drawn up into the syringe, it must be recognized that air bubbles within the syringe barrel and tip can occupy space that should be filled with the medication or contents of the vial. Cumulatively speaking, the amount of space occupied by air from air bubbles can result in a smaller volume of medication and, therefore, less medication dosage than prescribed. To remove air bubbles, first push the vial completely onto the needle so that the rubber closure is against the needle hub. Then pull the plunger down just slightly, which may temporarily increase the volume in the syringe or create a pocket of air at the top of the syringe. Tapping the syringe with your fingers or part of your palm in the area adjacent to the bubble will result in the bubble rising to the top of the syringe (**Figure 6-6**). Once this process is followed for all air bubbles, all of the air from the bubbles will reside at the top of the syringe or within the tip of the syringe or hub of the needle. It is important that the collected air then be ejected completely into the vial, as it will continue to occupy space within the tip of the syringe, hub of the needle, or shaft of the needle until completely ejected. The operator may be able to see the air ejected into the vial. Ejection of the bubbles should continue until solution is seen flowing through the needle tip. The final volume should then be readjusted to the desired volume.

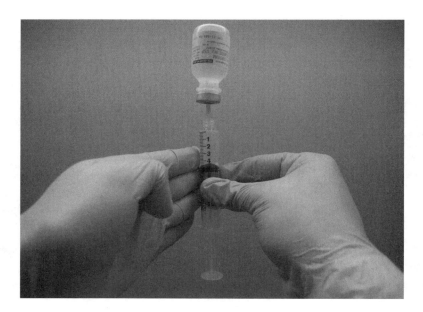

Figure 6-6 Removing Air Bubbles from a Syringe

TIP: *To aid in movement of air bubbles to the top of the syringe, hold all fingers close together and use the middle phalanx segment of the fingers to tap the syringe in the location of the bubble. Do not tap the syringe and rebound, but rather allow the fingers to remain on the syringe after tapping, which will maximize transfer of energy into the syringe. Bubbles should be completely ejected from the syringe and the needle.*

The final volume should be double-checked to ensure its accuracy. The syringe and attached needle can then be manipulated so that the vial is placed back onto the workbench surface using a "see-saw" motion opposite of the motion used earlier to invert the syringe and vial. At this point, the needle can be withdrawn from the vial. Needles should not be withdrawn from the vial with the vial in mid-air, as doing so increases the risk of needle sticks. The bottom of the vial should be firmly placed on the workbench surface and held with one hand prior to removing the needle with the opposite hand.

Withdrawing from an Ampule

Recalling that an ampule is an open system, the process used for withdrawing the contents of an ampule does not require milking. The contents of the ampule must first be accessed by tapping the neck of the ampule to move the contents from the neck into the body of the ampule. To break the neck of the ampule, firmly grasp the neck of the ampule with one hand while holding onto the body of the ampule with the other hand, aiming the thumbs toward each other. Face the ampule toward the one side of the workbench to prevent glass fragments from going toward the HEPA filter, which can compromise the integrity of the filter. Break the neck by applying pressure at the interception of the two thumbs, much like breaking a pencil. If the ampule does not break readily, rotate it by one-fourth turn and try again. Continue turning until the break point is found and the ampule can be readily broken. Some ampules are painted with a colored ring around the circumference of the ampule neck. This line does not indicate the point at which the neck should be broken; rather, the neck of the ampule should always be broken at the point where the neck and body of the ampule are connected. Care should be taken when breaking an ampule. In addition, opening an ampule that is still wet with alcohol should be avoided, as this could lead to injury.

> ▶ *Alert: Never break an ampule toward the HEPA filter. Ampules should be broken toward the side of the workbench.*

> ▶ *Alert: When using an ampule, withdraw the contents with a filter needle, then change to a regular needle.*

To withdraw the contents from the ampule, hold the ampule with one hand while holding the syringe with the other hand (**Figure 6-7**). The ampule can be held either horizontally or vertically, as solution will not escape if the ampule is held upright. Place the needle through the opening of the ampule, bevel downward, and pull on the plunger to draw up the contents, using a one-handed technique to manipulate the syringe. Care should be taken to prevent the needle from touching the edge of the ampule opening. Air bubbles can be removed in a similar fashion as described previously for a vial. When all of the ampule's contents are needed, place the ampule in a horizontal orientation and place the tip of the needle, bevel side down, into the cusp, or shoulder, of the ampule closest to the opening. Allow the contents to gather in this cusp while pulling the plunger continuously.

The most important, and required, step of withdrawing the contents from an ampule is using a filter needle. Recall that the presence of microscopic particles in the final admixture can result in patient harm or death. Breaking the neck of the ampule results in glass fragments falling into the solution. When withdrawing the

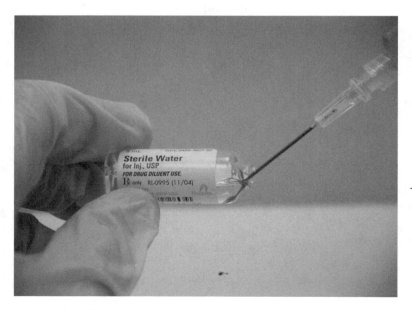

Figure 6-7   Ampule Manipulation

contents from an ampule, potential exists for shards of glass to enter into the syringe. Thus a filter needle must be used to prevent such shards from entering into the final admixture. After correcting the final volume within the syringe, recap the needle using the scoop method. Remove the filter needle from the syringe and place a new regular needle onto the syringe. The contents of the syringe can then be ejected into the final solution. The opened ampule and the removed neck should be disposed of into the sharps container after use.

At all times during the inversion and manipulation of the needle and syringe to withdraw the ampule's contents, every critical site must be exposed to the flow of first air. Aseptic technique becomes compromised when parts of the hand or other objects come between the critical sites and the first air from the HEPA filter during manipulations.

6. Inject into Solution

Most commonly, the contents of the syringe are ejected into the bag containing solution as prescribed. Prior to adding these contents to the bag, the operator should double-check the solution to ensure that it is the solution or medication prescribed. The additive port should have been disinfected in a previous step. The bag should be placed with the additive port facing the HEPA filter, sideways with the additive port closest to the HEPA filter, or vertically by hanging on a pole hook. The additive port must remain in constant contact with first air. When adding the contents of the syringe to a bag with a long exterior additive port, place the bag sideways and enter the port horizontally, or bend the port upward so that it is directly vertical and enter it vertically with the needle. When adding the contents to a hanging bag, the additive port must be downward. Be sure that no objects block the path of first air to the additive port.

Figure 6-8 and **Figure 6-9** depict various methods that can be employed when injecting a solution into the additive port. All methods shown allow for proper airflow of first air to the additive port, which is considered a critical site. The additive port on most bags will have a raised circle indicating where entry into the port should be targeted. The needle should then be inserted completely

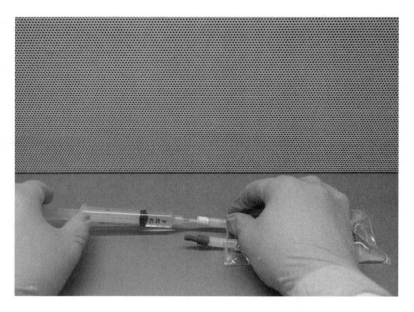

Figure 6-8 Horizontal Bag Placement

perpendicular to the surface of the port, with the needle remaining straight until the hub of the needle touches the surface of the port. It is not necessary to enter at a 45-degree angle, and doing so may risk penetration of the needle through the side of the port. The contents should be ejected into the bag.

At times, accumulation of the contents can occur within the shaft of the additive port. This buildup can result from small quantities remaining within the shaft of the additive port secondary to the small volume. Additionally, accumulation in the port can occur when the length of the needle is shorter than the additive port, which may prevent the contents from being directly injected into the main contents of the bag. To prevent accumulation within the port, after ejecting all contents, pull the hub of the needle away from the surface of the port so that the tip of the needle is just inside the port. Pull back the plunger, filling the syringe with contents of the bag, and eject to "flush" the port. This process is particularly important when adding small amounts of content, such as less than 1 mL, to a bag.

As described in the *Supplies and Equipment for Compounding and Administering Sterile Preparations* chapter, a "belly-button"

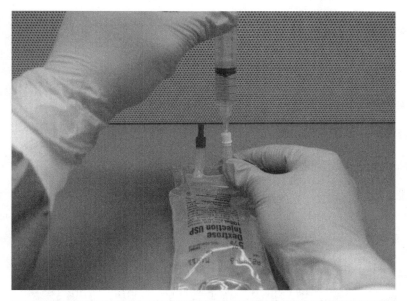

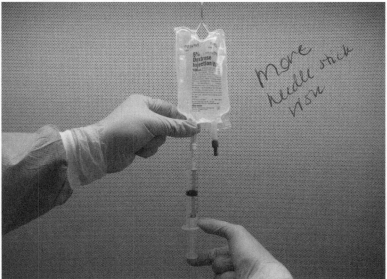

Figure 6-9 Vertical Bag Placement

bag has the additive port directly attached to a flat side of the bag, as opposed to having an extended additive port at one end of the bag. When adding the contents of the syringe to a "belly-button" bag, place the bag in a manner in which the additive port is closest to the HEPA filter, with no objects or parts of the bag interrupting the flow of first air to the port. These types of bags also often have a raised circle indicating where the point of entry should take place. The operator should use one hand to apply pressure to the bag thereby distending the "belly-button," making it easier to penetrate. The port should then be penetrated by entering it straight with the needle, while taking care to stop after the needle reaches the solution. Longer needles can go through the port and create a hole on the other side of the bag. Applying pressure to the bag as described previously can help prevent this problem. The contents should be ejected as described earlier. Because this type of bag does not contain a shaft as part of the additive port, flushing the port is not necessary.

7. Mix and Check the Final Admixture

Once the contents of the syringe have been added to the solution, the final preparation should be mixed. To do so, lay the bag on the workbench surface and place the hands on opposite sides of the bag. Gently apply pressure with the hands on the bag, alternating hands, to create a back-and-forth motion of the solution within the bag. Alternatively, the bag can be gently inverted several times, although it should never be shaken. Once the solution is mixed, it should always be checked for coring from the vial, particulate matter, and other incompatibilities. The checking process should be performed by raising the bag to the light and then observing it against contrasting backgrounds.

ALERT: *All final admixtures should be checked for particulate matter and incompatibilities as an essential step of the compounding process.*

8. Cover and Label Admixture

A sterile adhesive seal should be placed onto the additive port after all necessary contents have been added and after checking the final solution (**Figure 6-10**). Placement of such a seal can prevent contamination of the additive port and reveal tampering of the CSP.

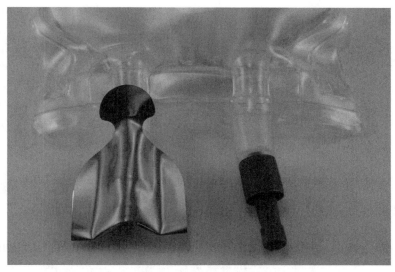

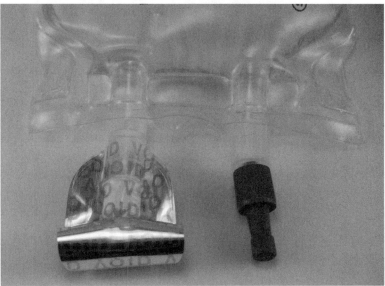

Figure 6-10   Additive Port Seal

Additionally, after the product is removed from the LAFW, the appropriate label should immediately be affixed to it—an important step to ensure that the bag does not get mixed up with other preparations and labeled incorrectly. A double-check should occur by the operator at this time to ensure that the contents added and the solution used match with the contents and volumes listed on the label. Any auxiliary labels should be affixed to the bag at this time, such as "refrigerate" or "protect from light" labels. Labels should be attached in a manner that does not preclude the contents of the bag from being identified. Some solutions, such as those prepared with nitroprusside, require protection from light to prevent degradation or chemical modification of the medication. For these types of medications, an amber sleeve should be added over the admixture bag at this time.

Reconstituting Medications for Parenteral Administration

Often, medications are manufactured as a "powder" for reconstitution, also called a dry powder. The solid form of the medication is contained within a vial and requires the addition of a diluent for its conversion to an aqueous form. This process is referred to as reconstitution. To reconstitute a product, the following steps should be followed:

1. Refer to the product packaging to determine which diluent should be used, such as sodium chloride or sterile water for injection.
2. Determine the concentration of the reconstituted drug. The product packaging or vial will provide guidance as to the volume of diluent that should be added to the vial. The volume of diluent added will affect the final concentration and, therefore, the volume needed to fulfill the prescribed dosage of the final preparation.
   a. This is an important step in the process, as many medications result in displacement of volume. For example, 9.5 mL of diluent may be added but result in a total volume of 10 mL. This issue is further discussed in terms of powder volume in the *Calculations for Parenteral Compounding* chapter.
   b. If the product packaging does not indicate a specific volume to be added or if there are no effects of displacement, then the volume of diluent added should be based on specific institutional standards. The resultant

concentration will be the total amount of medication in the vial (grams or milligrams) in the total volume of diluent added (milliliters).

3. Remove the vial covers and disinfect the closures of both the medication and diluent vials with sterile, lint-free alcohol wipes.

4. Disinfect the additive port of the bag with a sterile, lint-free alcohol wipe.

5. Remove the desired volume of diluent using the "milking" technique or use a vented needle.

6. Stabilize the vial on the workbench and insert the needle into the vial needing reconstitution. Do not invert the vial.

7. While the vial remains on the workbench surface, use the "milking" technique to add the contents of the diluent. This technique is referred to as "reverse milking" since diluent is being expelled out of the syringe and air is entering into the syringe. To do so, add some of the diluent from the syringe into the vial until slight pressure is felt. Then allow air from the vial to enter into the syringe to equalize the pressure. Repeat this process until all diluent from the syringe has been added and the amount of air in the syringe is equal to the amount of diluent added. To alleviate the potential for positive pressure, a slight amount of air can be optionally withdrawn from the vial prior to removing the needle. During the process, care should be taken to keep the needle from touching the powder or solution.

8. The contents of the vial will need some time to completely dissolve. Rolling the vial between the palms of the hands can provide the agitation and warmth needed to expedite the dissolution process. Complete dissolution ensures that the solution is homogenous and the concentration of the drug is the same throughout the solution. The vial should never be shaken.

9. Inspect the vial for particulate matter, complete dissolution, or other incompatibilities. If either particulate matter or signs of incompatibilities are present, the product should be immediately discarded.

10. Determine the volume of reconstituted drug to be removed. Draw up an equal amount of air into a syringe.

11. Insert the needle into the vial while avoiding the original puncture site.

12. Invert the vial using a "see-saw" motion and remove the desired volume of reconstituted drug into the syringe by using the "milking" technique and taking care to avoid positive pressure.

13. Remove air bubbles as previously described and verify the volume for accuracy.

14. Place the vial on the workbench and remove the needle from the vial.

15. Add the contents of the syringe into the bag for completion of the final preparation.

16. Label and seal the final preparation as previously described.

If a multidose vial (MDV) is being used, the final concentration, the initials of the person who performed the reconstitution, the expiration date, and the date and time of the reconstitution should all be documented. The rubber closure of the MDV should be inspected for physical integrity and wiped with a sterile, lint-free, 70% IPA wipe prior to reentering it each time. If contaminants or abnormal properties are suspected, the MDV should be discarded.

 ## Recapping Needles

Recapping of needles introduces an unnecessary risk of needle sticks to the operator. Needle sticks can easily occur during recapping when one hand is used to hold the needle cap while the needle is placed back into the cap. Thus it is recommended that needles not be recapped. Many institutions have established policies and procedures specifically addressing recapping of needles. Withdrawing a drug from an ampule requires changing the filter needle used to withdraw the solution and replacing it with a regular needle. The filter needle needs to be recapped in this situation so that it can be removed and replaced. Specific techniques for recapping have been accepted in practice as these techniques minimize the risk of needle sticks and promote attention to safety. If recapping will be employed, the needle cap should be placed facing the HEPA filter when the needle is being used. If the needle will be reused, this method will ensure that the cap, which will house the needle, does not become contaminated.

The most frequently used technique for recapping is known as the "scoop method." To perform this technique, face the cap sideways, with the opening of the cap facing the needle. Next, scoop the cap up with the needle. Care should be taken not to hold the needle cap, as this process should involve only the hand holding the syringe. Once the cap is on the needle, the syringe and needle should be angled upright, while shaking the cap onto the needle. The cap can then be pushed completely on, as the cap is completely covering the needle and no risk is involved at this point.

Capping a Syringe

Oftentimes, medications are administered directly from a syringe for parenteral use. In these situations, the final preparation needs to be contained within the syringe. Such preparations should not be sent with a needle attached; rather, the needle needs to be removed and the tip of the syringe capped with a syringe cap (**Figure 6-11**). When ready for administration, the syringe cap can be removed and the syringe directly attached to a compatible catheter; alternatively, an appropriate needle for administration can be attached.

Syringe caps are available to accommodate both the Luer Lock and slip-tip syringes. They are available in a sealed package in rows of two. When accessing the caps, the package should be opened facing the HEPA filter to ensure that first air passes over exposed caps. The cap comes in direct contact with the tip of the syringe, so it should be treated as a critical site. Not only should

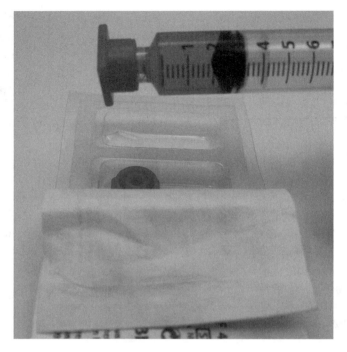

Figure 6-11   Capping a Syringe

the cap not be touched, but it should also stay in direct contact with first air at all times during manipulation.

Once the cap has been placed on the syringe, it should be tightened to ensure that it is secure. Any exposed syringe caps that are removed from the ISO Class 5 environment should be discarded.

 Priming an Infusion Set

On some occasions, infusion administration sets need to be attached to the set port of the prepared admixture prior to leaving the compounding facility, such as with chemotherapies. The individual administering the admixture will use the set to administer the drug to the patient, but first the tubing of the set must be primed, or filled with solution. When priming an infusion set, it is important to note that only drug-free solution should be used. Thus the tubing should be primed with solution from the bag before the drug is added to the bag. Priming with solution that already has chemotherapy added can create significant hazards.

> **ALERT:** *Only drug-free solution should be used to prime infusion sets.*

To prime the tubing of the infusion administration set, first ensure that the slide and roller clamps are closed completely. Next, insert the infusion set spike into the spike port, or set port, of the bag. The bag should be hanging to reduce the number of air bubbles introduced into the tubing. Squeeze the drip chamber on the infusion set a few times to fill the chamber halfway. Release the slide clamp, then slowly release the roller clamp. Allow the drug-free solution to flow through the tubing until it reaches the last 2 inches of the tubing. This 2-inch air pocket will ensure sterility of the solution within the tubing until it is time to be administered to the patient.

Vial Pressures

The interiors of unopened vials are typically at equal pressure to the atmosphere. The vial will make accommodations to maintain equal pressure within the vial throughout manipulations. For this reason, air needs to be added to the vial that is equal to the volume of solution to be drawn into the syringe. Doing so will maintain the vial at equal pressure.

 ### Positive Pressure

If the air added to the vial exceeds the volume of solution withdrawn, this will result in extra air in the vial and, in turn, positive pressure within the vial. As noted earlier, the vial will make accommodations to maintain the pressure equilibrium; in this case, the vial will push out the extra air. If a needle and syringe are inserted into the vial, the extra pressure will cause the plunger of the syringe to be pushed back and the extra air to be added to the syringe. If the vial has positive pressure and the syringe and vial are either removed from the vial or in the process of being removed, and the vial is inverted, then the solution from the vial will spray or drip out through the puncture of the rubber closure. The positive pressure in the vial needs to escape, which can be accomplished by either air escaping or solution escaping from the vial when a needle is inserted. In short, the vial attempts to regain equilibrium by pushing out either extra air or solution. If the vial is inverted, then the solution is closest to the route of escape, which is the puncture hole in the rubber closure—hence solution will spray or drip out. If the vial remains with positive pressure and is not equilibrated, then upon reentry with a new needle and syringe, air or solution will be pushed into the new syringe.

 ## NEGATIVE PRESSURE

If the amount of air removed from the vial exceeds the volume of solution removed, less air will remain in the vial than the original equal pressure condition. This is known as negative pressure, because the pressure inside the vial is negative compared to the pressure at equilibrium. If a vial has negative pressure, it becomes difficult to remove solution from it, especially as the amount of negative pressure increases. Again, the vial will attempt to regain pressure equilibrium. To do so, the vial needs more air within it. To achieve this, the vial will take in air or solution from the syringe, pulling up on the plunger. When withdrawing solution with the vial under negative pressure, much resistance will be felt when pulling the plunger. Thus negative pressure results in difficulty withdrawing the needed amount of solution. It is always recommended to use negative pressure when working with hazardous agents, such as chemotherapy, to avoid spraying or dripping of such agents secondary to positive pressure.

Negative pressure within the vial can be purposefully created, such as when working with hazardous agents, by drawing up less air than the volume of solution needed. For example, if 10 mL of solution is needed, drawing up 5 mL of air and adding it to the vial will result in negative pressure within the vial after the full 10 mL of solution is drawn into the syringe. Continuing this example, if only 3 mL of air is added to the vial, an even greater amount of negative pressure will result after the full 10 mL of solution is withdrawn.

ACCOMMODATING POSITIVE AND NEGATIVE VIAL PRESSURES

While it is best to avoid creating positive or negative pressure within the vial, with the exception of when working with hazardous agents, these scenarios become inevitable at times. Making accommodations for positive and negative pressures is a skill that requires practice. A skilled operator typically can tell whether the vial contains positive or negative pressure immediately upon entering it with a needle and syringe.

If a vial is found to contain positive pressure upon entry, the following steps can be used:

1. Withdraw the needle and syringe.
2. Eject all air contained within the syringe.
3. Reenter the vial with the needle and syringe.
4. Allow the extra air from the vial to push into the syringe until the syringe plunger completely stops moving. This will equilibrate the pressure in the vial.
5. Withdraw an additional small amount of air from the vial.
6. Withdraw the needle and syringe and eject all air contained within the syringe.
7. Determine the volume to be removed and add the same amount of air to the syringe.
8. Begin the normal process for withdrawing a solution from a vial.

If positive pressure is discovered during withdrawal of solution, the process can be stopped, solution added back to the vial, and the preceding steps followed. Alternatively, the plunger can be pressed to hold the volume needed in the syringe, followed by placing the vial on the workbench work surface and removing the needle and syringe. This will minimize the amount of spray that escapes the syringe because air is closest to the route of escape.

If negative pressure is found to exist in the vial upon entry with a needle and syringe, the following steps can be used:

1. Release the plunger to allow the vial to take in air that was originally placed in the syringe.
2. Wait for the plunger to come to a complete stop.
3. If all of the air in the syringe is completely taken into the vial, withdraw the needle and syringe. Then, draw up air into the syringe and reenter the vial. Allow the vial to take in as much air as needed until the plunger comes to a complete stop. If all of the air of the second syringe is completely taken into the vial, continue to add more air until the vial no longer needs air.
4. Determine the volume of solution needed and add that same amount of air to the syringe.
5. Begin the normal process for withdrawing solutions.

If negative pressure is discovered during the withdrawal process, the process can be halted, solution ejected back into the vial, and the preceding steps followed. Alternatively, if negative pressure is discovered in the midst of the preparation process, then the plunger can be held to the volume needed and, while keeping this place, the vial removed off of the needle without inverting the vial onto the workbench work surface.

Labeling

Labeling is required for all CSPs that are not intended for immediate use. According to USP Chapter <797>, immediate-use preparations should be labeled if not immediately and completely administered after preparation; the label should include the patient identification, names and amounts of ingredients, name or initial of the person who prepared it, and the exact 1-hour beyond-use time and date.

Proper labeling of a non-immediate-use CSP is an important step in the preparation process. Great care should be taken during this step, as mislabeling can easily occur. Labels should be placed on the final preparation immediately after removing the CSP from the LAFW. Doing so will prevent confusion and mix-up of final preparations, as the addition of medication to bags of solutions often cannot be visually differentiated.

The state board of pharmacy regulations for each state should be followed for determining the contents of the label. Additionally, label contents will vary depending on the use of the preparation, such as those CSPs used for home infusions, those administered in the inpatient setting, and those prepared from batch compounding.

For the inpatient setting, components of the label typically include the following items:

- Patient name
- Patient room number
- Additional patient identifiers (medical record number and/or visit number)
- Names and concentrations of all ingredients
- Volumes of all ingredients
- Total volume of preparation
- Instructions for administration
- Route and rate of administration
- Date of preparation
- Beyond-use date
- Preparer's signature
- Signature of pharmacist conducting verification

An example of a label that is used in an inpatient setting appears in **Figure 6-12**, although the structure and contents will vary between institutions.

CSPs also should bear auxiliary labels for the following purposes:

- Proper storage conditions: Labels should indicate preparations needing special storage conditions, such as "Refrigerate" or "Do not refrigerate." Storage conditions may also include "Protect from light." Labels indicating "Do not shake" should be placed on preparations that are affected by shaking.

```
┌─────────────────────────────────────────────────────────────┐
│                    General Hospital                           │
│  Doe, John                        5 West 5622-01              │
│  MRN 000545899                    Order # 021                 │
│  Visit # 000332243                Bag # 1                     │
│                                                               │
│  Vancomycin                       1000 mg                     │
│  NaCl 0.9%                         250 mL                      │
│  Total volume                      250 mL                      │
│  Rate                              250 mL/hr                   │
│                                                               │
│  Infuse IV over 60 min every 12 hr                            │
│                                                               │
│  Prepared: 12/7/13    by: JS        Checked by: DH            │
│  Use before: 1600 12/8/13                                     │
└─────────────────────────────────────────────────────────────┘
```

Figure 6-12 Example of a Label

- Administration alerts: Administration alerts, such as "For oral use only" or "For irrigation," are important to include on CSPs to avoid accidental administration of such medications intravenously. Alerts such as "In-line filter required" should also be included, if applicable.
- High-risk medications: Institutions often identify medications that are considered high risk due to the severe implications of medication errors associated with these particular medications or the potential for these medications to be involved in medication misadventures. All CSPs containing high-risk medications should be labeled as such—for example, "Insulin-containing preparation" or "High concentration of potassium chloride."
- Nonstandard concentrations: The Joint Commission's National Patient Safety Goals call for standard concentrations to be used in the institutional setting. This recommendation is intended to avoid confusion regarding the concentration, and resulting volume, of the medications that are administered. Although deviation from these standard concentrations is highly discouraged, in the event that diversion is necessary, the CSPs should clearly be labeled with an auxiliary label as such ("Nonstandard concentration").

■ Hazardous agents: Hazardous agents, such as chemotherapies, should be clearly labeled with auxiliary labeling. The
designated signage for hazardous agents should accompany written labels indicating "Chemotherapy" or "Hazardous agent."

Batch labeling differs from labeling for CSPs prepared on an
individual patient basis. Labels for batch compounding preparations should contain the names and volumes of all ingredients and
solutions, total volume, route of administration, storage conditions, lot or control number, and beyond-use date.[6,pp.138–139]

Batch Compounding

Batch compounding involves the creation of multiple preparations containing the same ingredients, which are prepared in one
extended process. Batch compounding can entail preparation of
multiple CSPs for multiple patients or compounding of multiple
CSPs for the same patient. Frequently used CSPs are compounded
in advance of the actual need for them.

When batch compounding is undertaken, specific documentation is required. Not only will the label for the preparations
contain different information compared to the labels for CSPs
individually prepared for institutional or home infusion use, but
master formula sheets must also be maintained. Information that
should be recorded includes the following elements:[6, pp. 192–193]

■ Name of the CSP
■ Names and amounts of all ingredients used to prepare the
CSP
■ Beyond-use date of the final preparation
■ Manufacturer name, expiration, and lot number for
ingredients
■ Signature of operator and supervisor performing checking
and release of the preparation
■ Packaging instructions
■ Labeling instructions
■ Control number and beyond-use date of the batch

- Storage instructions
- Number of preparations compounded
- Samples for assays, if applicable
- Quarantine period, if applicable

 ## Workflow Process

Distractions are common while workers are compounding sterile preparations. The risk of making a mistake secondary to a distraction or poor workflow is high and carries significant patient implications. Therefore, it is important that each CSP be prepared in an organized and consistent manner. Each individual is encouraged to establish an efficient and organized system of processing that will prevent errors and confusion. For example, if an operator is in the middle of adding a drug to four bags and is called away or interrupted before the processing is complete, would the operator unequivocally know which bags have drug added to them?

Either left-to-right or right-to-left processing of CSPs should be considered. In the right-to-left arrangement, all unused supplies are kept on the right side of the workbench; all used and finished supplies are kept on the left side, including bags that have been completed (**Figure 6-13**). For example, two trash piles should be created past the 6-inch line of demarcation in the LAFW. One trash pile is only for sharps; the second is for the outer packaging of syringes, needles, sterile alcohol wipes, and other materials. Keeping a trash pile on the workbench during preparation of CSPs prevents the need to take the hands out of the LAFW and then reenter it. During the compounding process, the operator's hands should not exit the LAFW unless absolutely necessary. The trash piles should be discarded after each preparation and be placed in the appropriate, designated waste container.

ALERT: *Hands should not be removed from the workbench during compounding. If it is required that hands be removed, then gloves must be disinfected prior to reentry into the workbench.*

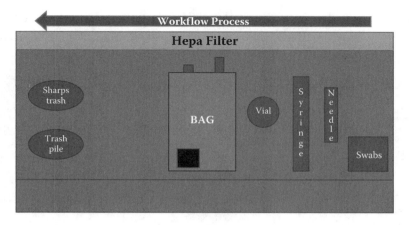

Figure 6-13 Work Flow

Once a bag has drug added to it, it should be flipped over, while ensuring that the additive port remains in contact with first air, and placed on the left side of the workbench, if using a right-to-left workflow process.

Implementing some type of organizational processing for preparing CSPs will prevent error and confusion. It also allows for more efficient processing of CSPs.

Conclusion

Poor work practices are frequently responsible for errors and contamination of CSPs. It is important that the operator does not get lulled into a false sense of security by compounding parenteral preparations in a controlled environment and by donning appropriate PPE. While these measures decrease the likelihood of contamination of CSPs, the most influential factor is aseptic technique. Personnel involved in compounding should diligently adhere to proper hand washing and disinfection techniques, donning of proper PPE, and utilization of aseptic technique to assume responsibility for the outcome of the final preparation. While these steps might seem cumbersome at times, these important practices should be an inherent part of compounding sterile preparations. Understanding the implications of not following these important procedures should motivate personnel to adhere to all recommendations and to be willing to self-assess and improve, such as with perfecting aseptic techniques. It is important to understand that aseptic technique is a skill that continues to evolve and takes much practice to do well. However, once good aseptic techniques become part of the skill set of the operator, improved efficiency can be achieved without compromising technique.

Review Questions

1. Which of the following syringe parts is considered a critical site?
   a. Ribs of the plunger
   b. Barrel of the syringe
   c. Flange of the syringe
   d. Tip of the plunger

2. Which of the following needle parts is considered a critical site?
   a. Shaft
   b. Tip
   c. Hub
   d. All of the above

3. Which of the following statements is true regarding aseptic technique?
   a. First air should constantly be in contact with critical sites, except during inversions (i.e., inverting the vial up and down during manipulations).
   b. If moving the hands between holding the vial and the syringe, passing the hands between the critical sites and the HEPA filter will result in blocked first air.
   c. Syringes and needles can be opened at the edge of the LAFW.

    d. When adding solution in a syringe to a bag, the additive port should face the operator.

4. Which of the following statements is true regarding milking of vials?
    a. Air equal to the amount of solution to be withdrawn should be added to the vial at one time.
    b. Negative pressure within the vial is necessary for milking.
    c. A small amount of air should be added until slight resistance is felt, followed by depressing the plunger to allow a small amount of solution to enter the syringe.
    d. Using a milking process decreases the risk of contaminating the final preparation.

5. List, in order, the personnel protective equipment that should be donned for compounding nonhazardous CSPs.

6. Hands and forearms should be washed for at least _____ seconds.

7. True or False: Negative pressure results from excess air residing inside the vial.

8. Which of the following items is required on a batch label, but not on a patient label for use in an institutional setting?
    a. Patient name
    b. Medical record number
    c. Lot number
    d. Room number

9. On which of the following occasions should gloves be disinfected using sterile 70% IPA?
    a. Each time hands exit the LAFW during preparation
    b. Before cleaning the LAFW
    c. Immediately after donning
    d. All of the above

10. Personal protective equipment should be replaced with new garb upon reentering the _____

CASE STUDIES *Case 1*

A new technician is being trained on sterile compounding and will be preparing both hazardous and nonhazardous drugs in a BSC and a HLFW, respectively. You are participating in training the technician on aseptic technique. Explain important concepts relating to aseptic technique and describe how this technique must be adjusted based on the primary engineering control utilized.

Case 2

An order is received for cisplatin, a chemotherapy, in normal saline to be administered intravenously to a patient who is in the outpatient infusion clinic. The medication will be directly administered to the patient, who currently has a peripherally inserted central catheter (PICC) line.

1. What are some preparation considerations for this particular order?
2. The pharmacy technician compounding the admixture is following the proper aseptic procedures, but is having difficulty finding the strength to withdraw the solution from the vial. What is the solution to this problem?
3. What are some administration considerations that should be accounted for during compounding?

References

1. Widmer AF. Replace hand washing with use of a waterless alcohol hand rub? *Clin Infect Dis.* 2000;31(1):136–140.
2. Weil DC, Chou T, Arnow PM. Prevalence of gram-negative bacilli in nares and on hands of pharmacy personnel: lack of effect of occupational exposure to antibiotics. *J Clin Microbiol.* 1984;20(5):933–935.
3. Centers for Disease Control and Prevention. Guideline for hand hygiene in health-care setting. *MMWR.* Available at: http://www.cdc.gov/mmwr/PDF/rr/rr5116.pdf. Accessed June 10, 2013.

4. Rotter M. Hand washing and hand disinfection. In: Mayhall CG, ed. *Hospital epidemiology and infection control.* 2nd ed. Baltimore, MD: Williams and Wilkins; 1999:1339–1355.

5. U.S. Pharmacopeial Convention. Chapter <797>: pharmaceutical compounding: sterile preparations. *United States Pharmacopeia 36/National Formulary 31.* Rockville, MD: U.S. Pharmacopeial Convention; 2013.

6. Buchanan EC, Schneider PJ. *Compounding sterile preparations.* Bethesda, MD: American Society of Health-System Pharmacists; 2009:138–139, 192–193.

CHAPTER 7

Principles of Compatibility and Stability

Hardeep Singh Saluja and Pamella S. Ochoa

 Where this icon appears, visit http://go.jblearning.com /OchoaCWS to view the corresponding video.

Chapter Objectives

1. Define stability and incompatibility as they relate to compounded sterile preparations.
2. Describe the types of incompatibilities seen with compounded sterile preparations.
3. List factors that influence the compatibility and stability of parenteral preparations.
4. List resources used to assign beyond-use dates.
5. Describe steps that can be utilized to prevent and identify incompatibilities or instabilities.

Key Terminology

Stability
Crystallization
Incompatibility
Precipitation
Precipitate

Solubility
Effervescence
Phase separation
Amorphous
Absorption
Adsorption
Epimerization
Decarboxylation
Photochemical degradation

Overview

Compatibility and stability are important aspects of the preparation, verification, and administration of compounded sterile preparations (CSPs). If products used for compounding sterile preparations are not compatible, it can result in various types of reactions that compromise the integrity of the final preparation. At times, incompatibilities can result in formation of particulate matter that can cause the patient serious harm, and even death, if infused. In acute settings, it is often necessary to administer multiple preparations concomitantly. The compatibility of drugs and final preparations must be considered in these circumstances. Stability is an important consideration when storing parenteral products and preparations. This factor influences the current standards for the types of containers used in drug storage and preparation, as well as the length of time that a CSP can be used following preparation. Knowledge of common incompatibilities, standards, and regulations regarding stability and practices for preventing problems related to compatibility and stability should be required of those preparing, verifying, and administering CSPs.

Stability

Stability is defined as "the extent to which a product retains, within specified limits, and throughout its period of storage and use (i.e., its shelf-life), the same properties and characteristics that it possessed at the time of its manufacture."[1] Instability results when a change or degradation in the active ingredients occurs.

Pharmacists should understand the importance of drug product stability, especially when compounding parenteral admixtures. The individual drug product supplied by the manufacturer undergoes extensive stability testing. This process involves exposing the drug to environmental factors such as various temperatures, pH, light, and moisture to determine the influence of each on drug stability. Drugs are manufactured and then packaged in suitable containers intended to protect them from degradation; however, once the product is removed from its original container and mixed with other ingredients, the stability of the drug and excipients is inevitably compromised. This occurs secondary to potential alteration of the individual components, which results in a preparation that is unique.[2] Various incompatibility reactions, such as physical or chemical incompatibilities, may occur within admixtures. For example, a physical incompatibility can change drug solubility, leading to precipitation, or, as with a chemical incompatibility, can cause formation of an undesirable product. Often, admixtures are refrigerated following compounding to prolong their stability; however, some drugs undergo crystallization or a change in color when refrigerated, such as mannitol and metronidazole, respectively. Other drugs are stable only when mixed in specific diluents, such as 0.9% sodium chloride (NS) or dextrose 5% water (D_5W). Thus it is important to consider information provided by the drug manufacturer regarding the stability of a particular preparation.

The United States Pharmacopeia (USP) recognizes five types of stability, illustrated in **Figure 7-1**.

> **TIP:** *Reference the drug manufacturer's recommendations when determining the stability of the product and final preparation.*

Incompatibility

Incompatibility is an undesirable reaction that can occur between two drug substances, a drug substance and an excipient used in the drug product, or a drug substance or excipient with the container used for drug product storage. Two of the incompatibilities

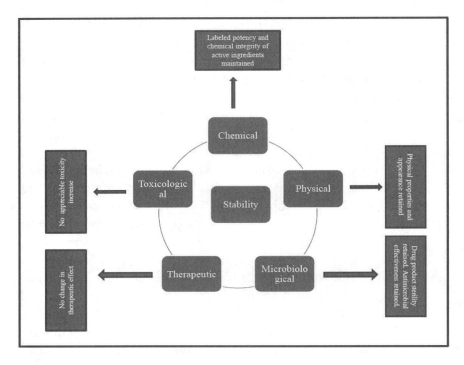

Figure 7-1 Five Forms of Stability and Their Acceptance Criteria

Adapted from U.S. Pharmacopeial Convention, Inc. Chapter <1191>, Stability considerations in dispensing practice. United States Pharmacopeia 36/National Formulary 31. Rockville, MD: U.S. Pharmacopeial Convention, Inc.; 2013.

mentioned in this section will be discussed in detail—namely, physical and chemical incompatibilities (**Figure 7-2**).

Drug substances can be susceptible to chemical or physical degradation that may decrease concentrations of the active ingredient and alter the therapeutic efficacy of the drug. Degradation can also result in production of undesirable products that can exert a toxicological effect. Therefore, a pharmacist should thoroughly understand which factors may alter the stability of a drug product and ensure that it remains stable during compounding, transportation, storage, and administration. A pharmacist should never make assumptions about drug stability, but rather should always rely on available scientific evidence.

 PHYSICAL INCOMPATIBILITY

Physical incompatibility refers to changes in the physical state of the drug substance, which may affect the physical properties of

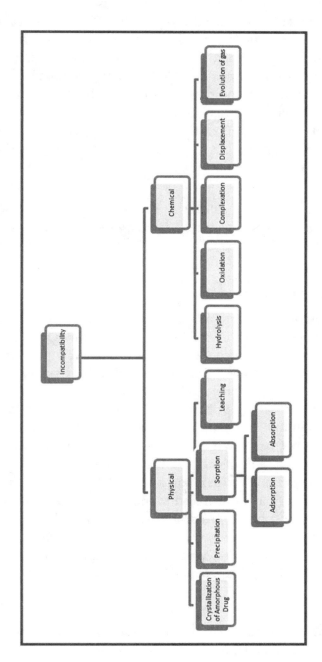

Figure 7-2 Types of Physical and Chemical Incompatibilities

the drug. For example, "drug solubility" is an important characteristic that influences the physical state of a drug. Any change in the solubility of a drug could affect the drug's efficacy and safety. Physical incompatibilities are manifested visually and, therefore, are the easiest to identify of all types of incompatibilities. For example, some incompatibilities can be observed as precipitation, cloudiness, changes in color and viscosity, phase separation, and effervescence. The following sections highlight the physical changes that can occur in a drug substance or excipient that can lead to physical incompatibilities.

> **TIP:** *Physical incompatibilities are the easiest to identify because they are manifested as incompatibilities that can be visually observed.*

Crystallization

The amorphous form of a drug usually exhibits higher solubility compared to its crystalline form.[3] Sometimes a poorly soluble drug is formulated in its amorphous physical state; however, this amorphous physical state may be thermodynamically unstable and tends to change to its more stable, crystalline state over time. Consequently, a pharmacist should pay close attention when reconstituting an amorphous drug. With time, the amorphous drug may change to a crystalline—or partly crystalline—form. It is important to understand that different physical forms of a drug (crystalline versus amorphous) will have different solubilities, which may in turn lead to incomplete drug solubilization upon reconstitution. If a drug that is incompletely solubilized is administered intravenously, it can result in serious patient consequences, even death. Mannitol, for example, readily undergoes crystallization at room temperature (**Figure 7-3**).

Precipitation

Precipitation is a process in which a solid, which was previously dissolved in liquid, is formed. Drug substances that are hydrophobic in nature are usually formulated with water miscible

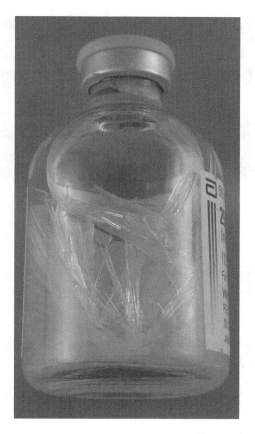

Figure 7-3   Mannitol Crystallization

co-solvents such as ethanol and polyethylene glycol. A drug will remain in solution as long as its concentration remains below the saturation solubility. Precipitation, however, tends to occur with a supersaturated solution. The factors that most commonly influence drug precipitation in a solution are temperature, change in pH, and chemical reaction between two components in a solution.

Calcium phosphate precipitation in parenteral nutrition (PN) admixtures, illustrated in **Figure 7-4**, is a common type of precipitation reaction, which will be discussed in detail later in this chapter. Drug precipitation also occurs when amikacin is mixed with heparin: A hazy mixture forms within minutes following the

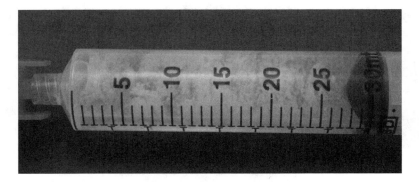

Figure 7-4   Calcium Phosphate Precipitation

addition of 250 mg of amikacin to 50 units of heparin in 100 mL D_5W. Amiodarone hydrochloride, an antiarrhythmic agent, at a concentration of 4 mg/mL in dextrose 5%, is reported to precipitate when mixed with aminophylline, cefazolin sodium, or heparin. Ceftriaxone sodium should not be concomitantly administered with solutions containing calcium, such as lactated Ringer's solution, to neonates younger than 28 days of age; such co-administration may lead to formation of a calcium ceftriaxone precipitate in the lungs and kidneys of the infants.[4]

Sorption and Leaching

Sorption occurs when drug molecules either adhere at the surface (adsorption) or penetrate into the matrix (absorption) of the container in which they are stored, the administration set used to deliver the drug, or the filter. The term "sorption" is used when both adsorption and absorption occur together. Drug sorption is dependent on the contact time and the surface area where the drug and the matrix come in contact. In general, a longer contact time and a larger contact surface area will lead to higher drug sorption. Additionally, storage or administration with polyvinyl chloride (PVC) can lead to drug loss, particularly with lipid-soluble substances such as some vitamins. Drugs such as diazepam, isosorbide nitrate, nitroglycerin, and amiodarone have shown loss of potency when stored in polyvinyl chloride (PVC) containers, compared to glass containers, due to sorption.[5, 6] When sorption is a concern with certain drugs, non-PVC or glass containers should be used.

> **TIP:** *Choose non-PVC or glass containers when sorption of drugs is a concern.*

Another important factor that can affect the pharmacologic activity of a drug is filtration. Apart from adsorption, absorption, and leaching, the three-dimensional (3D) structure of drugs, peptides, and proteins can be affected by filtration. This effect is of particular concern with high-molecular-weight drugs. When the drug passes through the small pores of the filter under sheer stress and pressure, the 3D structure of the drug could be altered, rendering the drug therapeutically inactive. Therefore, when filtering drugs, the pharmacist must ensure that the efficacy of the drug will be maintained after filtration or consult the drug manufacturer to obtain more information. The pharmacist should also obtain binding studies when filtering solutions that contain less than 5 mg of a drug. One must also exercise caution when selecting a filter, because some filters contain surfactants that make them hydrophilic. These surfactants can leach into the filtered solution and contaminate the preparation.[7]

Leaching occurs when substances, such as plasticizers, are extracted from the container and enter into the solution. For instance, PVC is a widely used polymeric matrix packaging for pharmaceutical materials. PVC contains phthalate esters, particularly DEHP [di-(2-ethylhexyl)-phthalate], that provide flexibility to the polymeric matrix. Because DEHP is not chemically bonded to the PVC, it may potentially leach from the matrix into the formulation within the container. DEHP has been reported to have toxic effects on animal models and is suspected to produce endocrine and reproductive disorders in humans.[5, 8–12] For example, release of DEHP occurs in appreciable amounts into formulations containing taxol and various other diluents when stored in PVC containers.[8]

CHEMICAL INCOMPATIBILITY

Chemical incompatibility refers to the loss of drug resulting from a chemical reaction. Chemical degradation can lead to loss of drug potency or production of toxic substances. Some chemical reactions may produce visible changes, such as changes in color, production of odor, or evolution of gas; many other chemical reactions do not produce any physical changes and cannot be detected with visual observation.

Because drugs have diverse chemical structures, they are susceptible to multiple degradation pathways such as hydrolysis, oxidation, epimerization, decarboxylation, dehydration, and photochemical degradation. The most common type of chemical degradation reaction for parenteral drugs is hydrolysis.

Hydrolysis

The term "hydrolysis" is derived from *hydro*, meaning "water," and *lysis*, meaning "breakdown." This type of reaction results from the cleavage of chemical bonds by water. If the chemical structure of a drug contains esters or β-lactam chemical bonds, it is most likely prone to hydrolysis. The rate of hydrolysis escalates with time relative to increases in temperature, with changes in pH, and in the presence of catalysts. For example, diazepam undergoes an acid-catalyzed hydrolysis at a pH less than 3. It is found to exhibit maximum stability within the pH range of 4 to 8.[13, 14] Additionally, as described in USP Chapter <797>, the extent of hydrolysis of a β-lactam antibiotic solution at room temperature for 1 day is equivalent to that of the same solution stored in cold conditions for about 3 to 5 days.[35]

Oxidation

Oxidation, another pathway of chemical degradation, results from the loss of electrons by atoms, molecules, or ions. Drugs that contain a hydroxyl group attached directly to an aromatic ring in their chemical structure are prone to oxidation. As with hydrolysis, the rate of oxidation is influenced by temperature and can be significantly altered in the presence of oxygen, ultraviolet (UV) exposure, or changes in pH, or in the presence of catalysts such as copper ions. Oxidation reactions can be prevented by adding anti-oxidants to the preparation, filling ampules' and vials' head space with nitrogen, employing amber-colored containers for storage, and adding a buffering agent to provide a stable pH environment.

Ascorbic acid, for instance, is readily oxidized in the presence of oxygen, with its rate of degradation increasing with higher exposures to oxygen. Allwood and Kearney reported that the oxygen present in ascorbic acid infusions and additives, along with the oxygen added during compounding, can account for 30 to 50 mg of ascorbic acid degradation. Therefore, it is recommended to remove all oxygen from bags that contain ascorbic acid. Also, the use of multilayered bags may prevent oxygen permeation into the solution.[2, 15] Ascorbic acid degrades into oxalic acid, a potentially toxic compound, which can react with cations such as calcium ions in parenteral nutrition admixtures, leading to the formation of insoluble calcium oxalate.[16] If insoluble calcium oxalate were infused into a patient, the result would be significant patient harm or death. Caution should be exercised when preparing products that are prone to oxidation, such as those containing ascorbic acid.

Complexation

Complexation refers to a chemical reaction between a ligand and a metal ion, such as aluminum (Al^{3+}), calcium (Ca^{2+}), or magnesium (Mg^{2+}), that results in formation of a coordination complex. Drugs such as tetracycline are known to form a complex in the presence of calcium.[17] Calcium gluconate is reported to be incompatible with tetracycline.[18] For this reason, tetracycline hydrochloride should not be mixed with calcium.

Displacement

Displacement refers to the replacement of one element by another in a compound. For example, cisplatin undergoes a displacement reaction with aluminum, resulting in a loss of drug potency and formation of a black metallic precipitate. The loss of drug potency is immediate; however, the black precipitate may take up to an hour to become visible.[19] Administration sets or needles

containing aluminum should be avoided with cisplatin preparation or administration; instead, stainless steel needles should be
used for this application.

Evolution of Gas

Gas formation may occur when an acidic drug solution is added
to a solution containing carbonate or bicarbonate. The chemical
reaction between the two results in the release of carbon dioxide;
however, the evolution of gas may not necessarily lead to an
incompatibility in the solution. For example, a ceftazidime formulation contains sodium carbonate and is supplied as a dry white to
off white powder. When ceftazidime is reconstituted with sterile
water for injection, it reacts with sodium carbonate, producing
carbon dioxide and a sodium salt of ceftazidime. Although leaking
or spraying may occur from the pressurized vials during reconstitution, the gas bubbles usually dissipate within a few minutes.[20] To
avoid gas formation during reconstitution, slowly inject the diluents into the vial, avoid vigorous shaking or agitation of the vial, and
swirl the contents gently during dissolution.

Factors Affecting Stability and Compatibility

The stability and compatibility of a drug are affected by both
intrinsic and extrinsic factors. Intrinsic factors include the chemical structure of the drug itself; extrinsic factors include the environment to which the drug is exposed, such as temperature, pH,
concentration, time, light, and mixing sequence.

TEMPERATURE

Pharmacists must understand the effect of temperature on drug
stability. It has been well documented that for every 10°C rise
in temperature, the rate of degradation increases exponentially.
Thus all pharmaceutical drug products should be stored according to the manufacturer's labeled requirements. The temperature
of the compounding and storage facility should be monitored
and recorded regularly—at least once daily—to ensure product

stability. The temperature should also be maintained and monitored in areas in which drug administration occurs.

For example, benzyl penicillin is reported to demonstrate temperature-dependent degradation. The rate of drug degradation has been found to increase with increases in temperature. Rapid degradation was reported with infusion bags that were maintained at 36°C compared to those maintained between 26°C and 21°C.[21]

Per USP Chapter <797>, if a sterile product is exposed for more than 4 hours to either temperatures that exceed its upper limit per the product labeling or temperatures greater than 40°C, then the product should be discarded.[35] For this reason, many CSPs are stored in refrigerated conditions. While refrigeration assists in extending the usability of a preparation, it can lead to crystallization or precipitation of drugs in some instances, as with mannitol or metronidazole. In the event that a preparation is refrigerated, it should be warmed prior to its administration to a patient to avoid the discomfort of infusing a cold preparation intravenously.

TIP: *If a CSP has been refrigerated, it should be allowed to warm for 30 to 60 minutes prior to its administration to a patient to avoid discomfort.*

pH

A change in pH can significantly affect drug solubility. Drugs are usually manufactured in a salt form to increase their aqueous solubility (e.g., phenytoin sodium, morphine sulfate). Salts of weak acids and strong bases are incompatible, both physically and chemically, with salts of weak bases and strong acids. Because changes in pH can alter the rate of drug degradation, pharmacists should use caution when mixing a drug solution with another solution that may change the final pH of the solution. For example, phenytoin sodium is soluble at a high pH. Mixing phenytoin with a solution such as D_5W causes a reduction in the pH of the admixture and, consequently, potential precipitation of free phenytoin.[22]

ALERT: *Salts of weak acids and strong bases are incompatible with salts of weak bases and strong acids.*

CONCENTRATION

In general, an increase in drug concentration will cause an increase in the rate of degradation because of an increase in the availability of ingredients to react. For example, the risk of calcium phosphate precipitation is higher in preparations made for infants than in those made for adults because of the small volume of the preparation (as little as 25 mL) and the high calcium and phosphate concentrations.[23] Drug concentration is also one of the primary limitations of preparing and storing drugs in syringes. For this reason, most drugs are diluted in bags of NS or D_5W prior to administration to a patient.

LIGHT

Drugs can undergo significant photo degradation in the presence of light. Like hydrolysis and oxidation, photo degradation can lead to the loss of drug potency or the formation of a secondary degradation product that can cause adverse effects if administered to a patient. In general, greater light intensity will cause greater photo degradation. Photo labile drugs must be protected from light to prevent their degradation.

For example, sodium nitroprusside formulations are a brown/light orange color. Upon exposure to light, nitroprusside undergoes discoloration; that is, a change in color to a dark brown/orange and blue occurs due to photo degradation. Therefore, the American Hospital Formulary Service (AHFS) recommends that storage containers and tubing used to administer sodium nitroprusside be wrapped with light-protective material.[24]

Similarly, because vitamins are prone to changes resulting from exposure to light, they should be added to parenteral nutrition immediately prior to administration. Vitamins, particularly vitamin A (retinol) and vitamin B$_2$ (riboflavin), are very susceptible to photo degradation. Vitamins should also be protected from light, especially UV light, which is known to cause more photo degradation of vitamins than does fluorescent light.[2, 25, 26]

> **TIP:** *Vitamins should be added to parenteral nutrition preparations just prior to patient administration to avoid degradation of vitamins over time.*

Drug formulations that are subject to photo degradation are manufactured in amber glass vials, as opposed to clear glass vials, to minimize the exposure of the drug to light. To prevent loss of drug potency, black, green or brown plastic sleeves should be placed over bags containing admixtures that are sensitive to light, such as preparations containing vitamins or nitroprusside.

> **ALERT:** *To prevent loss of drug potency, place light-protective sleeves over preparations that are sensitive to light.*

TIME

Pharmacists should frequently inspect the storage area and remove expired products periodically. In general, the "first in, first out" rule should be followed, such that the oldest stock is dispensed first. Special attention must be given to the storage and handling of the individual product. In consideration of the effect of time on CSPs, pharmacists should assign conservative beyond-use dates.

MIXING SEQUENCE

Drug stability can be influenced by the order in which drugs are admixed. For example, calcium and phosphate salts should not be added in close sequence. Separating the addition of these two products in an admixture can avoid calcium phosphate precipitation. The Food and Drug Administration (FDA) recommends that phosphate be added first into an admixture and that calcium be added last to avoid the increased propensity for precipitation when both of these components are present.

> **TIP:** *It is recommended that phosphate be added first into an admixture and calcium be added last to avoid precipitation.*

Calcium Phosphate Incompatibility

Calcium and phosphorus are available in various salt forms. Calcium gluconate, calcium chloride ($CaCl_2$), and potassium phosphate (K_3PO_4) are all sources of nutrition and electrolytes. As illustrated in the equation, when calcium salts are added to electrolytes containing phosphate, an end product of calcium phosphate is formed. This chemical reaction is physically manifested as precipitation, often observed as a haze in a prepared admixture.

$$3Ca[HOCH_2(CHOH)_4COO]_2 + 2K_3PO_4 \rightarrow Ca_3(PO_4)_2$$
(Calcium gluconate)   (Potassium phosphate)   (Calcium phosphate)

$$+ 6K[HOCH_2(CHOH)_4COO]$$
(Potassium gluconate)

Parenteral nutrition (PN) admixtures are administered intravenously to patients with a dysfunctional gastrointestinal tract. They provide nutrients, including calcium and phosphorus, to patients who are unable to take complete nutrition through the gastrointestinal (GI) tract. Pharmacists should understand that the PN admixture is a complex mixture that can contain as many as 50 different chemical components. Due to the complex nature of PN admixtures, a thorough understanding of the stability and compatibility of these CSPs is paramount. Stability generally refers to the loss or degradation of the admixed nutrients over time, whereas compatibility relates to the physical and chemical interaction between nutrients and/or containers. In both cases, the admixture is deprived of an essential nutrient, but the products of such reactions may also be harmful. PN admixtures usually contain macronutrients (proteins, carbohydrates, fats), micronutrients (electrolytes, trace elements, vitamins), and sometimes medications (insulin, ranitidine). Of the various interactions that are possible, the most dangerous involves the precipitation of calcium and phosphorus, which are the essential electrolytes added to meet the daily nutritional requirements via the PN admixture. In 1994, the FDA issued a safety alert reporting two fatalities associated with the incompatibility of calcium and phosphate salts in PN admixtures.[27, 28] Autopsy findings reported in the FDA safety alert revealed the cause of death to be "diffuse microvascular pulmonary emboli" containing dibasic calcium phosphate ($CaHPO_4$) from the PN admixture.[27]

The administration of PN, which often serves as the sole nutritional source for patients in the neonatal intensive care unit, presents unique therapeutic challenges. One of the most clinically significant issues relates to the ability to provide all essential nutrients at appropriate levels in a limited volume while avoiding incompatibilities and precipitation. If a particle-laden admixture is inadvertently infused into a patient, it can result in the development of a potentially fatal embolic syndrome. In 1992, the fatal consequence of accidental infusion of parenteral nutrition containing particulates in infants was poignantly demonstrated in postmortem examinations, which showed widespread granulomatous pulmonary arteritis.[23, 29] Thus sterile particulate matter that is intrinsically introduced by the manufacturer (e.g., from glass or plastic),[29] is extrinsically produced within the PN formulation (e.g., from an insoluble calcium phosphate product), or is poorly solubilized within injectables[30] may result in fatal emboli in patients receiving intravenous therapy.

The risk of calcium and phosphate incompatibilities is heightened in PN admixtures for neonates compared to preparations for adults for the following reasons:

- Volumes as small as 25 mL are infused to neonates, resulting in high calcium and phosphate concentrations of as much as 60 mg/dL and 46.5 mg/dL, respectively.

- The final amino acid concentrations are lower, often 4% or less, for neonates compared to adults.
- Calcium concentrations are higher in neonates. Concentrations can be as much as three times the amount per liter compared with admixtures for adults.
- Ambient temperatures are elevated. Neonates are sometimes kept in the incubator, where the temperature is 37°C—almost 12°C higher than the room temperature of 25°C. PN preparations are administered at room temperature; however, the tubing used to deliver the admixtures is inside the incubator at 37°C, which can lead to precipitation inside the tubing.

In PN admixtures, these factors can worsen the risk of precipitation, which may prove fatal upon infusion of the precipitate. This complex reaction is related to the availability of free dissociated forms of calcium and phosphate ions present in PN admixture at any given time. The compatibility of calcium and phosphate salts in PN admixtures is a concentration-dependent phenomenon highly dependent on pH that can be accentuated by other variables, such as temperature, amino acid concentration, and mixing sequence. Calcium gluconate is preferred over calcium chloride in PN admixtures because of the difference in ionization efficiency of the two compounds. Calcium gluconate in water is only partly ionized; as its concentration increases, its dissociation decreases. By comparison, dissociation of calcium ions is almost 90% from calcium chloride.[31, 32] Therefore, use of calcium gluconate limits the availability of calcium to react with phosphate ions in the PN admixture.

> **TIP:** *Calcium gluconate is preferred over calcium chloride in parenteral admixtures to minimize the potential for precipitation of calcium and phosphate.*

Another important factor that dictates calcium phosphate compatibility is pH. Usually, divalent and trivalent ions are known to cause incompatibility compared to monovalent ions. As the phosphate anion is trivalent, depending on pH, three different ions may exist:

1. Dihydrogen or monobasic phosphate ($H_2PO_4^-$)
2. Monohydrogen or dibasic phosphate (HPO_4^{2-})
3. Tribasic phosphate (PO_4^{3-})

Of these, only the monobasic and dibasic phosphate ions are relevant to PN given the typical pH profile of such formulations as encountered in neonates and adults, which is generally in the range of 5–7. For the practically insoluble tribasic calcium phosphate, $[Ca_3(PO_4)]_2$, to be present, pH values of greater than 10 are necessary and, hence, not relevant to PN formulations. Lower pH values (less than 6) favor the formation of the more water-soluble monobasic calcium phosphate, $Ca(H_2PO_4)_2$. The solubility of monobasic calcium phosphate in water is 18 g/L; however, higher pH values favor the formation of the less water-soluble dibasic calcium phosphate, $CaHPO_4$, with an aqueous solubility of 0.3 g/L (**Figure 7-5**).

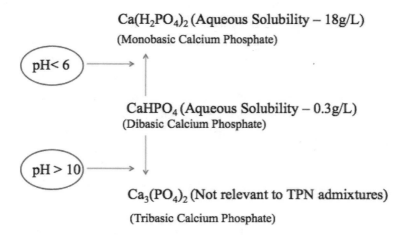

$Ca(H_2PO_4)_2$ (Aqueous Solubility – 18g/L)
(Monobasic Calcium Phosphate)

pH< 6

$CaHPO_4$ (Aqueous Solubility – 0.3g/L)
(Dibasic Calcium Phosphate)

pH > 10

$Ca_3(PO_4)_2$ (Not relevant to TPN admixtures)
(Tribasic Calcium Phosphate)

Figure 7-5   Different Forms of Calcium Phosphate and Their Solubilities

The Henderson-Hasselbalch equation can be used to calculate the prevalence of monobasic and dibasic calcium at different pHs:

$$pH = pK_a + \log ([A-]/[HA]$$
$$\downarrow$$
$$\text{\% ionized} = 100/[1 + \text{antilog} (pK_a - pH)]$$

(pK_a of dangerous dibasic phosphate = 7.2)

There is a 10-fold difference in the amount of dibasic calcium phosphate (pK_a = 7.2) at pH = 6 (6%) versus pH = 7.4 (60%). Thus the 60-fold difference in solubility between the "participating" calcium phosphate products means the likely calcium phosphate precipitate is dibasic calcium phosphate when the pH is elevated; in fact, this form has been identified in both postmortem and in vitro specimens.[27, 32] With an increase in pH above 6.4, a greater amount of insoluble dibasic calcium phosphate product forms. Once its limited solubility in solution is exceeded, precipitation occurs. The effects of pH on two adult PN admixtures—a fatal one (which favored dibasic calcium phosphate) and a nonfatal one (which favored monobasic calcium phosphate)—were reported with pH values of 6.68 versus 5.86, respectively.[27]

Another important factor that can affect calcium phosphate stability is temperature. Pharmacists should understand that low pH favors the formation of monobasic calcium phosphate, although a small fraction of dibasic calcium phosphate may be present in the admixture. The availability of free calcium ions from the salt form is enhanced with elevated temperatures of the neonatal incubator (37°C), which can ultimately lead to precipitation. Also, the solubility of calcium salts decreases with increases in temperature—a unique physical property of dibasic calcium phosphate. The fact is counterintuitive, as most inorganic salts becomes more soluble with increases in temperature.[23]

The clinical risks of precipitation can result in the following outcomes:

- Suboptimal delivery of calcium and phosphate
- Precipitation of a saturated solution, resulting in occlusion of the in-line filter of an indwelling catheter
- Microvasculature and/or pulmonary embolism

Amino acids in PN admixtures also influence calcium phosphate incompatibility. Amino acids can form soluble ion complexes with both calcium and phosphate in the PN admixtures. Because of the opposite charges of amino acids and ions of calcium and phosphate, negatively charged acidic amino acids can bind to positively charged calcium ions. Likewise, positively charged basic amino acids can bind to negatively charged phosphate ions. Thus amino acids influence compatibility in two ways. First, they limit the availability of calcium and phosphate ions to interact. Second, they form complexes that are soluble in PN admixtures.[23, 32]

In summary, the stability and compatibility of PN admixtures can be improved as follows:

1. Select the appropriate salt of calcium. Utilize calcium gluconate over calcium chloride in admixtures.
2. Maintain a low pH for the final admixture, preferably less than 5. This will discourage the formation of poorly soluble dibasic calcium phosphate.
3. Increase the amino acid concentration in the final preparation.
4. Store and administer preparations at lower temperatures.
5. Do not add calcium and phosphate salts in close sequence. Follow manufacturers' recommendations when using automatic compounding devices to prepare admixtures.
6. Calculate the solubility of calcium using the volume of the admixture at the time when calcium is added, rather than the volume of the final preparation.[7]

Preventing Incompatibility

Misadventures in parenteral preparations can result in microbial or particulate contamination and physicochemical incompatibilities. These errors not only affect the efficacy of the drug, but also heighten the risk of adverse effects, especially for patients who require intensive care.[33, 34] Occasionally, these patients may require administration of multiple IV drugs in addition to PN. As discussed in the *Supplies and Equipment for Compounding and Administering Sterile Preparations* chapter, Y-sites are convenient choices for administering multiple drugs while decreasing contact time of multiple ingredients. When concomitant administration via a Y-site or piggyback route may be necessary, care should be taken to ensure that the components of the various admixtures will not affect the efficacy of one another and that no incompatibilities will be manifested.

Many resources are available to assist in predicting incompatibilities. For example, package inserts of drug products are available from the manufacturer to provide guidance on maximum concentrations, pH, diluent compatibilities, and proper reconstitution, if applicable. Drug databases and reference sources with electronic databases enable different drugs or diluents to be entered to determine compatibility, much like the tool for determining drug interactions. Books and incompatibility charts, such as the *Handbook on Injectable Drugs* and the *King Guide to Parenteral Admixtures*, are frequently used to determine compatibility between different drugs or diluents. These resources provide information such as the maximum concentrations allowed for administration, storage conditions, compatibility, and stability. Primary literature can provide information on experimental studies that have been performed, which can be useful in situations in which limited information is available. These resources should be made available to personnel involved in compounding sterile preparations and should be readily referenced when ascertaining compatibility.

In the event that compatibility cannot be determined using these references, the operator can generally predict drug incompatibilities by using the steps outlined in **Figure 7-6**.

TIP: *Check compatibilities using reliable references, such as books, electronic sources, and incompatibility charts.*

STEP 1: VERIFY SOLUBILITIES

The solubility of all ingredients in the solvent, co-solvent, and active drug used in the preparation should be verified. A drug may

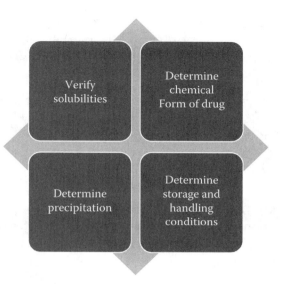

Figure 7-6   Factors for Preventing Drug Incompatibilities

precipitate if its concentration exceeds the saturation solubility for that drug in the solvent. Drugs are formulated into solutions using one or more solvents, known as co-solvents. If the composition of the solvents is changed, either by altering the ratio of the individual solvent or through addition of another solvent, precipitation may occur. Because most drugs have poor aqueous solubility, co-solvents such as ethanol or propylene glycol are added to improve drug solubility. For example, digoxin, an anti-arrhythmic agent, is practically insoluble in water.[36] It is formulated with 40% propylene glycol and 10% alcohol. The injection is buffered to pH 6.8–7.2 with 0.17% dibasic sodium phosphate and 0.08% citric acid. If this formulation is diluted with water, it may result in precipitation of the digoxin.[36] Therefore, digoxin may be administered undiluted. However, if dilution is required, the drug should be diluted at least fourfold in D_5W or NS prior to direct injection; otherwise, it may lead to drug precipitation.[37]

   Drug solubility may also be affected by dilution, especially for drugs that are soluble in a particular pH range. Most drug solutions contain buffers to maintain the pH of a solution; however, if the addition of a different solution significantly alters the pH,

precipitation may occur. For example, erythromycin lactobionate demonstrates pH-dependent stability. It is stable at pH 6–9
and undergoes almost 10% degradation every 8 hours outside
this pH range. Therefore, drugs that can alter the pH of the solution significantly, such as acidic or basic drugs, should not be
mixed with erythromycin lactobionate to prevent degradation
or precipitation.[38]

STEP 2: DETERMINE THE CHEMICAL FORM OF THE DRUG AND THE FINAL pH

Drugs are often developed into solutions for parenteral administration by formulating the drug into its salt form. In general, salts
of acidic or basic drugs have higher aqueous solubilities compared to their corresponding free acid or base form.[39, 40] The solubility of the salt form, however, depends on the pH of the medium.
A change in pH of the medium may lead to conversion of the salt
form to its free form, which can cause drug precipitation. Also,
a change in pH may lead to a different salt form with a different
solubility. As previously mentioned, dibasic calcium phosphate
is converted to monobasic calcium phosphate at a lower pH. The
solubility of the latter is 60 times greater than the solubility of
the former. Hence, a low pH is recommended in those admixtures containing calcium and phosphate to avoid the formation
of poorly soluble dibasic calcium phosphate.

STEP 3: DETERMINE RISK OF PRECIPITATION

Basic physical chemistry principles can be utilized to determine
the pH at which precipitation can occur. The following equations
can be used.

1. For salts of weak acids:
$$\text{pH (ppt)} = pK_a + \log\left(\frac{s - s_0}{s_0}\right)$$
   where pH (ppt) is the pH below which precipitation occurs
2. For salts of weak bases:
$$\text{pH (ppt)} = pK_a + \log\left(\frac{s_0}{s - s_0}\right)$$
   where pH (ppt) is the pH above which precipitation occurs

pK_a = acid dissociation constant for the drug

S = total solubility (expressed in moles per liter) of the drug in solution

S_0 = solubility (expressed in moles per liter) of the undissociated (or neutral) form of the drug

STEP 4: DETERMINE THE STORAGE, HANDLING, ADMINISTRATION, AND TRANSPORTATION CONDITIONS

Pharmacists must ensure that sterile preparations are stored, handled, and transported properly. All personnel involved in compounding parenteral preparations should assume responsibility for identifying conditions that might potentially compromise the integrity of the preparation as well as for maintaining proper conditions influencing compatibility. Policies and procedures should further clarify and outline the responsibilities of personnel in identifying and preventing compatibility issues related to storage, handling, administration, and transportation of CSPs.[41]

Compounding personnel can employ tactics such as the following to prevent incompatibilities:

1. Use a preparation shortly after compounding it.
2. Minimize the number of drugs in a single preparation.
3. Utilize references and resources to determine compatibility and stability.
4. Closely review products with high or low pH.
5. Closely review products containing calcium, phosphate, or magnesium.

Identifying Incompatibilities

An essential step, which should be performed as the final step in compounding of all admixtures by the operator, is visual inspection. After all components of an admixture are added, the preparation should be gently mixed, then visually inspected for particulates, haziness, gas formation, turbidity, crystal formation, changes in color of the admixture, solid matter such as coring from rubber vial closures, or other signs of incompatibility and particulate matter. Additional visual inspections should take place prior to the preparation being dispensed and prior to its administration to the patient.

It is important that steps be taken during compounding to ensure that incompatibilities are not masked. For example, intravenous lipid emulsions (ILEs) are an opaque white color, with an appearance similar to that of milk. When ILEs are added to total nutrition admixtures (TNA) they will mask precipitation or other incompatibilities. Thus ILEs should either be administered separately or should be added as the last ingredient to an admixture. Likewise, ingredients that contain color, such as intravenous vitamins, should be added at the end of compounding to prevent masking of incompatibilities.

ALERT: *Components that are opaque or colored should be added to an admixture last so as to prevent masking of incompatibilities.*

To best identify incompatibilities during visual inspection, the admixture should be held up to the light and the operator should try to see through the solution after mixing, which will help identify particulate matter, evolution of gas, and other incompatibilities. Following this, it is essential to check the admixture against a contrasting background. For example, precipitation in an admixture may not be apparent against a white background, but would readily be identified against a black background. As such, each preparation should be checked against a contrasting background prior to being dispensed.

TIP: *Always visually inspect the final preparation against light as well as against a contrasting background.*

Beyond-Use Dates and Expiration Dates

Pharmacists should clearly understand the difference between beyond-use dates (BUDs) and expiration dates. Expiration dates are determined by the manufacturer through extensive stability studies according to FDA regulatory requirements. According to USP Chapter <797>, "Expiration dates for the chemical and physical stability of manufactured sterile products are determined from results of rigorous analytical and performance testing, and they are specific for a particular formulation in its container and at stated exposure conditions of illumination and temperature."[35]

Expiration dates relate to products manufactured as a single entity or preparation, such as a drug in a vial or a bag of D_5W. The expiration date available from the manufacturer does not necessarily relate to microbiological purity of the product once the product has been opened or accessed. Furthermore, when sterile products are extemporaneously compounded, they are subject to conditions outside of those used for determining expiration dates. For example, the buffer capacity and antimicrobial properties for a system can significantly alter upon its dilution or if the preparation is stored inappropriately. As such, the stability of the CSP requires that a BUD be determined, serving as a date beyond which the compound will no longer be stored, transported, or administered to a patient and will be discarded appropriately. For instance, intravenous vitamin preparations have expiration dates assigned by the manufacturer; however, once added to a PN admixture, a BUD should be determined for the PN admixture based on the projected stability of the entire preparation.

Table 7-1 summarizes the differences between expiration dates and beyond-use dates.

DETERMINING BEYOND-USE DATES

Determining BUDs is necessary because CSPs are intended to be administered immediately following compounding or short-term storage. BUDs for sterile preparations should be based on

Table 7-1   Differences Between Expiration Dates and Beyond-Use Dates

Expiration Date	Beyond-Use Date
• Assigned by the manufacturer	• Assigned by a pharmacist
• Determined using extensive analytical testing	• Determined based on available scientific evidence or per manufacturer recommendations

professional experience and derived from information for the same or similar formulations.[35] Assignment of a BUD should take into consideration the amount of time that a CSP will maintain sterility for its risk level and the chemical stability of the active ingredients.[7] The date and time the admixture was compounded serves as the primary point from which the BUD is determined. USP Chapter <797> recommends determining and extrapolating BUDs using literature sources, direct testing, manufacturers' recommendations, and USP recommendations, as outlined here and illustrated in **Figure 7-7**.[35, 42]

Direct Testing or Literature

Product-specific data acquired from instrumental analysis are considered the most reliable source for determining BUDs.[35] For example, quantitative stability-indicating assays employing high-performance liquid chromatographic (HPLC) provide an accurate determination of a BUD. Preparation-specific analysis is strongly recommended if a BUD exceeding 30 days is assigned. Resources specifically geared toward determining stability and compatibility can be useful in determining BUDs. Reliable literature resources provide specific information regarding the storage of drugs in various environmental conditions as well as

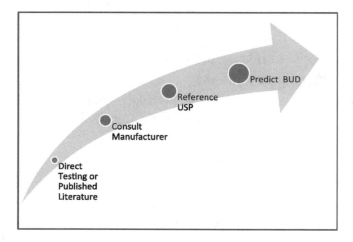

Figure 7-7   Steps for Determining Beyond-Use Dating

the longevity of the CSP based on direct product testing. These resources should be readily available to personnel compounding sterile preparations.

Manufacturer Information

Many manufacturers provide information on the stability of their products when compounded; this information is typically found on the product label or in the package insert. Because they also employ scientific experts to provide advice on stability-related issues for their products, manufacturers are often able to provide additional information if needed. Advice from manufacturers in assigning a BUD may be helpful, particularly in situations in which CSPs deviate from conditions in the approved manufacturer's labeling of the products.

USP Recommendations

USP Chapter <797> provides specific criteria for beyond-use dating, which should be followed by all personnel compounding sterile preparations. For example, USP Chapter <797> recommends that a BUD of 28 days be assigned to multidose containers with preservatives that have been opened or entered, unless otherwise specified by the manufacturer.[35] **Table 7-2** provides additional BUDs for single-dose and multidose containers as outlined by USP Chapter <797>. **Table 7-3** references the published limits for BUDs as given in USP Chapter <797>. Unless sterility testing is performed on CSPs, the assigned BUD cannot exceed these limits. If direct testing or reliable literature is not available for a particular CSP, then the pharmacist should follow the criteria mentioned in USP to assign a BUD. USP Chapter <1191>, "Stability Considerations in Dispensing Practice," is an excellent resource on general stability considerations for a pharmacist when determining the stability of an admixture.

Predicting BUDs

Pharmacists can obtain stability, compatibility, and degradation information for the drug itself and for drugs in a similar class and with a similar structure from the published data. This information

Table 7-2 Differentiating Beyond-Use Dates for Vials and Ready-to-Use Products

Description	Beyond-Use Date
Multidose vials	• 28 days from entering/opening the vial (or less per manufacturer)
Single-dose vials exposed to ISO Class 5 or cleaner	• 6 hours from entering/opening the vial (or less per manufacturer)
Any compounding equipment, container, or compounded sterile products exposed to air quality worse than ISO Class 5	• 1 hour from entering/opening the container • All remaining contents past 1 hour (or less per manufacturer) must be discarded
Ready-to-use products (commercially prepared)	• As indicated by the manufacturer label until entered/opened • BUD should not be extrapolated to extemporaneous preparations
Vial systems (e.g., ADD-Vantage, add-EASE, Minibag Plus, Vial-Mate)	• As indicated by the manufacturer until entered/opened

Source: Data from U.S. Pharmacopeial Convention. Chapter <797>: pharmaceutical compounding-sterile preparations. *United States Pharmacopeia 36/National Formulary 31.* Rockville, MD: U.S. Pharmacopeial Convention; 2013.

Table 7-3 Determining Beyond-Use Dates for Compounded Sterile Products

Risk Level	Controlled Room Temperature: 20°C to 25°C (68°F to 77°F)	Refrigerated: 2°C to 8°C (36°F to 46°F)	Frozen: −25°C to −10° C (−13°F to 14°F)
Immediate use	1 hour	n/a	n/a
Low with 12 hour or less BUD*	12 hours	12 hours	n/a
Low	48 hours	14 days	45 days
Medium	30 hours	9 days	45 days
High	24 hours	3 days	45 days

* Categorized as low with 12-hour or less BUD if the ISO Class 5 primary engineering control is not located within an ISO Class 7 buffer area.

Source: Data from U.S. Pharmacopeial Convention. Chapter <797>: pharmaceutical compounding-sterile preparations. *United States Pharmacopeia 36/National Formulary 31.* Rockville, MD: U.S. Pharmacopeial Convention; 2013.

can be used in determining a theoretically predicted BUD. Pharmacists, however, should pay close attention to the nature of the drug and its mechanism of degradation, packaging and storage conditions, and duration of therapy because the preparation is a unique system and must be treated as such. Remember that theoretically predicted BUDs are based on certain assumptions and, therefore, probabilities of making errors are high. Because the BUD is predicted based on published data, the likelihood of making an error will depend on differences between compositions, ingredient concentrations, and storage containers. If the pharmacist is unsure of the predicted BUD, and it is believed that predicting a BUD would result in a high degree of inaccuracy, the BUD can be determined experimentally. The probability of an inaccurate predicted BUD is heightened if the product is prepared from a non-sterile active ingredient or if the preparation is distributed to facilities other than a healthcare facility because it can be exposed to an uncontrolled environment.

Institutions should develop written policies and procedures addressing assignment of BUDs that should be followed by all personnel to ensure consistency. If experimental stability data for a particular compounded preparation are unavailable, the pharmacist should follow these institutional policies and procedures to conservatively assign a BUD to the preparation.[35]

Conclusion

Certain physical and chemical incompatibilities can have detrimental effects, such as patient harm, administration of a subtherapeutic dose, or production of a toxic or undesired product. Because of these significant implications, pharmacists should never assume that two ingredients are compatible and should always check each CSP for incompatibilities prior to it being dispensed and administered to a patient. Exercising caution and due diligence during compounding, storing, transporting and administering CSPs can prevent patient harm. Compatibility and stability cannot be assured by retrospective checks alone.

Thus pharmacists and compounding personnel should be familiar with and readily reference the resources available to them for preventing incompatibilities, assuring stability, and determining BUDs. All personnel involved in compounding, dispensing, and administration of CSPs are responsible for ensuring that the admixture is a quality preparation in an effort to protect patients from potential harm.

Review Questions

1. Define incompatibility and list five types of incompatibilities.
2. Which type of incompatibility is "sorption"?
3. What is the difference between sorption and leaching?
4. What is chemical incompatibility, and what is the most common type of chemical degradation reaction for parenteral drugs?
5. List the factors that can affect stability and compatibility of sterile preparations.
6. Tacrolimus, an immunosuppressant, should be stored in a glass or polyethylene container and not in a polyvinyl chloride (PVC) container. Why?
7. When reconstituting alefacept, a drug used for the treatment of severe chronic plaque psoriasis, foaming can occur. Which of the following measures can help prevent excessive foaming?
    a. Inject diluents slowly into the vial for reconstitution.
    b. Avoid shaking and vigorous agitation.
    c. Gently swirl the contents during dissolution.
    d. All of the above.
8. Cefoxitin vials are sealed under nitrogen to prevent exposure of the drug to oxygen. Can exposure of cefoxitin to oxygen lead to oxidation of the drug?
    a. Yes
    b. No

CASE STUDIES *Case 1a*

Ryan, a second-year pharmacy intern, has recently joined your hospital pharmacy. He has a very inquisitive mind and always backs up his decision with a rationale. He is currently assisting a pharmacy technician in setting up an automated compounder to make parenteral nutrition (PN) admixtures. Ryan observed that there were two vials on the shelf for calcium administration (calcium chloride and calcium gluconate). The pharmacy technician used the calcium gluconate vial to prepare the PN admixture. Ryan asked the pharmacy technician why he used calcium gluconate and not calcium chloride. The pharmacy technician was not sure of the answer so he directed Ryan to you about this concern.

Do you think Ryan has a legitimate concern and, if so, why?

Case 1b

After his initial discussion with you about calcium phosphate precipitation, Ryan realized how important it is to use the right calcium salt. But Ryan was not completely sure if selecting the right salt is the only thing that can avert precipitation. The next day, he researched issues related to calcium phosphate and came up with a recommendation that should be followed to avoid precipitation.

What were Ryan's recommendations?

Case 2a

You recently received some vials of cefotaxime in your pharmacy, and you ask Ryan to help store them in the pharmacy. Ryan recently learned about the importance of drug storage in his pharmacy class. He comes to you to confirm the storage conditions for the medication. You used this opportunity to develop critical thinking in Ryan and ask him to find out more information on storage conditions of cefotaxime.

What did Ryan find during his search?

Case 2b

You were happy with Ryan's findings. Your next challenge to Ryan was to examine the effect of pH on the stability of cefotaxime. What were Ryan's findings?

References

1. U.S. Pharmacopeial Convention. Chapter <1191>: stability considerations in dispensing practice. *United States Pharmacopeia 36/National Formulary 31.* Rockville, MD: U.S. Pharmacopeial Convention; 2013.
2. Allwood MC, Kearney MC. Compatibility and stability of additives in parenteral nutrition admixtures. *Nutrition.* 1998;14(9): 697–706.
3. Hancock BC, Parks M. What is the true solubility advantage for amorphous pharmaceuticals? *Pharm Res.* 2000;17(4):397–404.
4. Ceftriaxone. *Lexi-Drugs Online.* Hudson, OH: Lexi-Comp, Inc. Available at: http://online.lexi.com/lco/action/doc/retrieve/docid /patch_f/6745. Accessed February 8, 2013.
5. Martens HJ, De Goede PN, Van Loenen AC. Sorption of various drugs in polyvinyl chloride, glass, and polyethylene-lined infusion containers. *Am J Hosp Pharm.* 1990;47(2):369–373.
6. Weir SJ, Myers VA, Bengtson KD, Ueda CT. Sorption of amiodarone to polyvinyl chloride infusion bags and administration sets. *Am J Hosp Pharm.* 1985;42(12):2679–2683.
7. Buchanan EC, Schneider PJ. *Compounding sterile preparations.* 3rd ed. Bethesda, MD: American Society of Health-System Pharmacists; 2013.
8. Waugh WN, Trissel LA, Stella VJ. Stability, compatibility, and plasticizer extraction of taxol (NSC-125973) injection diluted in infusion solutions and stored in various containers. *Am J Hosp Pharm.* 1991;48(7):1520–1524.
9. Latini G, Verrotti A, De FC. DI-2-ethylhexyl phthalate and endocrine disruption: a review. *Curr Drug Targets Immune Endocr Metabol Disord.* 2004;4(1):37–40.
10. Latini G. Monitoring phthalate exposure in humans. *Clin Chim Acta.* 2005;361(1–2):20–29.
11. Latini G, Del VA, Massaro M, et al. Phthalate exposure and male infertility. *Toxicology.* 2006;226(2–3):90–98.
12. Latini G, Ferri M, Chiellini F. Materials degradation in PVC medical devices, DEHP leaching and neonatal outcomes. *Curr Med Chem.* 2010;17(26):2979–2989.

13. Diazepam. *Facts & Comparisons*. Available at: http://online
.factsandcomparisons.com. Accessed February 25, 2013.

14. Newton DW, Driscoll DF, Goudreau JL, Ratanamaneichatara
S. Solubility characteristics of diazepam in aqueous admixture
solutions: theory and practice. *Am J Hosp Pharm*. 1981;38(2):
179–182.

15. Allwood MC. Factors influencing the stability of ascorbic acid
in total parenteral nutrition infusions. *J Clin Hosp Pharm*. 1984;
9(2):75–85.

16. Das G, V. Stability of vitamins in total parenteral nutrient solutions. *Am J Hosp Pharm*. 1986;43(9):2132, 2138, 2143.

17. Albert A, Rees CW. Avidity of the tetracyclines for the cations
of metals. *Nature*. 1956;177(4505):433–434.

18. Tetracycline hydrochloride, calcium gluconate. King Guide database. Napa, CA. Available at: http://www.kingguide.com/kgpa2
/x2.asp?DRUG=TETRACYCLINE+HYDROCHLORIDE&D2
=CALCIUM+GLUCONATE. Accessed February 25, 2013.

19. Rose-Williamson K. Cisplatin: delivering a safe infusion. *Am J
Nurs*. 1981;81(2):320–323.

20. Ceftazidime. *Facts & Comparisons*. Available at: http://online
.factsandcomparisons.com. Accessed February 25, 2013.

21. Vella-Brincat JW, Begg EJ, Gallagher K, et al. Stability of benzyl-
penicillin during continuous home intravenous therapy. *J Anti-
microb Chemother*. 2004;53(4):675–677.

22. Phenytoin. *Facts & Comparisons*. Available at: http://online
.factsandcomparisons.com. Accessed February 25, 2013.

23. Singh H, Dumas GJ, Silvestri AP, et al. Physical compatibility of
neonatal total parenteral nutrition admixtures containing organic
calcium and inorganic phosphate salts in a simulated infusion
at 37 degrees C. *Pediatr Crit Care Med*. 2009;10(2):213–216.

24. Nitroprusside. *Facts & Comparisons*. Available at: http://online
.factsandcomparisons.com. Accessed February 25, 2013.

25. Allwood MC. The influence of light on vitamin A degradation
during administration. *Clin Nutr*. 1982;1(1):63–70.

26. Allwood MC, Martin HJ. The photodegradation of vitamins A
and E in parenteral nutrition mixtures during infusion. *Clin Nutr*.
2000;19(5):339–342.

27. Hill SE, Heldman LS, Goo ED, et al. Fatal microvascular pulmonary emboli from precipitation of a total nutrient admixture solution. *J Parenter Enteral Nutr.* 1996;20(1):81–87.

28. McKinnon BT. FDA safety alert: hazards of precipitation associated with parenteral nutrition. *Nutr Clin Pract.* 1996;11(2): 59–65.

29. Puntis JW, Wilkins KM, Ball PA, et al. Hazards of parenteral treatment: do particles count? *Arch Dis Child.* 1992;67(12):1475–1477.

30. Lehr HA, Brunner J, Rangoonwala R, Kirkpatrick CJ. Particulate matter contamination of intravenous antibiotics aggravates loss of functional capillary density in postischemic striated muscle. *Am J Respir Crit Care Med.* 2002;165(4):514–520.

31. Henry RS, Jurgens RW Jr, Sturgeon R, et al. Compatibility of calcium chloride and calcium gluconate with sodium phosphate in a mixed TPN solution. *Am J Hosp Pharm.* 1980;37(5): 673–674.

32. Parikh MJ, Dumas G, Silvestri A, et al. Physical compatibility of neonatal total parenteral nutrient admixtures containing organic calcium and inorganic phosphate salts. *Am J Health Syst Pharm.* 2005;62(11):1177–1183.

33. Bertsche T, Mayer Y, Stahl R, et al. Prevention of intravenous drug incompatibilities in an intensive care unit. *Am J Health Syst Pharm.* 2008;65(19):1834–1840.

34. Lesar TS, Briceland L, Stein DS. Factors related to errors in medication prescribing. *JAMA.* 1997;277(4):312–317.

35. U.S. Pharmacopeial Convention. Chapter <797>: pharmaceutical compounding: sterile preparations. *United States Pharmacopeia 36/National Formulary 31.* Rockville, MD: U.S. Pharmacopeial Convention; 2013.

36. Digoxin. *Facts & Comparisons.* Available at: http://online.factsandcomparisons.com. Accessed February 25, 2013.

37. Digoxin. *Lexi-Drugs Online.* Hudson, OH: Lexi-Comp, Inc. Available at: http://online.lexi.com/lco/action/doc/retrieve/docid/patch_f/6745. Accessed February 8, 2013.

38. Erythromycin lactobionate. *Facts & Comparisons.* Available at: http://online.factsandcomparisons.com. Accessed February 25, 2013.

39. Serajuddin AT. Salt formation to improve drug solubility. *Adv Drug Deliv Rev.* 2007;59(7):603–616.

40. Sweetana S, Akers MJ. Solubility principles and practices for parenteral drug dosage form development. *PDA J Pharm Sci Technol.* 1996;50(5):330–342.

41. Thompson JE. *A practical guide to contemporary pharmacy practice.* 3rd ed. Baltimore, MD: Lippincott Williams & Wilkins; 2009.

42. Cohen MR. Safe practices for compounding of parenteral nutrition. *J Parenter Enteral Nutr.* 2012;36(2 suppl):14S–19S.

CHAPTER 8

Preparation of Hazardous Drugs for Parenteral Use

Helen T. Wu

Chapter Objectives

1. Describe hazardous-drug handling guidelines.
2. Explain environmental controls for compounding hazardous drugs.
3. Discuss the role of primary engineering controls in compounding hazardous drugs.
4. Define closed-system vial-transfer devices.
5. Identify the personal protective equipment used specifically for compounding hazardous drugs.
6. Describe proper procedures for cleaning, disinfection, decontamination, and disposal of hazardous drugs.
7. Outline important patient safety measures for hazardous-drug ordering and dispensing.

Key Terminology

Hazardous drug
Asepsis

USP Chapter <797>
ASHP Technical Assistance Bulletin
Environment control
Negative-pressure room
ISO class number
Primary engineering control (PEC)
Biological safety cabinet (BSC)
Compounding aseptic containment isolator (CACI)
Closed-system vial-transfer devices (CSTD)
PhaSeal
Personal protective equipment (PPE)
Sodium hypochlorite solution
Chemotherapy spill kit

Overview

Preparation of hazardous drugs presents unique considerations beyond those for nonhazardous drugs, such as issues related to personnel safety and exposure. Hazardous drugs, including antineoplastic agents, certain antiviral agents, immunosuppressants, hormones, biological modifiers, and others, may cause harm to healthcare workers if not handled appropriately. It is important to maintain the sterility of compounded sterile preparations (CSPs) involving hazardous drugs, while minimizing exposure to healthcare workers. Accuracy in dosing and related calculations is also of importance with many hazardous drugs, as administering excessive or deficient doses can lead to unnecessary exposure or detrimental effects vis-à-vis disease progression.

This chapter reviews pertinent issues associated with safe handling of hazardous drugs. Important references for hazardous drug preparations include United States Pharmacopeia Chapter <797> and the American Society of Health-System Pharmacists' (ASHP) published guidelines on the safe handling of cytotoxic agents.[1,2] These references provide standards to guide preparation of hazardous drugs and outline important safety considerations to protect both the operator and the patient. All personnel involved in the preparation, verification, transportation, and administration of hazardous CSPs should be knowledgeable about safe practices for hazardous agents.

Hazardous Drugs and Exposure Risks

The federal *Hazard Communication Standard* (HCS) defines a health hazard as a chemical for which there is evidence that acute or chronic health effects may occur following exposure. HCS identifies the following substances as hazardous agents: carcinogens, toxic or highly toxic agents, reproductive toxins, irritants, corrosives, sensitizers, and agents that produce target organ effects.[3]

In 1990, the American Society of Health System Pharmacists (ASHP) first used the term "hazardous drug" in reference to drugs that involve risks from occupational exposure. Like HCS, ASHP defines hazardous drugs as those that may cause genotoxicity, carcinogenicity, teratogenicity, fertility impairment, and serious organ or other toxicity at low doses, in either animal models or treated patients. In 2004, the National Institute for Occupational Safety and Health (NIOSH) revised the ASHP's criteria for hazardous drugs with similar definitions. USP Chapter <797> defines hazardous drugs as those which have a potential to cause cancer, developmental or reproductive toxicity, or harm to organs, either in animal studies or in humans.

According to NIOSH's *List of Antineoplastic and Other Hazardous Drugs in Healthcare Settings*, hazardous drugs may include antineoplastic agents (chemotherapy), antiviral agents, biological modifiers, immunosuppressants, hormones, and other agents. These agents provide therapeutic benefits for patients; however, studies have shown that healthy workers who are exposed to these drugs may experience adverse effects, such as adverse reproductive outcomes and cancer.[4]

Occupational exposures to hazardous drugs have been associated with both short-term toxicity and reproductive risks. Short-term toxicities from hazardous drug exposure may include rash, allergic reactions, hair loss, and skin and nail problems.[1] Many hazardous drugs have also been shown to be teratogenic and embryotoxic. Personnel of reproductive capability who are compounding hazardous drugs must confirm in writing their understanding of the risks involved in this activity.[1] Some drugs are spermatotoxic, causing concerns for male workers. In females, reported adverse effects from exposure to hazardous drugs include menstrual dysfunction, infertility, and ectopic pregnancy. Fetal loss, low birth weight, birth defects, and children with learning differences have also been reported.[5-8] Increased incidence of cancers linked to occupational exposure has been reported as well. Exposure surfaces contaminated with moderate amounts of cyclophosphamide, for example, pose a calculated risk between 1.4 and 10 cancers per year per 1 million workers.[9]

Exposure routes may include the following:

- Inhalation: inhaling air contaminated with a hazardous drug
- Dermal absorption: touching contaminated surfaces with bare skin
- Ingestion: transferring contaminants from hands into the mouth through food or drink
- Accidental injection: involving a needle stick or glass cut

Sources of contamination may include vial surfaces, work surfaces contaminated during routine compounding, drug administration and waste handling, and poor technique during compounding, handling, and transporting. Therefore, caution must be taken at every step—from handling of hazardous drugs to administration of the CSP to the patient—to minimize contamination and, ultimately, direct exposure. Because such risks clearly exist, standards of safe handling of hazardous drugs must be set and followed closely to ensure operator safety.

Exposure of healthcare workers to hazardous drugs was recognized as a problem in the 1970s. Since then, numerous guidelines for handling hazardous drugs have been developed. Professional and governmental organizations that set standards for handling hazardous drugs include the American Society of Health Systems Pharmacists, Oncology Nursing Society (ONS), Occupational Safety and Health Administration (OSHA), and

United States Pharmacopeial Convention (USP). OSHA, part of the U.S. Department of Labor, is the main federal agency charged with the enforcement of safety and health legislation. NIOSH is part of the Centers for Disease Control and Prevention (CDC), and is the U.S. federal agency responsible for conducting research in occupational safety and health matters. In 2004, a NIOSH alert was issued after assessing the extent of occupational exposure to chemotherapy and other hazardous drugs in healthcare settings. The alert makes recommendations to improve safety programs in an effort to reduce this exposure. Of note, the NIOSH alert on hazardous drugs addresses workers in all healthcare settings, so it is applicable beyond hospital settings. The NIOSH alert does not have the power of legal enforcement; however, the principles in the alert can be enforced by OSHA. A 1990 ASHP Technical Assistance Bulletin provided extensive recommendations on equipment and work practices, which are most applicable to pharmacy practice; it also updated existing guidelines. OSHA, NIOSH, and ASHP all recommend essentials for safe handling of hazardous drugs, including environmental controls (ventilation), personal protective equipment (PPE), work practice controls (training programs), and administrative controls to reduce occupational exposure to hazardous drugs.

In 2007, USP released Chapter <797>, "Pharmaceutical Compounding: Sterile Preparations," which became effective in 2008. While useful as a reference for compounding hazardous drugs, USP Chapter <797> is an enforceable standard that establishes many of the NIOSH recommendations as requirements. Specifically, it mandates compliance with environmental conditions, engineering controls, and training standards for workers as well as for protection of the final preparation. In today's pharmacy practice, USP Chapter <797> standards, as adjuncts to state pharmacy board regulations, must be adhered to.

Environment Control[1,2]

Minimizing exposure to hazardous agents is an important goal of environmental control. While those workers preparing hazardous

janitors, laundry, personnel

drugs are at highest risk of exposure, environmental controls should minimize exposure to other personnel as well. As such, the locations where hazardous drugs are stored and compounded should be specially designated and isolated areas.

For easy identification, all hazardous drug containers should be labeled with a distinct and consistent design (see **Figure 8-1** and **Figure 8-2**). Hazardous drugs should be stored separately from other drugs in an area with sufficient general exhaust ventilation to dilute and remove any airborne contaminants. Per USP Chapter <797>, storage of hazardous drugs should take place within a contained area, such as a negative-pressure room that is properly vented. The negative-pressure room should be at a lower pressure than the adjacent spaces—as with the clean room, for example. The net flow of air into the room prevents the escape of hazardous drug into the workplace. Air from the negative-pressure room must be properly ventilated to the outside; proper ventilation of the room is essential for workers' protection.

ALERT: *As a safety mechanism, all hazardous containers should be labeled with a distinct and consistent design.*

Hazardous drugs should be compounded in a controlled area that is devoted to that purpose alone and is restricted to

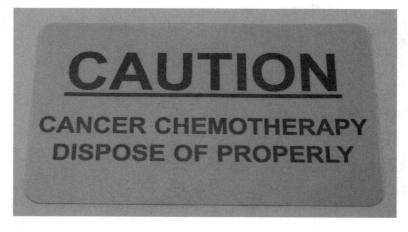

Figure 8-1 Chemotherapy Label

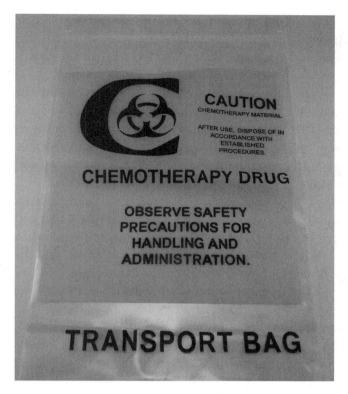

Figure 8-2 Chemotherapy Transport Bag

authorized personnel. USP Chapter <797> requires hazardous drugs be prepared in a primary engineering control (PEC), which should be placed in an International Standards Organization (ISO) Class 7 area that is physically separated from other preparation areas.

Primary Engineering Controls for Compounding Hazardous Drugs

As discussed in the *Primary and Secondary Engineering Controls* chapter, a primary engineering control (PEC) is a device that provides an ISO Class 5 environment for the exposure of critical sites when compounding CSPs. Such devices include, but are not limited to, laminar airflow workbenches (LAFW), biological safety cabinets (BSC), compounding aseptic isolators, and compounding aseptic containment isolators (CACI).

An appropriate BSC or CACI is needed for compounding hazardous drugs. The BSC or CACI must be able to maintain an ISO Class 5 air quality environment under dynamic operating conditions. The airflow for PECs for compounding nonhazardous drugs may be recirculated into the room; however, the PEC for compounding hazardous drugs should be completely vented to the outside through high-efficiency particulate air (HEPA) filtration to minimize airborne exposure. The purpose of maintaining an ISO Class 5 environment is to prevent microbial contamination of CSPs; however, a controlled environment is also in place to protect workers by preventing the escape of hazardous drug aerosols or residue.

A BSC is a ventilated cabinet for compounding sterile preparations. BSCs have an open front with inward airflow for personnel protection, downward HEPA-filtered laminar airflow for product protection, and HEPA-filtered exhausted air for environmental protection.

Various types of BSCs are available, and it is important to understand the differences between Class I, Class II, and Class III models. Class I BSCs are "fume hoods" that protect the operator, but do not ensure asepsis. Class I BSCs are not appropriate for aseptic compounding and, therefore, should not be used for compounding hazardous drugs.

Class II BSCs protect personnel, as well as the CSP and environment. These BSCs include four different types: A1, A2, B1, and B2. In Class II B2 BSCs, airflow is drawn from external air and exhausted to the atmosphere through a HEPA filter without recirculation. A best practice recommendation for PECs for compounding hazardous drugs is to use a Class II BSC, type B2, in a negative-pressure clean room, and 100% vented to outside. Class II BSCs have an open front and depend on an air barrier to prevent hazardous drug contamination from escaping the cabinet. The air barrier is formed by drawing air from the buffer area around the BSC. Given that air is pulled into the BSC, poor air quality in the buffer area may compromise the ISO Class 5 compounding environment.

Class III BSCs are completely contained units of gas-tight construction. Operation of these BSCs is conducted through attached rubber gloves and viewed through a fixed window. Class III BSCs are maintained under negative pressure and use HEPA-filtered air for intake. Exhausted air is also HEPA filtered; however, depending on the design, the exhausted air may be vented to the outside or recirculated into the compounding room. Class III BSCs are essentially isolators.

The various types of isolators differ in myriad ways, such as positive pressure versus negative pressure, airflow dynamics, aseptic versus containment, and recirculation of air versus complete venting to the outside. Ideally, for hazardous drug preparation, a CACI with unidirectional airflow that is completely vented to the outside should be utilized. For maximum safety, this unit should be situated in the ISO Class 7 negative-pressure clean room reserved for hazardous drug preparation. If this is not possible, at a minimum, it should be situated in a separate negative-pressure room with adequate air exchange.

> **TIP:** *A CACI with unidirectional airflow that is completely vented to the outside is an ideal choice for hazardous drug preparation.*

Of note, total exhaustion of air to outside, as with a CACI, is required if the hazardous drug to be compounded is known to be volatile. Therefore, when mixing volatile hazardous drugs, a ventilated cabinet that recirculates air inside the cabinet or exhausts air back into the room environment should not be used.

Personal Protective Equipment[1,2]

In addition to environmental and engineering controls, PPE is required during any activity that might potentially involve contact with hazardous drugs, such as receiving and shelving products, compounding, administration, spill cleaning, drug waste disposal, and handling of patient waste. During sterile compounding, barrier garments must be worn to prevent the shedding of human skin and hair cells and the deposition of mucus or respiratory residue into the compounding area. USP Chapter <797> specifies that compounding garb must include the following items: dedicated shoes or shoe covers, face masks, head and facial hair covers, a non-shedding gown with sleeves that fit snugly around the wrists and that is enclosed at the neck, and sterile powder-free chemotherapy gloves. Eye protection is also recommended and should consist of a face shield or goggles that prevent spills or splashes from reaching the eyes. The proper order of donning PPE for hazardous drug compounding is outlined in **Table 8-1**.

ALERT: *Additional PPE is required when preparing hazardous drugs.*

GLOVING

Gloving plays an important role in PPE. Gloves for manipulation of hazardous drugs should be certified and labeled as "chemotherapy gloves." When working with hazardous drugs, workers should always practice "double gloving," which provides extra protection to the operator during compounding.

ALERT: *Double gloves should be donned when compounding hazardous drugs.*

Table 8-1 Proper Donning of PPE for Preparing Hazardous Drugs

1. Shoe covers
2. Hair cover
3. Beard cover
4. Face/eye protection
5. Hand hygiene
6. Gown
7. Gloves

Source: Data from U.S. Pharmacopeial Convention. Chapter <797>: pharmaceutical compounding: sterile preparations. *United States Pharmacopeia 36/National Formulary 31*. Rockville, MD: U.S. Pharmacopeial Convention; 2013.

Inner and outer pairs of chemotherapy gloves should be powder free and made from latex, nitrile, polyurethane, neoprene, or other materials that meet the American Society of Testing and Materials (ASTM) standard. As with standard processing of CSPs, gloves should be sanitized with sterile 70% isopropyl alcohol (IPA) or other appropriate disinfectant before performing any aseptic compounding activity. Outer gloved hands must be sterilized with sterile 70% IPA at the following times:

- Prior to entering the ISO Class 5 space (LAFW or BSC), such as to put materials into the PEC
- At the start of each batch prior to compounding
- Anytime the hands of the operator reenter the ISO Class 5 area
- Periodically during prolonged periods of compounding within the ISO Class 5 area

It is important that hands be washed before donning and after removing gloves to prevent product and surface contamination as well as to prevent exposure to the operator. Gloves should be changed every 30 minutes during compounding, immediately when damaged or contaminated, or whenever the operator exits the PEC environment. Sterilization of gloves should occur prior to reentering the PEC and with each change of gloves. Gloves should also be changed after administering hazardous drugs or when the operator leaves the immediate administration area. Outer gloves must be changed after wiping down the final preparation but before labeling or removing the preparation from the BSC to minimize spread of hazardous contamination. After completing each preparation, outer gloves must be removed and placed in a containment bag while in the BSC or isolator. Used gloves should then be disposed of as contaminated waste. It is recommended that specific procedures for their removal be established and followed at each institution.

In a CACI, a pair of gloves must be worn inside the fixed-glove assembly. In an isolator, fixed gloves or gauntlets must be surface cleaned after compounding is completed to avoid spreading hazardous drug contamination to surfaces. Clean inner gloves should be used to decontaminate the surface of the final preparation, place the label onto the final preparation, and place the into the pass-through of the isolator. Fresh gloves should be donned to complete the final check, place the preparation into a clean transport bag, and remove the bag from the pass-through.

TIP: *To facilitate double gloving, alcohol can be applied to the first pair of gloves to provide a slippery surface for donning the second set of gloves.*

GOWNING

Gowns should be worn during compounding, administration, cleaning spills, and handling waste from patients who were recently treated with hazardous drugs. Disposable gowns of material tested to be protective against the hazardous drugs should be donned for each activity.

The gown used in handling hazardous drugs should be a lint-free polyethylene-coated gown with long sleeves, a solid front, closures in the back, and knitted, tight-fitting wrist cuffs. Proper donning of gloves in conjunction with the chemotherapy gown is important to protect the operator from accidental sprays and spills. Gown cuffs should be placed over the inner, first set of non-sterile chemotherapy gloves. A second outer pair of sterile chemotherapy gloves is then worn over the first pair and pulled over the wrist cuff of the gown.

When working within the CACI, the operator's hands should be washed (gloving is optional) and then placed into the glove/gauntlet arms. A set of sterile chemotherapy gloves can then be placed over the fixed glove/gauntlet gloves using the sterile glove donning process. Proper introduction of items into the CACI ante-chamber and working zone chamber should follow.

Coated gowns must be worn no longer than 3 hours during compounding and must be changed immediately when damaged or contaminated. Gowns worn for barrier protection in the compounding of hazardous drugs must never be worn outside the immediate preparation area. Gowns used during compounding are considered contaminated waste and should be contained and disposed of as such. It is important to wash hands after removing and disposing of gowns to remove any hazardous contamination.

Compounding Sterile Hazardous Agents

PREPARATION TECHNIQUE

As discussed in the *Aseptic Technique and Compounding Manipulations* chapter, manipulation within a BSC must account for laminar airflow in a vertical direction. Thus it is important that the path of first air to critical sites never be blocked during the preparation process, such as by situating objects above the direct compounding areas or positioning hands between the HEPA filter and critical sites.

Because of the hazardous nature of cytotoxic drugs, preparation considerations are of utmost importance to protect the operator. When withdrawing chemotherapy from the vial, negative pressure should always be used. Slight negative pressure can be used to draw up large volumes. Maintaining the same air-to-volume ratio while withdrawing the solution increases the potential for sprays and leakage resulting from positive pressure. Drawing up less air into the syringe than is to be withdrawn from the vial will maintain negative pressure and decrease the risk of accidental exposure. Increasing negative pressure is created as the amount of air added to the syringe, and subsequently to the vial, decreases compared to the amount of solution to be withdrawn. For example, negative pressure would result if 7 mL of air is drawn into the syringe and injected into the vial when 10 mL of solution is to be withdrawn from a vial. If only 3 mL of air is drawn into the syringe and injected into the vial, when 10 mL of solution is needed, this would create even greater negative pressure.

> **TIP:** *Always use negative pressure when withdrawing cytotoxic drugs from a vial.*

The size of the syringe is also a consideration when preparing hazardous admixtures. Syringe sizes should not be too small for the volume to be withdrawn from the vial. As a rule of thumb, a three-fourths rule should be followed—that is, the volume of solution to be withdrawn should not exceed three-fourths of the syringe capacity. For example, if using a 20-mL syringe, no more than 15 mL of solution should be drawn into the syringe. While the three-fourths rule is widely used, some institutions utilize a more conservative one-half rule. Drawing up too-large of volumes into syringes increases the risk of accidental spills or sprays.

> **TIP:** *When working with cytotoxic drugs, the volume of solution that is withdrawn should not exceed three-fourths of the syringe capacity.*

The compounding techniques described by Wilson and Solimando remain the standard for mixing of hazardous drugs.[10] When performed accurately, these techniques minimize the risk of drugs escaping from the containers. Although care can be taken during the preparation process, exposure to chemotherapy can still occur. Vapors and sprays that are not seen with the naked eye may result in unnecessary exposure to the operator and those administering the drug. Closed-system vial-transfer devices provide optimal protection from accidental exposures and vapors both during preparation and administration of hazardous drugs.

Closed-System Vial-Transfer Devices

Many adjunct devices have been developed to reduce the generation of hazardous contamination during the compounding process. Today, however, the use of closed-system vial-transfer devices (CSTDs) is considered best practice for compounding hazardous drugs. Such a device mechanically prohibits the escape of hazardous drugs, contaminants, and vapors into the environment, but provides additional operator protection as well. USP Chapter <797> defines CSTDs as "vial transfer systems that allow no venting or exposure of hazardous substances to the environment." USP Chapter <797> further states that CSTDs must be used within an ISO Class 5 environment of a BSC or CACI. In facilities that prepare a low volume of hazardous drugs, the use of two tiers of containment (e.g., a CSTD within a BSC or a CACI that is located in a non-negative-pressure room) is acceptable. During compounding, a CSTD is locked onto the top of a drug vial to exert a protective effect. In addition to their use during compounding, CSTDs are utilized during administration of hazardous drugs. For administration, the device is locked onto the patient's IV catheter for either IV infusion or IV push. Using CSTDs during medication administration will provide protection to nurses administering the medication. Studies have demonstrated the effectiveness of these devices in reducing hazardous contamination for both inpatient and outpatient compounding as well as with drug administration. The use of CSTDs also significantly reduces surface contamination of hazardous agents compared to standard practice.[11-16]

One well-known brand of CSTD is PhaSeal, which is compatible with all standard-size syringes, vials, and administration sets. PhaSeal was the first CSTD cleared by the Food and Drug Administration (FDA) with an indication to reduce exposure to hazardous drugs. This system contains several parts, such as the protector, injector, connector, administration components, and application components. The multicomponent system uses a double membrane to enclose an injection cannula as it moves into a drug vial, Luer Lock, or infusion-set connector. The following website address contains additional information on CSTDs as well as explanations and demonstrations on how to use different devices of the PhaSeal system.[17]

http://www.bd.com/pharmacy/phaseal/

Cleaning, Disinfection, and Decontamination[1,2]

In addition to the proper PEC cleaning procedures, appropriate preparation of materials to be used for compounding must be done before their introduction into the BSC or CACI. Such preparations may include wiping the compounding surface with a residue-free disinfecting agent (e.g., sterile 70% isopropyl alcohol).

In addition to cleaning and disinfection, decontamination must be performed when preparing or administering hazardous drugs. Any chemotherapy surface contamination will create potential harm for healthcare workers. Therefore, the work surfaces must be decontaminated and cleaned on a regular basis. Per ASHP guidelines, decontamination may be defined as cleaning or deactivation. The use of sterile alcohol for disinfecting the BSC or isolator will not deactivate any hazardous drugs and may result in the spread of contamination rather than any actual cleaning. The Material Safety Data Sheet (MSDS) recommends sodium hypochlorite solution as an appropriate deactivating agent for many hazardous drugs. A widely used commercial product is Surface Safe, which provides a system for decontamination and deactivation using sodium hypochlorite, a detergent, and thiosulfate as a neutralizer.

(bleach)

The work surfaces should be cleaned and decontaminated before and after each activity and at the end of each shift. **Figure 8-3** shows an appropriate decontamination sequence of workflow.

Because the various engineering devices differ in terms of their design, personnel must follow the manufacturers' recommendations carefully to ensure proper operation during cleaning, disinfection, and decontamination. The following is an example of a cleaning and disinfecting procedure:

don't learn steps

- At the beginning of each shift, use Surface Safe (or equivalent) two-step applicator kit (two packets per kit) to properly clean and decontaminate the surface areas. Each pair of packets provides enough solution to treat approximately 2 square feet. Two to four packet pairs may be necessary for each cleaning of the BSC.
- Step 1: Use Packet 1 containing 2% sodium hypochlorite (soap solution serves as an oxidation agent).
  - Apply the premoistened pad to the entire surface.
  - Discard the used pad in the chemotherapy waste container and then proceed to Step 2.

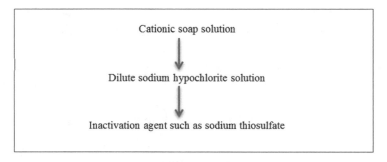

Cationic soap solution

↓

Dilute sodium hypochlorite solution

↓

Inactivation agent such as sodium thiosulfate

Figure 8-3 Hazardous Drug Decontamination Sequence

- Step 2: Use Packet 2 containing 1% sodium thiosulfate + 0.9% benzyl alcohol (for chemical degradation and mutagenic deactivation of many commonly used hazardous drugs; also eliminates residual chlorine from Packet 1).
  - Apply the premoistened towelette to the entire area treated with Packet 1.
  - Discard the used pad in the chemotherapy waste container.
- After Step 2 is complete, all treated surfaces must be rinsed with sterile water for irrigation (SWFI) to remove all cleaning residue. When plastic 500-mL bottles of SWFI are opened and used, they must be discarded within 24 hours. Bottles should be labeled with the date and time of opening, the date and time due to expire, and staff initials.
- For all surfaces, a residue-free disinfecting agent (e.g., sterile 70% isopropyl alcohol) should be used to wipe all inside surfaces, starting from the back and working toward the front. Side panels should be wiped from top to bottom using a left side–to–right side motion, then allowed to dry. All sides must be cleaned.
- All wipes and supplies must be considered contaminated and placed in appropriate hazardous waste receptacles.

Many chemotherapy vials come directly from the manufacturer with surface contamination present on the vial. All chemotherapy vials should be decontaminated with sodium hypochlorite wipes prior to shelving the product. When chemotherapy vials are initially unpacked and wiped down, full PPE should be utilized, just as if chemotherapy were being prepared. It is also a best practice recommendation for all healthcare workers to thoroughly wash their hands after removing PPE.

Chemotherapy Spills[1, 2]

To decrease the risk of spills occurring during transport, it is recommended that chemotherapy preparations be placed in a chemotherapy transport bag and remain in the bag until administration. Chemotherapy spills may occur at any time during preparation, transport, or administration. Consequently, spill kits should be readily available in all areas where these preparations are present.

> **TIP:** *Chemotherapy spill kits should be readily available in all locations in which cytotoxic drug preparation, transport, and administration occur.*

Chemotherapy spill kits are used for the containment and cleanup of spills involving cytotoxic drugs. All staff handling chemotherapy should be trained in spill management and use of spill kits. A chemotherapy spill kit should include the following items:

1. Supplies to absorb a spill of about 1000 mL
2. Appropriate PPE, including two pairs of disposable chemotherapy gloves, chemotherapy gowns, shoe covers, and face shield
3. Absorbent, plastic-backed sheets or spill pads
4. Disposable toweling
5. At least two sealable, thick plastic, hazardous waste disposal bags
6. One disposable scoop for collecting glass fragments
7. One puncture-resistant container for glass fragments
8. Decontamination supply

Once a spill has occurred, containing it is the most important step before cleaning. The spill can be contained by draping a chemotherapy mat or absorbent pad over the spill area. If the spill is less than 5 mL, it may be cleaned by staff responsible for the spill. If the spill is greater than 5 mL, it is best practice to call environmental services to handle the spill. If the spill involves direct contact with a patient or healthcare worker, the contaminated clothing should be removed and the skin immediately washed with soap and water for 20 minutes. If chemotherapy splashes into the eyes, the eyes should be rinsed with water continually for 15 minutes. An eye wash or eye bath should be located in all areas where splash risk may occur. Immediate medical attention should be provided.

Small spills can be cleaned up by wiping the area with disposable towels and disposing of all contaminated materials as chemotherapy waste. If glass is present, it may be cleaned up with the hard plastic scoop supplied in most spill kits. Any contaminated linen should be placed in a chemotherapy-labeled bag for special cleaning. As with the decontamination that occurs during cleaning of BSCs, spills should be decontaminated with sodium hypochlorite and neutralized with sodium thiosulfate.

Proper Disposal of Hazardous Drugs[1,2]

Containment is the key to properly handling hazardous drug waste. During compounding, all material contaminated with hazardous drugs should be disposed of inside the PEC and sealed appropriately before placing it in the hazardous drug waste container. Examples include gloves, syringes, adapters, tubing, wipes, and other materials used in the compounding process.

All hazardous drug waste must be disposed of according to policies and procedures established by each institution's Department of Environmental Health and Safety and state regulations. Chemotherapy waste must be handled separately from other hospital waste. A licensed medical waste contractor should be retained to remove this waste on a regular basis. In general, the contractor incinerates hazardous drug waste at a licensed facility. All staff should be trained to ensure that full PPE is worn when handling hazardous waste. Contaminated materials can include ampules, vials, bags, bottles, tubing, unused doses, chemotherapy mats used on work surfaces, and body fluids containing chemotherapy. All materials used in preparation and administration of chemotherapy must be disposed in a labeled and sealable chemotherapy container. To protect all healthcare workers from possible needle sticks with hazardous drugs, all sharps should be placed in a puncture-proof and properly labeled chemotherapy container. Any container with cytotoxic waste needs to be closed to minimize the escape of any hazardous vapors.

Patient Safety: Policy and Procedure for Ordering Hazardous Drugs

Implementation of and adherence to institutional policies and procedures protect both the patient and the healthcare worker. Because of the narrow therapeutic window and significant toxicity of chemotherapy drugs, institutions must develop policies and procedures that deal specifically with chemotherapy drug ordering, order processing, and dispensing.

When processing a chemotherapy order, both clinical information and patient-related parameters must be checked to ensure correctness of the order. Upon receiving a chemotherapy order, the pharmacist should look for the patient's diagnosis to confirm selection of an appropriate treatment protocol. All treatment protocols should be referenced, and pharmacists should not accept a chemotherapy order if the reference is not indicated. Once the selection of an appropriate protocol is confirmed, the pharmacist should check whether there are any contraindications and whether the dose prescribed is appropriate for the patient. For example, a patient with severe renal dysfunction will not be a candidate for methotrexate therapy. To evaluate appropriate dosing, organ function and relevant lab test results must be evaluated. Pharmacists should always check renal function, liver function, and blood counts before dispensing chemotherapy medications.

All chemotherapy orders should include the following patient parameters: current total body weight, height, body surface area, and drug allergies. Chemotherapy is usually dosed by body weight (mg/kg) or body surface area (mg/m^2). An average adult weight is considered 70 kilograms, with an average body surface area (BSA) being 1.73 m^2. If a patient's weight or BSA differs significantly from these average numbers, the pharmacist needs to make sure there is no incorrect information reported. On the chemotherapy order, the dose by weight and total dose need to be written clearly. In addition to chemotherapy drugs, appropriate premedication should be ordered to prevent chemotherapy drug–induced toxicities. Most chemotherapy agents cause significant nausea and vomiting, so orders for antiemetics often accompany chemotherapy orders. Thus the pharmacist should check whether appropriate antiemetic agents are ordered. Some chemotherapies may induce allergic or infusion-related reactions. Because of this risk, the pharmacist should check whether appropriate emergency medications have been ordered.

A multiple-checkpoint system for verifying final preparations should be in place to ensure patient safety. At a minimum, two pharmacists must be involved in the verification process. For example, one pharmacist should perform calculations and verify dose volumes, diluents, drugs, route, and expiration dates using the original order. A second pharmacist, who was not involved in the original processing of the order, should double-check calculations, ensure the right drugs and diluents were used, verify dose volumes and route, and check expiration dates. This second check should use the original order for reconciliation of the preparation process and the intent of the original order. Both pharmacists should document their reviews.

Personnel Education and Training for Hazardous Compounding

The qualifications of each individual involved in ordering and handling of chemotherapy drugs must be closely evaluated. Any pharmacist who specializes in the field of oncology should be encouraged to complete the Board of Pharmaceutical Specialty certification in oncology (BCOP). Institutions should develop competency programs that assess their employees' ability to effectively understand all policies and procedures related to handling and verification of hazardous drugs. For pharmacy departments, the competency program should be offered to both pharmacists and pharmacy technicians, albeit with different emphasis on the minimum required competency. For pharmacists, competency programs should include didactic training that addresses medication order entry, reference sources, and skills to review problem orders and complex protocols. For pharmacy technicians, training in aseptic technique, safe handling of chemotherapy agents, and cleaning and disinfecting of the compounding area should be included.

Because of the risk of exposure that is inherent to handling of hazardous agents, all personnel should be certified as competent to perform chemotherapy drug handling. This competency should be verified by a written evaluation, by media-fill testing to verify aseptic technique, by observation of simulated chemotherapy preparation utilizing fluorescein dye as a surrogate marker for chemotherapy, and by observation of compounding technique during normal working conditions. Competency should be verified for all new technicians and at least annually for all currently certified technicians.

Patient or Caregiver Training[1]

Patients and their caregivers should be informed about how to handle hazardous drugs at home if a patient will be receiving infusions with hazardous agents in this setting. Information on how to handle, contain, and dispose of hazardous drug wastes should be part of the education provided. The patient or caregiver should have the knowledge of how to respond immediately to an emergency or critical situation such as an IV catheter breakage or displacement, tubing disconnection, clot formation, flow blockage, and equipment malfunction. Training programs should include a hands-on demonstration and practice with actual items that the patient or caregiver is expected to use. When handling patient waste during or shortly after hazardous drug infusions, the caregiver must wear proper PPE. All waste must be contained and returned to the institution for proper disposal. It is important that the patient and caregiver understand that no hazardous drug waste should be disposed in the household waste.

Conclusion

To minimize exposure to hazardous drugs and ensure patient safety, hazardous drugs must be handled carefully and appropriately. Targeted regulations and processes for preparing, verifying, transporting, and administering hazardous drugs should be implemented. Policies and procedures should be developed to address these needs, and standards established for education and training of personnel involved in handling of hazardous drugs. It is the responsibility of those involved in the preparation process to ensure that safe practices are employed, in addition to ensuring the accuracy and sterility of the final preparation. Although many guidelines have been developed by different organizations, no one set of guidelines can address all the needs of every health-care facility. Consequently, healthcare professionals must exercise their professional judgment, experience, and common sense when applying the guidelines to their unique work setting. In addition, federal, state, and local regulations, as well as the requirements of appropriate accreditation agencies, all need to be considered.

Review Questions

1. List guidelines that are commonly used for handling of hazardous drugs.
2. List drugs that are classified as hazardous.
3. Describe routes through which healthcare workers may be exposed to hazardous drugs.
4. Describe the best recommendation for environmental control for storing and compounding hazardous drugs.
5. Describe the best recommendation for primary engineering controls for compounding hazardous drugs.
6. Describe the personal protective equipment needed for hazardous drug compounding.
7. Describe the proper decontamination procedures for PECs used to compound hazardous drugs.
8. Describe proper handling of a chemotherapy spill.

CASE STUDIES *Case 1*

PL is a newly trained pharmacy technician who is working in the chemotherapy compounding area. While PL was taking a break this morning, 10 boxes of chemotherapy drugs were received. At the end of PL's break, and while he was still in the break room, PL was asked to unpack the chemotherapy drugs and store them on the shelf. PL then went to the receiving area in his scrubs, opened all the boxes, and transported the drugs to the IV room in a cart. You are PL's supervising pharmacist. Which advice would you offer him?

Case 2

The pharmacy was short-staffed today because the employee who typically transports chemotherapy called in sick. In her absence, PL helped transport hazardous drug preparations that he compounded. He exited the room designated for chemotherapy compounding without taking off his gloves, chemotherapy gown, or shoe covers. He was ready to leave the pharmacy with the preparations placed in a cart. As his supervising pharmacist, what advice would you offer him?

References

1. U.S. Pharmacopeial Convention. Chapter <797>: pharmaceutical compounding: sterile preparations. *United States Pharmacopeia 36/National Formulary 31*. Rockville, MD: U.S. Pharmacopeial Convention; 2013.
2. American Society of Health-System Pharmacists. ASHP guidelines on handling hazardous drugs. *Am J Health Syst Pharm*. 2006;63:1172–1191.
3. U.S. Department of Labor, Occupational Safety and Health Administration. Hazard Communication 1910.1200. Available at: http://www.osha.gov/pls/oshaweb/owadisp.show_document? p_table=STANDARDS&p_id=10099. Accessed January 29, 2013.
4. National Institute for Occupational Safety and Health. NIOSH alert: preventing occupational exposures to antineoplastic and other hazardous drugs in health care settings. Available at: http://www.cdc.gov/niosh/docs/2004-165/pdfs/2004-165.pdf. Accessed January 29, 2013.
5. Hemminki K, Kyyronen P, Lindholm ML. Spontaneous abortions and malformations in the offspring of nurses exposed to anesthetic gases, cytostatic drugs, and other potential hazards, based on registered information of outcome. *J Epidemiol Community Health*. 1985;39:141–147.
6. Selevan SG, Lindbohm ML, Hornung RW, et al. A study of occupational exposure to antineoplastic drugs and fetal loss in nurses. *N Engl J Med*. 1985;313:1173–1178.

7. Valanis BG, Vollmer WM, Labuhn KT, et al. Occupational exposure to antineoplastic agents and self-reported infertility among nurses and pharmacists. *J Occup Environ Med.* 1997;39:574–580.

8. Valanis BG, Vollmer WM, Steele P. Occupational exposure to antineoplastic agents: self-reported miscarriages and stillbirths among nurses and pharmacists. *J Occup Environ Med.* 1999;41:632–638.

9. Sessink PJ, Kroese Ed, van Kranen HJ, et al. Cancer risk assessment for health care workers occupationally exposed to cyclophosphamide. *Int Arch Occup Environ Health.* 1995;67:317–323.

10. Wilson JP, Solimando DA Jr. Aseptic technique as a safety precaution in the preparation of antineoplastic agents. *Hosp Pharm.* 1981;16(11):575–576, 579–581.

11. Nygren O, Gustavasson B, Strom L, et al. Exposure to anti-cancer drugs during preparation and administration: investigations of an open and a closed system. *J Environ Monitor.* 2002;4:739–742.

12. Sessink PJ. How to work safely outside the biological safety cabinet [Abstract]. *J Oncol Pharm Pract.* 2000;6:15.

13. Connor TH, Anderson RW, Sessink PJ, et al. Effectiveness of a closed-system device in containing surface contamination with cyclophosphamide and ifosfamide in an i.v. admixture area. *Am J Health-Sys Pharm.* 2002;59:68–72.

14. Vandenbroucke J, Robays H. How to protect environment and employees against cytotoxic agents: the UZ Gent experience. *J Oncol Pharm Pract.* 2001;6:146–152.

15. Spivey S, Connor TH. Determining sources of work-place contamination with antineoplastic drugs and comparing conventional IV drug preparation with a closed system. *Hosp Pharm.* 2003;38:135–139.

16. Wick C, Slawson MH, Jorgenson JA, Tyler LS. Using a closed-system protective device to reduce personal exposure to antineoplastic agents. *Am J Health Syst Pharm.* 2003;60(22):2314–2320.

17. Carmel Pharma. PhaSeal eLearning module. Available at: http://static.phaseal.com/eLearning/index.html. Accessed January 29, 2013.

CHAPTER 9

Multiple Product Preparations for Parenteral Nutrition

Gordon S. Sacks

Chapter Objectives

1. Compare and contrast the advantages and disadvantages of the two delivery methods for parenteral nutrition.
2. Identify the two types of vascular access for administration of parenteral nutrition.
3. Discuss the potential hazards associated with aluminum contamination of the parenteral products used in compounding parenteral nutrition.
4. Distinguish between the two methods used for compounding parenteral nutrition.
5. Explain the recommended guidelines for labeling of parenteral nutrition preparations.
6. Justify the most appropriate testing method to confirm the integrity of compounded parenteral nutrition.
7. Describe the factors that affect the stability, compatibility, and physical characteristics of parenteral nutrition formulations.
8. List the appropriate beyond-use dates for medium-risk preparations stored at room temperature (20–25°C) and under refrigerated conditions (2–8°C).

Key Terminology

Total nutrient admixture (TNA)
2-in-1 admixture
Injectable lipid emulsion (ILE)
Phlebitis
Coring
Automated compounding device (ACD)
Maillard reaction
Gravimetric analysis
Refractometry
Beyond-use date

Overview

Patients often require parenteral preparations that contain more than one sterile product within the same container. These multiple product preparations are used for numerous therapeutic purposes and vary in their content. Most commonly, multiple product preparations are administered for nutritional purposes, such as with parenteral nutrition. Parenteral nutrition (PN) formulations are extremely complex preparations that may contain as many as 50 different components, including carbohydrates, amino acids, fats, electrolytes, vitamins, and trace elements. Two different delivery methods exist for PN formulations: the traditional dextrose–amino acid formulation (2-in-1) and the total nutrient admixture (TNA) system, also known as a 3-in-1 or all-in-one admixture. The TNA system incorporates injectable lipid emulsions (ILEs) into the same container with electrolytes, vitamins, and trace elements, giving it a milky white appearance. In the 2-in-1 system, the dextrose and amino acid base solution contains other prescribed micronutrients combined in one single container. Because ILEs are administered separately as a piggyback infusion with the 2-in-1 formulation, the final preparation will not appear milky white, but rather will be yellow from the addition of multivitamins in the preparation. The decision to utilize one system versus the other is dictated by the types of patients served, convenience, compatibility/stability issues, and logistical issues related to the ordering process and labeling format.

Advantages and Disadvantages of the 2-in-1 System

Historically, ILEs have been administered as a separate infusion directly from the manufacturer's container concurrently with 2-in-1 formulations. Advantages of using this method include that a smaller filter size (0.22-micron) can be used with administration of the dextrose–amino acid base solution to remove pathogenic microorganisms, such as *Staphylococcus epidermidis, Escherichia coli,* and *Candida albicans,* from the PN administration catheter.[1]

When considering the addition of medications to PN formulations, a 2-in-1 system usually confers much greater stability than a TNA system. Stability of PN formulations refers to the ability of additives, including medications, to maintain their chemical integrity and pharmacologic activity. An example of instability would be the photo degradation of some vitamins (e.g., cyanocobalamin, folic acid, pyridoxine) in PN formulations due to excessive light exposure.[2]

In contrast, compatibility issues with PN formulations typically involve precipitate formation, such as crystalline matter, or phase separation of oil and water, as in a TNA. Thus the presence of ILEs in a TNA can determine the stability of the medications as well as the overall compatibility characteristics of the PN formulation. When studies of medications included in 2-in-1 and TNA formulations were performed using simulated Y-site administration, incompatibilities ranged from formation of precipitates to haziness, discoloration, and emulsion disruption with frank separation of oil and water phases.[3,4] **Table 9-1** summarizes the Y-site compatibility of selected medications with 2-in-1 and TNA formulations.[5]

Another benefit of 2-in-1 PN is the decreased risk for divalent or trivalent cations, such as magnesium or iron, to destabilize the PN formulation. These same conditions present in a TNA system can neutralize the negative surface charge of ILEs, causing aggregation of lipid particles into large lipid globules and emulsion destabilization.

Finally, 2-in-1 formulations are more attractive in pediatric patients because pediatric amino acid products have much lower final pH (approximately 5.3) and can irreversibly destabilize or "crack" the emulsion.[6]

Table 9-1 Compatibility of PN with Selected Medications via Y-Site Administration

Medication	Admixture Type	
	2-in-1	TNA
Acyclovir 7 mg/mL D_5W	I	I
Amikacin 5 mg/mL D_5W	C	C
Amphotericin B 0.6 mg/mL D_5W	I	I
Ampicillin 20 mg/mL 0.9% NaCl	C	C
Butorphanol 0.04 mg/mL D_5W	C	C
Cefazolin 20 mg/mL D_5W	I	C
Ceftazidime 40 mg/mL D_5W	C	C
Cimetidine 12 mg/mL D_5W	C	C
Ciprofloxacin 1 mg/mL D_5W	I	C
Cyclosporine 5 mg/mL D_5W	I	I
Dopamine 3200 mcg/mL D_5W	C	I
Dobutamine 4 mg/mL D_5W	C	C
Famotidine 2 mg/mL D_5W	C	C
Fentanyl 12.5 mcg/mL D_5W	C	C
Fentanyl 50 mcg/mL undiluted	C	C
Ganciclovir 20 mg/mL D_5W	I	I
Gentamicin 5 mg/mL D_5W	C	C
Haloperidol 0.2 mg/mL D_5W	C	I
Heparin 100 units/mL undiluted	C	I
Hydromorphone 0.5 mg/mL D_5W	C	I
Insulin 1 unit/mL D_5W	C	C
Lorazepam 0.1 mg/mL D_5W	C	I
Midazolam 2 mg/mL D_5W	I	I
Morphine 1 mg/mL D_5W	C	C
Morphine 15 mg/mL undiluted	NA	I
Ofloxacin 4 mg/mL D_5W	C	C
Ondansetron 1 mg/mL D_5W	C	I
Potassium phosphates 3 mmol/mL undiluted	I	I
Ranitidine 2 mg/mL D_5W	C	C
Sodium bicarbonate 1 mEq/mL undiluted	I	C
Tacrolimus 1 mg/mL D_5W	C	C
Ticarcillin/clavulanate 30/0.1 mg/mL D_5W	C	C
Tobramycin 5 mg/mL D_5W	C	C
Trimethoprim/sulfamethoxazole 0.8/4 mg/mL D_5W	C	C
Vancomycin 10 mg/mL D_5W	C	C
Zidovudine 4 mg/mL D_5W	C	C

C = compatible, I = incompatible, NA = no data available.

By the early 1980s, there was a heightened awareness of the risk for proliferation of pathogenic organisms, both bacterial and fungal, in ILEs administered as separate infusions. This recognition led the Centers for Disease Control and Prevention (CDC) to develop specific guidelines restricting the administration time when ILEs are given separately as a piggyback infusion to no more than 12 hours from the moment the manufacturer's original container is opened.[7] In an effort to simplify PN administration procedures, it was proposed that ILEs be admixed directly into the PN formulation to provide a total daily infusion in one large container. Thus the concept of the TNA was created, and this new delivery mode was recognized as offering several major advantages relative to 2-in-1 systems.

ALERT: *Injectable lipid emulsions should be administered within 12 hours of opening the original container.*

Advantages and Disadvantages of the TNA System

Use of the TNA system involves a single container for infusion over 24 hours, which offers an increased convenience for administration and a reduced risk for microbial contamination resulting from fewer manipulations or entries into the central venous catheter. Although there were initial concerns about increased microbial growth with this approach because the ILEs (as a component of the TNA) were hanging for greater than 12 hours, the risk of infection actually proved to be decreased: The hypertonic and acidic environment created from the addition of ILEs to the PN formulation inhibited the growth of most microorganisms.

Additional advantages of this system include a more efficient preparation for pharmacy personnel, especially if automated technology is used. Because all of the components are combined into a single container, there are fewer supply and equipment expenses, resulting from the need for only one infusion pump and administration tubing set. The TNA system is especially welcomed by the home-care community because of its more convenient storage, administration, and overall cost savings. Finally, there may be improved fat clearance in some patients from infusing ILEs over 24 hours, as compared to the less than 12 hours' infusion when ILEs are administered as a separate piggyback infusion.

Table 9-2 identifies the primary advantages and disadvantages associated with the TNA delivery mode for PN.[8]

Table 9-2 Advantages and Disadvantages of the Total Nutrient Admixture System

Advantages

- All components aseptically compounded by the pharmacy
- Preparation is more efficient for pharmacy personnel, especially if automated
- Less manipulation of the system during administration
- Less risk of contamination during administration
- Inhibited or slower bacterial growth if contamination does occur, compared to separate injectable lipid emulsion (ILE) administration
- Less nursing time needed for one container per day and no piggyback ILE to administer
- Less supply and equipment expense—only one infusion pump and IV tubing
- More convenient storage, fewer supplies, easier administration in home care settings
- Dextrose and venous access tolerance may be better in some situations
- Possible applications in fluid-restricted patients because ILE 30% is restricted to use in TNA
- May be more cost-effective overall in certain settings
- Fat clearance may be better when ILE is administered over more than 12 hours

Disadvantages

- Larger particle size of admixed ILE precludes use of a 0.22-micron (bacteria-eliminating) filter, and requires a larger pore size filter of 1.2 microns
- Admixed ILE is less stable and more prone to separation of lipid components
- Formulations are more sensitive to destabilization with certain electrolyte concentrations
- Formulations are more sensitive to destabilization with low concentrations of dextrose and amino acids
- Lower pH amino acid formulations may destabilize the ILE portion of the admixture

- Formulation may be unstable when the final concentration of ILE is low

- Difficult to visualize precipitate or particulate material in the opaque admixture

- Certain medications are incompatible with the ILE portion of the admixture

- Catheter occlusion is more common with daily ILE

- Less stable over time than dextrose–amino acids PN formulations with separate ILE

Peripheral Parenteral Nutrition

PN formulations are usually administered as highly concentrated, hypertonic, and hyperosmolar solutions. These preparations are administered through a large-diameter central vein, where they can be diluted by a rapid blood flow so as to prevent any vein damage. The preferred anatomic sites for central access to the vascular system include the subclavian, jugular, and femoral veins. The usual position of the central venous catheter is the superior vena cava. Because this vessel is located near the body's vital organs and blood supplies, catheter placement is verified by radiograph. Both the 2-in-1 and TNA systems can be infused through a central venous access device.

If a peripheral vein is used for administration of PN, the formulation given must be less hypertonic. Peripheral parenteral nutrition (PPN) formulations have osmolarities of approximately 700–900 mOsm/L.[9,10] Concentrations of electrolytes, such as calcium and potassium, should be decreased to minimize the risk of phlebitis and damage to peripheral veins. For some institutions, this may equate to a calcium concentration of 5 mEq/L and a potassium concentration of 40 mEq/L or less. ILEs are typically infused via the same line and administered over 24 hours, with the container being replaced every 12 hours to comply with the 12-hour hang time limit. It has been suggested that daily infusion of ILEs through the same peripheral line may provide a venous lumen–protective effect. The limitation of low osmolarities for PPN administration results in relatively dilute formulations in large-volume quantities (i.e., 2.4–3 L) to deliver close to the necessary nutrient requirements. As a result, patients who cannot tolerate large fluid volumes (e.g., those with congestive heart failure or end-stage renal disease) are poor candidates for this modality.

When final concentrations of amino acids are less than 4%, dextrose less than 10%, and ILEs less than 2% (conditions that might be observed with PPN formulations), TNA stability has been shown to be compromised.[6] Coalescence of sub-micrometer droplets into large fat globules often occurs before the 30-hour beyond-use date is reached. Thus the use of a TNA system for PPN formulations is unsafe and 2-in-1 formulations with separate piggyback infusions of ILEs must be used as the preferred modality for nutrient provision.

Formation of insoluble dibasic calcium phosphate precipitates is also a much greater risk in low-osmolality formulations, such as PPN.[10] Reports of significant respiratory failure and death have been noted, especially among patients receiving incompatible formulations found to contain dibasic calcium phosphate precipitates. Extreme care must be taken by the compounding pharmacist to ensure that concentrations of calcium and phosphate are verified against published product-specific solubility curves.

> **ALERT:** *Concentrations of calcium and phosphate must be verified against published product-specific solubility curves to prevent incompatible formulations.*

Aluminum Contamination

Several of the small-volume parenteral products used in compounding have been shown to be contaminated with aluminum. This phenomenon arises primarily from the introduction of raw materials adulterated with aluminum as well as the leaching of aluminum over time from glass containers and elastomeric closures.[11] Products found to be the most highly contaminated include specific amino acids, calcium and phosphate salts, and some trace elements and vitamin products. Under normal conditions, the gastrointestinal tract acts as an effective barrier and allows less than 1% to reach the systemic circulation after aluminum ingestion. However, when aluminum bypasses the gastrointestinal tract through contamination of parenteral products, the only mechanism available to prevent aluminum toxicity is renal excretion through the kidneys. As a result, infants and neonates with immature renal function and adults with significant kidney impairment are especially vulnerable to developing aluminum toxicity. Alterations in bone formation and mineralization, encephalopathy, reduced parathyroid hormone secretion, and impaired neurologic development have been observed in pediatric patients, adults patients receiving long-term PN, and patients with renal dysfunction.[12]

In 2004, the Food and Drug Administration (FDA) mandated that manufacturers of products used in compounding PN disclose on the label the aluminum content of their small- and large-volume parenteral products.[13] The safe upper limit for aluminum in large-volume parenteral products (i.e., amino acids, concentrated dextrose, ILEs, and sterile water for injection) was set at 25 mcg/L, whereas labels on small-volume parenteral products (i.e., electrolyte salts) and pharmacy bulk packages (i.e., parenteral multivitamins) had to state that "no more than 25 mcg/L of aluminum" was provided at product expiration. The FDA also determined that 4–5 mcg/kg/day was the upper limit of acceptable aluminum exposure in humans.

ALERT: *Aluminum contamination is a concern with PN. Exposure to aluminum should not exceed 4–5 mcg/kg/day.*

Parenteral Nutrition Preparation Methods

According to United States Pharmacopeia (USP) Chapter <797>, the procedures and requirements for compounded sterile preparations (CSPs) must be followed when compounding PN formulations. PN is classified as a "medium-risk level" CSP when it is prepared from crystalline amino acids and commercially available monohydrated dextrose, ILEs, electrolytes, multiple vitamins, trace elements, and sterile water. It carries a higher level of risk because it requires the mixing of multiple small doses of different sterile products into one large bag.[14] When PN is compounded using powdered amino acids, however, it is classified as a high-risk level CSP because its preparation involves the use of non-sterile ingredients and carries the highest risk for contamination by microbial, chemical, or physical matter. As a result, high-risk level CSPs must undergo some type of sterilization process prior to administration.

All risk-level compounds should be prepared in an environment in which particulate matter and microorganisms are minimized, and the air quality must meet certain standards. Pharmacies must be designed specifically to meet the standards, which require an ante-room and a buffer area to separate the general environment from the area of compounding. Levels of cleanliness and limits of particulate matter are defined for all areas by International Standards Organization (ISO) classifications. PN formulations prepared from sterile products are compounded in an ISO Class 5 environment, which means that there are no more than 3520 circulating particles of size 0.5 micrometer per cubic meter. Additional discussion and classification of environmental controls can be found in the *Primary and Secondary Engineering Controls* chapter.

Both automated and manual methods of PN compounding are available. The preparation of PN formulations by the manual method involves the transfer of separate nutrients, with the aid of sterile solution transfer sets and via syringe and needle delivery, into one final sterile container that provides a 24-hour supply of nutrients. These formulations may also be mixed into empty 1-liter bags. During preparation of PN using the manual method, transfer sets are connected to large-volume parenteral products that are typically hung in a laminar airflow workbench. Contents of the manufacturers' partial-fill bags or bottles flow into a final large empty container with the use of gravity. Small-volume parenteral products and components stored in pharmacy bulk packages are typically drawn up into syringes and admixed into the final container using a syringe and needle. This process can be quite labor intensive and requires multiple manipulations of infusion containers, syringes, and needles, all of which increase the risk for extrinsic contamination of the final admixture. When using syringes and needles, there is also a danger of introducing particulate matter from the elastomeric or rubber tops of vials (i.e., "coring") into the final infusion container.[8]

With the advent of automated technology, the PN compounding process became more accurate, less time-consuming, and more cost-effective, with a decreased risk for touch contamination. These automated compounding devices (ACDs) use dedicated computer software interfaced with bar-code technology to test for source-solution errors, rely on electronically stored curves to predict calcium/phosphate incompatibilities, and perform end-product verifications to confirm compounding accuracy. With improved accuracy, PN formulations can also be customized to meet patient-specific requirements compared to the practice of using volumes of convenience (i.e., 250- or 500-mL volumes for dextrose) with the manual method. Currently in the United States, there are two commercially available ACDs: ExactaMix Compounding Systems (Baxter Healthcare Corporation, Deerfield, IL) and Pinnacle TPN Management System (B. Braun Medical Inc., Bethlehem, PA).

In addition to manual or automated methods used for compounding PN formulations, manufacturer-premixed PN formulations are available in a variety of forms for central and peripheral vein administration. These products may already contain a standard amount of electrolytes or may be electrolyte free. Parenteral multivitamins and trace element solutions must still be added to these products to make them nutritionally complete. These products are also manufactured in multichamber bags that must be mixed or "activated" just prior to administration to combine the dextrose and amino acid components. Commercially available formulations of dextrose and amino acids already mixed together are not possible because the temperatures required for sterilization would result in the "browning" or Maillard reaction—that is, a chemical reaction between intravenous dextrose and certain amino acids, such as lysine. The occurrence of the Maillard reaction is identified by the presence of a brownish discoloration of a final 2-in-1 formulation.[15]

Labeling Parenteral Nutrition Formulations

The American Society for Parenteral and Enteral Nutrition (A.S.P.E.N.) has developed safe practice guidelines that outline best practices for labeling parenteral nutrition.[9] **Figure 9-1** provides an example template.

Because PN formulations are complex pharmaceutical preparations with multiple ingredients, their labels must display the ingredients in the most straightforward way possible. Each label must also list other required elements, including the route of administration, date and time for administration, infusion rate (expressed in mL/hr over 24 hours), beyond-use date, and dosing weight. The dosing weight is included so that anyone can determine whether the nutrient doses are appropriate by reading the PN label. A healthcare organization must standardize all labels so that each PN component is listed (i.e., base solutions, electrolyte additives, micronutrients, medications) in the amount per day for adult patients to avoid any misinterpretation. For neonatal or pediatric patients, nutrient doses should be labeled as amount per kilogram per day. Optional columns on the label may be included to reflect amount/day or amount/100 mL.

All ingredients should be listed in the same sequence and same units of measure as on the PN order. Electrolytes should be ordered as the complete salt form rather than the individual ion. Each individual macronutrient and micronutrient ordered should also be listed with its corresponding dose. If ILEs are to be infused separately, a separate label should be used on this product to reflect the amount per day, administration rate, and infusion duration.

For home/alternative-site PN labels, a list of patient/caregiver additives should be included on the label; these additives should be easily identified and differentiated from the other PN

Institution/Pharmacy Name   **Address and Pharmacy Phone number**

Name _____   Dosing Weight _____   Location _____
Administration Date/Time _____   Do Not Use Afer: Date/time _____

Base Formula	Amount/day	(Amount/L)
Dextrose	**g**	(g/L)
Amino acids[a]	**g**	(g/L)
Lipid[a]	**g**	(g/L)

Electrolytes

Sodium chloride	**mEq**	(mEq/L)
Sodium acetate	**mEq**	(mEq/L)
Potassium chloride	**mEq**	(mEq/L)
Potassium acetate	**mEq**	(mEq/L)
Potassium phosphate	**mmol of P**	(mmol/L)
(mEq of K)		(mEq/L)
Sodium phosphate	**mmol of P**	(mmol/L)
(mEq of Na)		(mEq/L)
Calcium gluconate	**mEq**	(mEq/L)
Magnesium sulfate	**mEq**	(mEq/L)

Vitamins, trace elements and medications

Multiple vitamins[a]	**mL**	
Multiple trace elements[a]	**mL**	
Insulin	**Units**	(Units/L)
H_2 - antagonists[a]	**mg**	
Rate mL/hour	Volume mL	Infuse over___hours

Formulation contains _____ mL plus _____ mL overfill

Discard any unused volume after 24 hours

Central Line Use Only

[a] Specify product name.

g = gram.

Reproduced with permission *JPEN J Parenter Enteral Nutr* 2004;28(suppl): S39-S70.

Figure 9-1A   Standard PN Label Template – Adult Patient

Institution/Pharmacy Name, Address and Pharmacy Phone Number

Name _____ Dosing Weight _____ Location _____
Administration Date/Time _____ Do Not Use Afer: Date/time _____

Volume   Amount/kg /day   Amount/day

Intravenous fat emulsion[a] (%)   ___ mL   ___ gram/kg ___ gram

Infusion rate _____mL/hour Infuse over hours

May contain overfill - Discard any unused volume after 12 hours

For peripheral or central line administration

[a] Specify brand name

Reproduced with permission from *JPEN J Parenter Enteral Nutr* 2004;28(suppl): S39-S70.

Figure 9-1B Standard ILE Label Template - Adult, Neonate or Pediatric Patient

components. Highlighting or attaching an asterisk may be used to identify the additives that are added just prior to administration.

Compounding personnel should have a standard procedure for verifying the contents of the finished product, by comparing the finished labeled PN product to the original order. Using a double-check procedure for verification of contents is considered best practice.

Quality Assurance for PN Compounding

End-product testing of PN formulations must be performed to ensure the accuracy and precision of the final compounded preparation. In light of the complex nature of PN formulations, several different processes exist to identify flawed and unsafe compounding practices. When multiple additive containers are used to manually compound PN formulations, all empty containers must be presented to a pharmacist for visual confirmation of the amount of each ingredient prior to its addition into the final container. Alternatively, syringes with prescribed volumes of each ingredient can be positioned on the LAFW surface next to the vial from which the contents were withdrawn. A pharmacist can then verify the contents and volumes of each syringe prior to all ingredients being added to the final container. Proxy methods of verification for addition of ingredients, such as the syringe pull-back method, are not recommended and should not be used without the presence of the actual original-source containers (including medication diluents).[16]

Most ACDs use gravimetric and volumetric methods to verify the accuracy of the compounding process. In gravimetric analysis, the volume of each component added to the final PN container is measured. If the weight of the final preparation is considerably different from the theoretical weight calculated by the ACD, a warning message alerts personnel to the possibility of a compounding error. Some ACDs are capable of determining the weight of each individual component as well as the final product. Gravimetric analysis can also be used as an independent quality control measure for automated or manual compounding methods. Individual additive containers with narrow margins of safety (e.g., concentrated potassium chloride solutions) can be weighed by an analytical balance to assess the accuracy of delivery to the final PN formulation.[9]

Refractometry is an alternative technique that can establish whether a PN formulation was prepared correctly. The refractive indices of dextrose and amino acids can be measured and compared to established values for known concentrations of these macronutrients. If the measured values vary significantly from the expected results, the PN formulation may have been erroneously compounded. Inability to measure a refractive index of ILEs prevents the use of this technique to assess the integrity of TNA formulations. Refractive indices are also indirect measurements of dextrose or amino acid concentrations, so chemical analysis can be used to directly measure the final content of these individual components of PN formulations.[9]

Implementation of technology and automation is recommended for the safe compounding of sterile products.[16] Some ACDs use numbered, color-coordinated tubing sets and barcode verification for source containers and patient formulations to reduce the risk of errors. Guidelines recommend that personnel who operate ACDs should also trace each tubing set from the source container to the port where it is attached during the initial daily setup and with each change of a source container.[16] ACD tubing changes must occur at appropriate time intervals as per manufacturer recommendations; if such changes are not made, mortality from infections transmitted through contaminated solutions can result.[17]

ALERT: *Personnel who operate ACDs should trace each tubing set from the source container to the port where it is attached during the initial daily setup and with each change of a source container.*

Despite the optimal use of ACDs, reports of unsafe compounding procedures continue to occur. An incorrect mixing sequence of PN components and an elevated pH of the final PN admixture were critical issues in the fatal events that prompted the 1996 FDA safety alert.[18] Four patients died of unexplained respiratory distress due to the deposition of dibasic calcium phosphate crystals in the pulmonary vasculature. The calcium and phosphate concentrations did not exceed the solubility limit in the *final* PN formulation. However, the calcium gluconate salt form was added when only 46% of the PN volume had been pumped into the final container and before the 70% dextrose injection was included; thus the final pH values for the lethal formulations were much higher than anticipated. As pH rises, the danger of calcium phosphate precipitation due to the increased formation of dibasic calcium phosphate increases in tandem. Lack of in-line filtration, failure to agitate the PN formulation sufficiently prior to administration, and the short time frame between completion of the compounding process and the beginning of PN administration were all factors that contributed to the formation of an insoluble dibasic calcium phosphate precipitate.[19]

> **TIP:** *Calcium and phosphate salts should not be added in close sequence when preparing PN. Separating the addition of these two products in an admixture can avoid calcium phosphate precipitation.*

Compatibility and Stability of PN Formulations

Every effort must be made to ensure that PN formulations are compatible and stable to avoid patient-related complications. As mentioned previously, precipitation is central to the concept of incompatibility, whereas the inability of PN components to maintain their chemical integrity is indicative of instability. General factors that influence the stability of PN formulations include temperature, pH, exposure to light and oxygen, composition, and compounding sequence.

Temperature can play a key role in the risk for precipitation of specific electrolytes. As temperature is increased, the calcium salts (chloride or gluconate) are dissociated more completely and more calcium ions become available for precipitation. Therefore, an increase in temperature increases the possibility that dibasic calcium phosphate precipitates might form. Furthermore, room temperature accelerates the degradation of several amino acids (e.g., tryptophan, arginine, methionine) when compared to refrigeration temperatures.[9]

Changes in pH can dramatically influence the characteristics of a final PN formulation. While a higher pH confers greater stability for ILEs, the converse is true for calcium and phosphorus solubility.

Degradation of selected vitamins and amino acids can be hastened by exposure to oxygen and fluorescent lights. Consequently, light protection of the final admixture is usually recommended for neonatal patients exposed to high levels of ultraviolet light in the treatment of neonatal jaundice.[8]

Stability of PN formulations is also greatly affected by the specific doses and nutrient combinations it contains. Concentrated dextrose solutions should never be added directly to ILEs because their acidic pH can destabilize emulsions in TNAs. Instead, dextrose should first be mixed with amino acid solutions because of their ability to act as a buffer and enhance stability. Excess cation amounts, such as divalent calcium and magnesium, can decrease or neutralize the negative surface charge exerted by the egg phospholipid emulsifying agent in ILEs. This effect would remove the repulsive force, thereby allowing fat droplets to aggregate; the ultimate result would be irreversible separation of the oil and water phases, producing an unstable TNA.[20]

TIP: *To enhance stability of a TNA, mix concentrated dextrose and amino acids together prior to admixing other additives and ILEs.*

Compounding personnel should always inspect the physical appearance of the final PN formulation.[9] Although micro-precipitates and incompatibilities cannot be seen by the naked eye, large particle contaminants or precipitates are the most likely particulates to immediately harm the patient, and they can easily be detected before the product is dispensed. For PN formulations without ILEs, the product should be inspected against a dark background for the presence of particulates, such as fibers from alcohol wipes, cores of additive vials, or insoluble precipitates. Compounding personnel should also look for any signs of crystallization or for haziness of the product. For PN admixtures with lipid emulsions, compounding personnel should examine the bag for any signs of a cracked emulsion, such as separation of components into an oil layer or fat droplets. Finally, access to and use of any ACD equipment for PN preparation should be available only to personnel who have been appropriately trained and demonstrated competency in this area to ensure the continued safety of compounding operations.[16]

> **TIP:** *ILEs should be added last when preparing TNAs. Because the addition of ILEs causes the CSP to become an opaque, milky-white color, the presence of ILEs makes it difficult to identify incompatibilities in the final preparation.*

> **ALERT:** *All preparations should be checked against a contrasting background for incompatibilities.*

Storage and Use of PN Admixtures

A beyond-use date should appear on every PN label. The concept of a beyond-use date is similar but clearly different from an expiration date. Whereas expiration dates are based on rigorous tests of the chemical stability of manufactured sterile products, beyond-use dates reflect the risk level of the CSP with consideration given to the time and temperature at which the preparation will be stored. According to USP Chapter <797> standards, a beyond-use date for a PN admixture prepared for inpatient administration is 30 hours based on storage at room temperature and a medium risk level.[14] In the home-care environment, the beyond-use date can be extended to 9 days as long as PN admixtures are stored at 2–8°C (36–46°F) until use. The 30-hour time limit still applies once the PN infusion is initiated. Further discussion on beyond-use dates is presented in the *Principles of Compatibility and Stability* chapter.

Conclusion

PN formulations are extremely complex admixtures that may contain as many as 50 components, so tremendous care must be taken to ensure the safe preparation and delivery of this intricate therapy. Despite the successful use of PN formulations for more than four decades, adverse events continue to occur that may result in serious patient harm or even death. Several components of PN solutions have been found to contain variable amounts of aluminum that are inherently present in certain raw materials or intrinsically introduced during the manufacturing process. Physicochemical incompatibilities have resulted from improper admixing practices and administration of unsafe PN formulations. Standardized templates for labeling PN formulations must be used to avoid misinterpretation of the PN contents, volume, and infusion rate. It is the responsibility of pharmacists involved in the preparation and delivery of PN formulations to have an in-depth understanding of the principles associated with safe administration of these CSPs.

Review Questions

1. Current FDA guidelines mandate that in patients with impaired kidney function, including premature neonates, maximum daily intake of aluminum (Al) should *not* exceed
   a. 1–2 mcg/kg/day
   b. 3–4 mcg/kg/day
   c. 4–5 mcg/kg/day
   d. 6–7 mcg/kg/day

2. Which of the following is an advantage of the TNA system over the 2-in-1 system?
   a. Allows the use of a larger pore size filter (1.2 micron)
   b. Improved stability with low concentrations of dextrose and amino acids
   c. Preparation is more efficient for pharmacy personnel
   d. Increased medication compatibility of medications with the ILEs portion of the admixture

3. Which of the following is a limitation of peripherally administered parenteral nutrition (PPN) formulations?
   a. Categorized as a high-risk level compounded sterile product

b. Requires large-volume quantities to deliver the necessary nutrient requirements

c. Increases the difficulty of visualizing precipitates or particulate matter

d. Prevents the use of an automated compounding device for preparation

4. According to USP Chapter <797>, what is the assigned risk level for a PN formulation prepared from powdered amino acids?

a. Low

b. Medium

c. High

d. Extremely high

5. Which of the following must be added to commercially available premixed PN formulations so these products are nutritionally complete?

a. Electrolytes

b. Branched-chain amino acids

c. Parenteral multivitamins

d. Glycerol

6. What is the *most* appropriate method for the product label to identify a PN formulation as containing dextrose 150 g per day in a total volume of 1000 mL?

a. Dextrose 15% (percentage of the final concentration after admixture)

b. Dextrose 150 g per day (grams per day)

c. Dextrose 150 g per liter (grams per liter of PN admixed)

d. Dextrose 30% water, 500 mL (percentage of the original concentration and volume)

7. Which of the following is an example of an automated compounding device using volumetric analysis to ensure the accuracy of the compounding process?

a. Direct measurement of the final PN dextrose concentration

b. Measuring the refractive index of the PN dextrose content

    c. Performing daily ACD tubing changes

    d. Weighing the final PN admixture

8. According to USP Chapter <797>, what is the beyond-use date for a PN admixture stored under refrigerated conditions (2–8°C)?

    a. 30 hours

    b. 3 days

    c. 9 days

    d. 14 days

CASE STUDY

A pharmacy technician in training is preparing a TNA formulation. You are the pharmacist who will be providing verification of the final preparation. The technician has placed all vials of the components of the preparation within the laminar airflow workbench (LAFW). Next to each vial is the syringe with the appropriate volume drawn into the syringe. The dextrose, amino acids, and lipid emulsions have not been added yet. Which directions, regarding the sequence of adding all components, will you provide to the technician?

The technician adds the ingredients of the parenteral nutrition as you suggested. You will now be verifying the preparation prior to its distribution to the patient for administration. What should you look for during the verification process?

References

1. Bethune K, Allwood M, Grainger C, Wormleighton C. Use of filters during the preparation and administration of parenteral nutrition: position paper and guidelines prepared by a British Pharmaceutical Nutrition Group Working Party. *Nutrition.* 2001;17:403–408.
2. Smith JL, Canham JE, Wells PA. Effect of phototherapy light, sodium bisulfite, and pH on vitamin stability in total parenteral nutrition admixtures. *J Parenter Enteral Nutr.* 1988;12:394–402.

3. Trissel LA, Gilbert DL, Martinez JF, et al. Compatibility of medications with 3-in-1 parenteral nutrition admixtures. *J Parenter Enteral Nutr.* 199;23:67–74.

4. Trissel LA, Gibert DL, Martinez JF, et al. Compatibility of parenteral nutrient solutions with selected drugs during simulated Y-site administration. *Am J Health Syst Pharm.* 1997;54:1295–1300.

5. Sacks GS. Drug–nutrient considerations in patients receiving parenteral and enteral nutrition. *Prac Gastroenterol.* 2004;XXVIII(7):39–46.

6. Driscoll DF. Lipid injectable emulsions: 2006. *Nutr Clin Pract.* 2006;21:381–386.

7. Pearson ML. Hospital Infection Control Practices Advisory Committee: guidelines for prevention of intravascular device-related infections. *Infect Control Hosp Epidemiol.* 1996;17:438–473.

8. Barber JR, Sacks GS. Parenteral Nutrition Formulations. In: Mueller CM, ed. *The A.S.P.E.N. adult nutrition support core curriculum.* 2nd ed. Silver Spring, MD: A.S.P.E.N.; 2012:245–264.

9. Mirtallo J, Canada TW, Johnson D, et al. Safe practices for parenteral nutrition. *J Parenter Enteral Nutr.* 2004;28(suppl): S39–S70.

10. Joy J, Silvestri AP, Franke R, et al. Calcium and phosphate compatibility in low-osmolarity parenteral nutrition admixtures intended for peripheral vein administration. *J Parenter Enteral Nutr.* 2010;34:46–54.

11. Klein GL. Aluminum contamination of parenteral nutrition solutions and its impact on the pediatric patient. *Nutr Clin Pract.* 2003;18:302–307.

12. Klein GL. Aluminum in parenteral solutions revisited—again. *Am J Clin Nutr.* 1995;61:449–456.

13. Department of Health and Human Services, Food and Drug Administration. Aluminum in large and small volume parenterals used in total parenteral nutrition. *Federal Reg.* 2000;65(17):4103–4111.

14. U.S. Pharmacopeial Convention. Chapter <797>: pharmaceutical compounding: sterile preparations. *United States Pharmacopeia 36/National Formulary 31.* Rockville, MD: U.S. Pharmacopeial Convention; 2013.

15. Newton DW. Introduction: physicochemical determinants of incompatibility and instability of drugs for injection and

infusion. In: Trissel LA, ed. *Handbook on injectable drugs.* 3rd ed. Bethesda, MD: American Society of Hospital Pharmacists; 1983:xiii–xv.

16. Proceedings from the ISMP Sterile Preparation Compounding Safety Summit: guidelines for SAFE preparation of sterile compounds. Horsham, PA: Institute for Safe Medication Practices; October 2011. Available at: http://http://www.ismp.org/Tools/guidelines/IVSummit/IVCGuidelines.pdf

17. Anonymous. Two children die after receiving infected TPN solutions. *Pharm J.* 1994;252:596.

18. Hill SF, Heldman LS, Goo ED, et al. Fatal microvascular pulmonary emboli from precipitation of a total nutrient admixture solution. *J Parenter Enteral Nutr.* 1996;20:81–87.

19. Newton DW, Driscoll DF. Calcium and phosphate compatibility: revisited again. *Am J Health-Syst Pharm.* 2008;65:73–80.

20. Driscoll DF. Stability and compatibility assessment techniques for total parenteral nutrition admixtures: setting the bar according to pharmacopeial standards. *Curr Opin Clin Nutr Metab Care.* 2005;8:297–303.

CHAPTER 10

Considerations for Intravenous Drug Therapy in Infants and Children

Sherry Luedtke

Chapter Objectives

1. Describe methods for preparing dilutions for parenteral medications for use in infants and children.
2. List factors to consider in the development of standard concentrations for use in infants and children.
3. Identify parenteral drug additives and contaminants to avoid in infants and children.
4. Describe the influence of intravenous (IV) access and volume restrictions on drug preparation and dispensing in children.
5. Differentiate the capabilities of large- and small-volume infusion devices.
6. Develop practices in parenteral drug preparation that minimize the risk for medication errors in children.

Key Terminology

Geometric dilution
Standard concentration
Benzyl alcohol

Propylene glycol
Methylparaben
DEHP
Central venous catheter (CVC)
Percutaneous central venous catheter (PCVC)
Intraosseous (IO) catheter
Microbore tubing
Macrobore tubing
Dead space
Small-volume pump
Large-volume pump
Smart pump
Extravasation
Infiltration
Vesicant
Phlebitis
Thrombophlebitis

Overview

The preparation of parenteral medications for the pediatric patient poses numerous challenges. Medications for infants and young children do not merely require smaller doses; rather, their selection and preparation must consider the limits associated with available drug formulations, infusion volumes, parenteral access, catheter and tubing sets, and infusion devices. An understanding of these limitations is essential for accurate preparation and safe delivery of drugs via the parenteral route.

Dilutions

One of the greatest challenges faced in the preparation of parenteral medications for infants and young children is the lack of "pediatric-friendly" formulations. The concentrations of most medications have been developed for delivery of adult dosages. To obtain a concentration that allows one to accurately measure the small doses needed for a young infant, preparations must be

Table 10-1   Drugs Commonly Requiring Dilution
in Infants and Children

Aminophylline
Amphotericin
Clonidine
Dexamethasone
Digoxin
Famotidine
Filgrastim
Heparin
Hydralazine
Hydrocortisone
Levothyroxine
Methylprednisolone
Phenobarbital
Sodium bicarbonate

diluted from commercially available "adult" formulation via geometric dilution. Typically, a 2-, 5-, or 10-fold dilution is employed.
For example, if a drug comes in a formulation of 100 mg/mL and a
dose of 2 mg is needed for an infant, the 100 mg/mL solution will
typically be diluted by 10-fold to achieve a 10 mg/mL solution and,
therefore, to be able to accurately measure 2 mg (0.2 mL) of drug.
Intravenous digoxin, for example, commonly requires dilution
for measurement of the small doses necessary for young infants.
Digoxin is commercially available in a 100 mcg/mL IV solution.
Most institutions require the use of a diluted solution (10 mcg/
mL) for preparation of doses less than 10 mcg. **Table 10-1** lists
medications that are commonly used in neonates and children
and require dilution for accurate measurement.

The accuracy of preparing drugs with dosing volumes less
than 1 mL is of greatest concern, because small errors of even
0.1 mL dosing volume can result in a significant overdose or
underdose. Most institutions recommend 0.2 mL as the minimal
dose volume that should be dispensed for parenteral administration to a pediatric patient. Thus the dilution factor used to prepare a medication is often dictated by this minimal dose volume

(approximately 0.2 mL). In addition, medications that require a specific infusion time may require further dilution to provide an adequate volume to be infused over that given time. If a dose volume of 0.2 mL is to be infused over an hour, for example, many institutions will dispense it in a final volume of 2–3 mL to ensure an accurate infusion rate, depending on the infusion device employed (see the discussion of infusion devices later in this chapter).

ALERT: *Care should be taken when preparing drugs with dosing volumes less than 1 mL, as small errors can result in significant dosing variances.*

The use of geometric dilutions for preparation of neonatal and pediatric formulations adds not only an extra step in the process of preparation, but also an additional risk for error. Numerous cases of fatal overdoses have occurred due to dilution errors that resulted in 10- to 100-fold overdoses of drugs.[1,2] Unfortunately, these errors are not isolated cases, because most institutions prepare a diluted solution or "batch" that is used for all patients throughout the institution receiving the given medication. One error in preparing a dilution, therefore, impacts every infant or young child receiving the same medication dispensed from that batch.

In an effort to reduce such medication errors, institutions should develop policies and procedures for medication dilution concentrations and steps for preparation, double-check policies for verifying dilutions, and methods for documenting and tracking dilution batches.[3,4] The Institute for Safe Medication Practices' (ISMP) *Guidelines for Sterile Product Preparation* recommends that preparation labels (for the dilution product) and formulation records/worksheets be available when preparing dilutions for children. Many institutions utilize dilution logs or records to reduce the risk of errors (**Figure 10-1**). Pertinent information should be documented on these logs, such as the drug name, base solution, patient-specific dose, preparation calculations, final volume of the preparation, and dose form to be used (concentration and container).[3,4]

Example Formulation Record/Dilution Card

Drug Name: _____

Date	Batch/ Control #	Dilution Prepared	Manufacturer's Lot /Exp Date	Dilution Exp Date	Quantity Prepared	Prepared By	Checked By

Preparation Calculations:

Figure 10-1   Example Formulation Record/Dilution Card

Standard Concentrations

Traditionally, it was common practice to individualize concentrations of continuous infusions of drugs for use in pediatric patients based on body weight using a method referred to as the "Rule of Six"; however, in 2003, The Joint Commission issued National Patient Safety Goals (NPSGs) in an effort to standardize and limit the number of concentrations of drugs.[5,6] The use of standard concentrations can reduce the medication error risk that inherently exists when numerous concentrations are available. Standard concentrations also allow for adoption of drug libraries for programming into smart pump infusion devices, as described in the *Supplies and Equipment for Compounding and Administering Sterile Preparations* chapter. The American Society of Health Systems Pharmacists (ASHP) policy statements support the use of standard concentrations.[7] In addition to ASHP, the ISMP and the Vermont Oxford Group (a nonprofit group advocating for improved care of neonates) have drafted a standard concentrations list for adoption as national standard concentrations (**Table 10-2**).[8] Unfortunately, we remain far away from the adoption of national standard concentrations, and institutions

Table 10-2   Recommended Standard Concentrations of Neonatal Drug Infusions

Drug	Type(s) of Infusions	Recommended Concentrations
Acyclovir	Intermittent infusion	7 mg/mL
Alprostadil	Continuous infusion	10 mcg/mL
Amphotericin B	Intermittent infusion	0.1 mg/mL
Amphotericin B liposomal	Intermittent infusion	1 mg/mL
Cefazolin	Intermittent infusion	100 mg/mL
Cefotaxime	Intermittent infusion	100 mg//mL
Clindamycin	Intermittent infusion	6 mg/mL
Digoxin	Intermittent infusion	20 mcg/mL
		100 mcg/mL
Dobutamine	Continuous infusion	2000 mcg/mL
Dopamine	Continuous infusion	1600 mcg/mL
Epinephrine	Continuous infusion	10 mcg/mL
Fentanyl	Continuous/intermittent infusion	10 mcg/mL
Fluconazole	Intermittent infusion	2 mg/mL
Furosemide	Continuous/intermittent infusion	2 mg/mL
		10 mg/mL
Gentamicin	Intermittent infusion	2 mg/mL
		10 mg/mL
Heparin (in 0.45% NaCl)	Continuous infusion for line patency	0.5 unit/mL
Insulin (regular)	Continuous infusion	0.1 unit/mL
		0.5 unit/mL

Metronidazole	Intermittent infusion	5 mg/mL
Midazolam	Continuous	0.5 mg/mL
	Intermittent infusion	1 mg/mL (preservative free)
Morphine	Continuous and intermittent infusion	0.1 mg/mL
	Intermittent infusion	0.5 mg/mL
Norepinephrine	Continuous infusion	16 mcg/mL
Phenobarbital	Intermittent infusion	10 mg/mL
		65 mg/mL
Vancomycin	Intermittent infusion	5 mg/mL

Source: Institute for Safe Medication Practices, Vermont Oxford Network. Standard concentrations of neonatal drug infusions, 2011. Available at: http://www.ismp.org/Tools/PediatricConcentrations.pdf. Accessed May 10, 2013.

continue to struggle with the issue of limiting the numbers of drug concentrations used within their pediatric populations.[9]

The lack of universal acceptance of the recommended standard concentrations is partly due to the wide ranges of practice within a pediatric unit and the need to administer drugs for patients at the extremes of weight. Neonates weighing only 350 grams require vastly different doses and fluids restrictions than adolescents cared for on the pediatric unit who may weigh up to 150 kg. In addition, the infusion devices and pump technology utilized may restrict the ability to run infusions at the low rates necessary for some of the recommended standard concentrations, particularly when dosing an extremely low-birth-weight infant (see the discussion later in this chapter).

The United States Pharmacopeia's (USP) Safe Medication Use Expert Committee (SMU EC) developed guidelines for institutions regarding the selection of standard concentrations.[10] Standard concentrations adopted by an institution should be adequate for infusion in 80–90% of a patient population, with exceptions to these standards being made for extreme outliers. The concentrations available in commercially available premixed solutions are preferred, as is the use of a standard adult concentration that meets the needs of the majority of children.[10] Standard concentrations should allow for measurable infusion rates, but should not provide excessive fluid overload; moreover, when feasible,

concentrations selected should support the use of simple calculations for infusion rates (e.g., 10 mcg/mL, 1 unit/mL).[10] The
standard concentrations chosen must be tolerated via the respective route of administration, such as with peripheral and central
catheters. Although the SMU EC has recommended premixed
solutions in a sodium chloride base solution in lieu of dextrose
solutions to allow for broader use across patient populations, concerns have been raised that such solutions will provide sodium
overload particularly to premature infants.

Additive/Contaminant Toxicity

In addition to concerns about the concentrations of many of the
available parenteral medications, the pharmacist must also be
cognizant of the additives present in these solutions. Many parenteral drug formulations contain additives designed to stabilize
or extend the expiration of the product that can be toxic, particularly to a neonate or young infant.

BENZYL ALCOHOL

Benzyl alcohol is a preservative commonly used in parenteral
drug solutions. In adults, benzyl alcohol is metabolized to benzoic acid, followed by conjugation to form hippuric acid, which
is then excreted in the urine. Newborns, due to their immature
conjugation pathways, are unable to metabolize the benzoic acid,
so it may accumulate and cause significant toxicity.[11] The accumulation of benzoic acid has resulted in severe metabolic acidosis,
respiratory depression and central nervous system depression,
convulsions, paralysis, and death in premature infants.[12-16] Exposure of premature infants to saline flush solutions containing
benzyl alcohol has been associated with increased mortality and
incidence of cerebral palsy.[17-19]

The American Academy of Pediatrics (AAP) and the Food
and Drug Administration (FDA) have recommended avoiding
agents containing benzyl alcohol as a preservative in infants
and young children.[20,21] The exposure limit of benzyl alcohol in
infants and young children is unclear; however, many sources

recommend that it should not exceed a daily intake of 5 mg/kg/day, with toxicity occurring at amounts exceeding 100 mg/kg/day, cumulatively.[21,22] Drugs containing benzyl alcohol that require continuous infusions or intermittent administration, such as saline and heparin flush solutions, are of particular concern for exceeding exposure limits.

> **ALERT:** *Benzyl alcohol exposure in infants and young children should not exceed a cumulative dose of 100 mg/kg.*

PROPYLENE GLYCOL

Propylene glycol (PG) is an alcohol solvent agent commonly used in parenteral medications. Rapid infusion of solutions containing high concentrations of PG can result in hypotension, arrhythmias, and seizures in adults and children.[23,24] Drugs containing PG, such as intravenous sulfamethoxazole-trimethoprim and phenytoin, have specific guidelines for dilution and slow infusion to avoid these complications.

Adults metabolize PG to pyruvic acid and lactic acid, which are subsequently eliminated in the urine.[25] The metabolism and renal elimination of PG in neonates are prolonged, however, resulting in accumulation of PG. The recommended limit of PG exposure in an adult is 25 mg/kg/day, while the limit for neonates is unknown.[25] Propylene glycol toxicity in neonates has resulted in hyperosmolality with subsequent seizures and cardiac arrest, as well as lactic acid–associated hemolysis, seizures, central and respiratory depression.[26–28] Similar to the case with benzyl alcohol, drugs administered via continuous infusions (e.g., midazolam) and frequent intermittent injections are likely to pose the greatest risk of reaching the cumulative limits for PG toxicity.

METHYLPARABEN

Methylparaben, another commonly used preservative agent, has been shown to displace bilirubin from albumin with frequent exposure via flush solutions.[30] This effect may increase the risk for kernicterus encephalopathy in neonates with high bilirubin levels. Less is known about the potential toxicities of the other preservative agents found in parenteral drug products.

In the ideal world, only preservative-free agents would be used for all pediatric patients; however, it is virtually impossible to accomplish this due to the overall lack of availability of preservative-free drug alternatives, the higher costs of such agents, and the continuous struggle with drug shortages. In light of this reality, it is recommended that institutions make every attempt to provide parenteral drugs in a preservative-free form to limit overall exposure.[21,22] The most concerning drugs, for which the limitation of additives is essential, are those in which repeated dosing leads to cumulative exposure. These include flush solutions (heparin, normal saline), continuous infusions, and drugs requiring repeated dosing. When shortages of preservative-free agents exist, priority for the use of preservative-free solutions should be given to the most immature patients, neonates and young infants less than 2 months of age.

Aluminum

Aluminum is one of the most common contaminants found in parenteral drugs. During the manufacturing process, aluminum may leach out of glass containers and other sources during production and packaging. Further contamination may occur during drug preparation and administration at the local level via transfer tubing sets, needles, and syringes; this risk is further influenced by the duration of time the solution remains in contact with each of the sources of contamination.[30–32] In an attempt to limit human exposure, FDA regulations limit manufacturer product contamination of large-volume parenteral (LVP) products to 25 mcg/L of aluminum, while requiring labeling of small-volume parenteral (SVP) products with the maximum amount of aluminum contained in the product.[33,34] Aluminum concentrations have been found to be high in albumin solutions, dextrose solutions, intravenous calcium and phosphorus salts, and admixed parenteral nutrition solutions. The recommended maximum exposure amount of aluminum for an individual is 5 mcg/kg/day.[33,34]

Aluminum accumulation has been associated with several toxicities, including metabolic bone disease or osteomalacia, anemia, and encephalopathy.[35] These toxicities are of particular concern in neonates due to their immature renal function (which limits their ability to eliminate aluminum), larger relative exposure to aluminum per body mass with commercially available parenteral solutions, need for high calcium and phosphorus supplementation, and need for prolonged parenteral nutrition therapy. Reports of neonatal osteopenia, rickets, and fractures associated with aluminum toxicity are most common, although neurologic sequelae may occur as well.[35,36]

Despite regulations intended to limit aluminum contamination and exposure in parenteral compounded sterile preparations (CSPs), it is often impossible to provide necessary therapy, particularly nutritionally, without exceeding the limit of 5 mcg/kg/day. Nevertheless, measures to limit contamination of parenteral solutions should be employed, such as selecting products with the least amount of aluminum contamination, rotating stock on shelves to limit the time for aluminum to leach from metal rings of glass vials into solution and selecting products in plastic or polyethylene containers.[37]

ALERT: *The maximum recommended amount of aluminum exposure for an individual is 5 mcg/kg/day.*

DEHP

Di-ethylhexyl phthalate (DEHP) is a chemical used to make polyvinyl chloride (PVC) plastic soft and flexible. DEHP is found throughout the hospital environment in plasticized products and devices used for providing care, including respiratory therapy devices (oxygen tubing, endotracheal tubes), blood transfusions, feeding tubes, and tubing sets for medication administration.[38–40] DEHP leaches out of PVC products easily and, therefore, can contaminate a medication infusion delivered via a DEHP-containing product. From the medication perspective, IV bags and IV tubing sets are the most common sources of DEHP exposure.[40–42]

Animal studies have shown DEHP exposure to be particularly toxic to the reproductive system, with other reported toxicities affecting respiratory, renal, and liver function.[43–49] The smaller the size of the infant or child, the greater the relative exposure to DEHP from contaminated solutions. Those individuals at most risk for DEHP toxicity are premature infants. Premature infants are vulnerable to the effects of DEHP not only because of their small size and the vulnerable stage of development of their organs, but also because of their high exposure to DEHP products over a prolonged hospitalization.[50–52]

The FDA has issued a public health notification that DEHP-free devices be considered for all products used for premature infants.[53] Many hospitals have gone to completely DEHP-free products for use in the neonatal intensive care unit (NICU), although these products are slightly more expensive than the DEHP-containing alternatives. Solutions stored in DEHP-containing bags that have been shown to have the greatest risk of leaching are those with high lipid content and those with prolonged contact with IV bags or tubing (i.e., parenteral nutrition solutions, continuous infusions). DEHP-free IV bags are available from several different manufacturers. Premixed IV solutions are an additional source of DEHP exposure, so avoidance of premixed solutions and compounding of preparations in DEHP-free bags is preferred for infants.

Intravenous Access Limitations

Infusion of medication to the patient requires access to the venous circulation. Intravenous injection or infusion of medications should be administered only into the venous circulation, not arterially, to avoid complications such as severe pain, parathesias, and arterial vasospasm that could lead to loss of limbs. Medications may be infused into the venous system via several pathways, with the most common being peripheral or central venous access.

PERIPHERAL ACCESS CONSIDERATIONS

Peripheral access, or a peripheral IV, is obtained by inserting a needle and catheter into one of the peripheral veins. The veins in the extremities—particularly in the hand, forearm, or antecubital fossa—are preferred sites for peripheral access. Larger veins are easier to access, allow for the use of larger-bore IVs, and have a lower risk of thrombophlebitis; however, smaller veins at sites most distal to the patient are preferred to limit the area involved should any complications occur. A peripheral IV is inserted using a needle over which a catheter or small tube is passed and threaded into the vein. The needle is then removed, and the catheter is secured in place. Such a catheter can be used to administer medications or fluids, or to draw blood. Peripheral IVs usually remain in place for a few days and, therefore, are indicated for short-term infusion of medications. Complications of peripheral IVs may include thrombophlebitis, extravasation, infiltration, and bleeding and bruising at the access site.

Obtaining and maintaining IV access in infants and young children can be challenging. Veins in infants and young children are small and more fragile than their adult counterparts, increasing their risk of phlebitis and infiltration. In addition, numerous attempts are often required to obtain peripheral IV access in infants and young children,[54,55] which can further weaken and damage the vessel wall and increase these risks. Peripheral IV access can be inserted in the typical sites utilized in adults (e.g., antecubital, hand), but may also be obtained in less obvious places (e.g., scalp and foot veins). Infiltrations and extravasations in these areas can result in severe tissue damage and leave permanent scarring.

Ensuring line patency and preventing infiltration and thrombophlebitis with peripheral lines is imperative. Limiting drug solution osmolarity through peripheral lines is recommended to reduce the risk of complications. Some sources suggest that osmolarities of 900–1100 mOsm/L may be tolerated in some patients, while others recommend a maximum of 600 mOsm/L.[56–60] Many drugs have excessive osmolarities (greater than 8000 mOsm/L) and require further dilution prior to administration (**Table 10-3**).[61,62] Because the osmolarity of a drug solution is directly related to dose and concentration, reduced concentrations of drugs are infused through peripheral lines. Drug solutions with a pH outside the normal physiologic range (7.35–7.45) also have

Table 10-3   Osmolalities of Select Parenteral Drugs in Children

Agent	Concentration	Osmolality (mOsm/kg)
Alprostadil	0.5 mg/mL	17,230
Ampicillin	100 mg/mL	504
Cefotaxime	250 mg/mL	740
Ceftriaxone	250 mg/mL	895
Clindamycin	50 mg/mL	859
Dextrose	5%	272
	10%	600
	30%	1900
Digoxin	0.25 mg/mL	8144
Dobutamine	12.5 mg/mL	82
Dopamine	40 mg/mL	374
Fentanyl	0.05 mg/mL	275
Furosemide	10 mg/mL	282–2280*
Gentamicin	40 mg/mL	169
Indomethacin	1 mg/mL	290
Midazolam	5 mg/mL	205
Morphine	10 mg/mL	59
Penicillin G	2×10^5 mg/mL	547
Phenobarbital	15 mg/mL	14,479
Phenytoin	50 mg/mL	8207–8397*

*Varies by manufacturer.

Source: A.S.P.E.N. Board of Directors and the Clinical Guidelines Task Force. Guidelines for the use of parenteral and enteral nutrition in adult and pediatric patients. *J Parenter Enteral Nutr.* 2002;1SA.

increased risks of thrombophlebitis.[63–66] If the pH of the solution cannot be altered, its infusion through peripheral lines should be avoided. In addition, agents that are inherent chemical irritants tend to result in high rates of thrombophlebitis or venous irritation. Penicillins, cefotaxime, and amphotericin are common irritants for which reducing the concentration may help in maintaining peripheral access.[66] Finally, the use of peripheral lines for infusion of vesicant drugs, which are known to cause severe extravasation injuries, should be limited, particularly in infants. Extravasation injuries can result in severe tissue damage involving a large surface area in infants and young children. Institutions are required to develop specific guidelines regarding maximum drug concentrations based on osmolarity for infusion in pediatric patients via peripheral route.[7]

CENTRAL ACCESS CONSIDERATIONS

Due to the difficulty of maintaining peripheral access in young children, the use of central venous catheters (CVCs) is necessary for prolonged IV therapy. Central venous access is obtained via insertion of catheters into large veins such as the subclavian, internal jugular, or femoral veins. Because of the use of larger veins, central venous access is associated with fewer problems such as extravasation and infiltration, and it allows for administration of more concentrated solutions, higher osmolarities, and faster infusion rates. Central venous catheters may be inserted centrally or via a peripheral location. Devices that are placed peripherally (peripherally inserted central catheter [PICC]) are intended for relatively short-term use (2–6 weeks) and may be inserted at the bedside, while permanent CVCs are indicated for longer durations and require surgical placement. There are several methods of obtaining central access, all of which require either a trained/certified individual or surgical intervention for placement.

Typical CVCs used in children include Broviac, Hickman, and Groshong catheters. In addition, the umbilical vein can be catheterized immediately after birth in newborns with an umbilical venous catheter (UVC), which can function like other CVCs. For UVCs, PICCs, and CVCs, the tip of the catheter is threaded into a central vein (e.g., superior vena cava, inferior vena cava) where blood flow is much faster; thus these devices tolerate higher osmolarities (1500–2000 mOsm/L), drug concentrations, and solution pHs than are allowable in a peripheral line. Regardless of the type of access device, the tip of a CVC is placed into a large vessel within the central circulation of the patient. Although central venous access offers many advantages for medication administration, they are also associated with more serious complications such as central line infections and sepsis, deep venous thrombosis, arrhythmias, embolisms, and pneumothorax.

ALERT: *Be sure to check the osmolarity of a solution to determine if it can be administered via peripheral or central line and then verify the type of line that the patient has.*

As a pharmacist, it is important not only to be knowledgeable about the type of access device utilized to prepare the appropriate drug solution, but also to select the appropriate syringe size in which to dispense the drug. Some CVCs, particularly PICCs, have limits for syringe size (e.g., specify use of 5- to 10-mL syringes) for delivery and infusion of medications to avoid excessive pressure within the line that could result in rupture and embolization of the catheter.[67,68] Institutions may develop standards for dispensing medications in recommended syringe sizes for drug delivery. Alternatively, nursing guidelines may specify procedures for administration of drugs to avoid excessive line pressure for drug doses less than 1 mL (e.g., prime the line with the drug and then flush the drug through using a larger syringe size).

Central catheters come in a variety of lengths, number of lumens, lumen sizes, and number of access ports. The size of the large veins used for central access allows for catheters to have several lumens, or channels, through which medications can be infused. Central catheters can have single, double, or triple lumens, meaning there may be as many as three separate channels within a catheter in which drugs can be infused. Each of these lumens has its own access port through which a drug is injected or infused. An understanding of the characteristics of an access device aids in decisions regarding drug Y-site compatibility, infusion times, and flush volumes. Because IV access is often limited in infants and young children, catheters with multiple ports may allow for Y-site administration of drugs and reduced need for alternative IV access sites. Knowledge about the number of lumens, as well as lumen size and length, is necessary to determine the time for drug delivery to reach the central circulation and the need for and volume of flush solutions to push the drug through the line (see the discussion later in this chapter). CVCs and PICC lines require the addition of heparin (0.5–1 unit/mL) to intravenous solutions (e.g., IV fluids and total parenteral nutrition

[TPN]) to prevent catheter occlusion.[69] CVCs and PICC lines require heparin lock solutions of varying concentrations (0.5–10 units/mL) to maintain line patency when not in use.[71,72]

> **ALERT:** *When heparin flushes are used to maintain catheter patency in younger infants, a concentration of 10 units/mL is typically used. The heparin concentration for flushes used for older infants, children, and adults is 100 units/mL. Care must be taken to ensure the correct flushes are selected to avoid overdosing of heparin in young infants.*

INTRAOSSEOUS ACCESS

Intraosseous (IO) access devices are employed in infants and young children in emergency situations when peripheral access is unobtainable and there is not time to attempt CVC placement. These catheters are inserted into the anteromedial surface of the tibia, thereby gaining access to the highly vascularized long bone marrow. IO catheters are intended for short-term use (less than 6 hours) until IV access can be obtained. Intraosseous lines can be utilized like a CVC for delivery of IV solutions and drugs. Typical agents infused through an IO catheter include IV fluids, resuscitation medications, insulin, and narcotics.[73–75] Because they function like a CVC, IO lines can tolerate osmolarities and drug concentrations as used for a CVC.

Drug Volume and Infusion Rate Limitations

Drug dose volumes, particularly in neonates, are very small. Even when drug solutions are diluted to allow for a measurable volume, dose volumes in neonates are often less than 1 mL. A 1-kg premature infant may be allowed a total fluid daily volume of only 100 mL or approximately 3–4 mL/hr (including all medications, feedings, and other solutions), whereas a term infant may be allowed up to 450 mL of total daily fluid volume (approximately 20 mL/hr). Particularly in infants, drug volumes must be minimized to free up fluid volume for nutritional therapy. Thus standard concentrations of drugs for neonates should be developed at each institution to limit fluid volumes and appropriate-size syringes must be employed for drawing up these small doses.

The potential for errors in drug dosing and drug delivery is greatest when dose volumes are less than 1 mL. Delivery of the drug to the patient depends on the volume of the dose, the site where the dose is injected, and the infusion rate of the solution through the line in which the drug is being injected.[76,77] Small dose volumes (less than 1 mL) can have extremely delayed infusion if injected into a primary infusion line infusing at a rate of 3–4 mL/hr, particularly if injected into a port distal from the patient. Studies have shown that drug infusion can be delayed for as long as 12 hours in such situations.[78–80] A simple approach to limit this problem is to always inject small doses at a port close to the patient.

Ideally, the infusion of such small dose volumes should be delivered utilizing a syringe pump. Syringe pumps are designed to accurately deliver very small volumes from syringes at a rate independent of the primary fluid rate. They are used with microbore tubing sets, which hold a total volume of 0.3–0.4 mL, as compared to a standard tubing set, which typically contains more than 17 mL of volume. If the dose volume is 0.3 mL, a syringe pump can be programmed to deliver that dose over 30 minutes at a rate of 0.6 mL/hr. If a standard tubing set (macrobore) was employed with a primary infusion rate of 3–4 mL/hr, it could take as long as 6 hours to deliver that same dose. The separate infusion of drug doses with the syringe pump also avoids the problem of sudden drug boluses should the primary fluid rate be increased. Drugs with high specific gravities also have the potential to layer out and be lost if standard macrobore tubing sets and low infusion rates are employed.

TIP: *Always inject small doses, such as those less than 1 mL, into a port close to the patient to limit problems with delayed infusion of small-volume doses.*

> **ALERT:** *Small-volume doses should be administered using a syringe pump.*

Dead Space

When dose volumes are small, as with pediatric doses, there are numerous places where the drug can be hidden or lost within an IV set, referred to as "dead space." A dead space site familiar to most practitioners is within the hub of a needle. A priming volume or "needle volume" is generally added to syringes when needles are used for drug administration to avoid the drug being lost within the dead space. When small dose volumes are used, the amount lost in this space can be a significant percentage of the drug. Most institutions have adopted needleless systems, thereby eliminating concerns regarding needle priming volumes.

Similarly, dead space and drug loss can occur within numerous parts of an infusion set, including stopcocks, Y-site injection ports, T-connectors, and in-line filters.[78–80] Drugs can be lost within the microbore tubing (0.3–0.4 mL) if the line is not flushed.[76] In addition, if a drug is infused via a CVC, the dead space in the catheter itself can delay drug delivery to the central circulation.[79–81]

To ensure the entire drug dose is delivered to the patient, pharmacy and nursing personnel must work together to develop policies regarding how drugs will be prepared and subsequently administered. Some institutions prepare all medications with a priming volume equal to the anticipated dead space in the tubing sets; others dispense medications in the exact volumes and flush the lines after the drug infusion is complete. There are pros and cons for each method. Pharmacists must be knowledgeable about their institution's policies and procedures for infusion of small dose volumes to ensure that patients are not underdosed.[82,83]

Dead space also becomes an issue during the preparation of dilutions. If a small dose volume (less than 0.1 mL) is drawn from a large-volume solution into a syringe and then a dilution solution is drawn up into that same syringe, a small volume of extra drug will be pushed into the syringe from within the dead space of the syringe itself.[78] Although this amount may be insignificant in older patients with large dose volumes, it can result in a significant overdose in infants and children. Significant overdoses of digoxin and morphine, for example, can occur if the syringe dead space is not accounted for during preparation of the dilutions.[84,85]

> **ALERT:** *Overdoses can occur if dead space is not accounted for when compounding sterile preparations for pediatric patients.*

Infusion Devices and Drug Preparation

Parenteral drugs may be administered by slow IV push, intermittent infusion, and continuous infusion. Intravenous push medications are prepared in syringes, allowing the syringe to be connected to the IV access port for direct injection. Medications for IV push administration should be prepared in concentrations that can be readily administered and with appropriate priming volumes if applicable. A flush is administered after the injection is administered to ensure the drug is cleared from the catheter, catheter port, and IV tubing set.

Drugs for intermittent infusion are administered via slow infusion over a set time period and can be infused by gravity or with an infusion pump. Medications for continuous infusion require close titration of infusion rates and are to be delivered via an infusion pump device for more precise control and titration of infusion rates. Depending on the volume of medication and the infusion rate, intermittent and continuous infusions may be prepared in either minibags or syringes. Syringes are typically used for preparation and delivery of medications intended for infants and young children because of their small dose requirements, fluid restrictions, and slow infusion rates. Minibags are used when larger doses are required and volume restrictions do not exist.

Large-volume pumps are computer-controlled infusion pumps that are used to deliver IV fluids, TPN, and intermittent drug doses in children. Large-volume pumps deliver fluids or drug solutions from IV bags or bottles utilizing macrobore tubing at recommended infusion rates ranging from 0.1 to 999 mL/hr, although the accuracy at rates less than 2 mL/hr varies between manufacturers and models of large-volume pumps. The pump controls the infusion rate by placing pressure on the tubing to milk the line (peristalsis), resulting in pulsatile flow. Numerous models of large-volume pumps exist that offer variations in the number of pump lines, safety features, alarms, power supplies, and displays. Large-volume pumps are usually used in older children for intermittent doses and for delivery of IV fluids and TPN—all situations in which small variations in the pulsatile flow are insignificant. Because macrobore tubing is used, dead space issues must be considered when monitoring drugs infused via a large-volume pump.

Small-volume pumps or syringe pumps are preferred for infusing small volumes at precise rates in infants and young children. Syringes are used for delivering intermittent and continuous infusions of medications via syringe pumps using microbore tubing. The rate of infusion for a syringe pump is controlled by computerized variations in pressure placed on the plunger of the syringe, thereby achieving infusion rates ranging from 0.01 to 10 mL/hr. The pressure that a syringe pump can generate reflects the pump force and syringe characteristics. Because syringes vary in diameter and surface area between manufacturers, decisions regarding the adoption of syringes by an institution must be made jointly by pharmacy and nursing staff. The size of syringe in which to dispense a drug dose should take into consideration the rate of infusion needed to deliver the prescribed dose. Although syringe pumps can deliver low infusion rates, their accuracy decreases when large syringes are used for infusion rates of less than 1 mL/hr.[86-92] Many syringe pumps display error messages when practitioners attempt to infuse drugs at very low rates using large syringes. The use of a 10-mL syringe will allow for an accurate infusion rate down to 0.1 mL/hr, although variations exist between pumps.[86,87] It is preferred that continuous infusions of drugs such as vasopressors, insulin, and other drugs that require tight titration control be dispensed in small syringe sizes (10 mL or less).[86,87] Smaller-size syringes must be used to accurately deliver drugs at rates of less than 0.1 mL/hr. The degree of accuracy below this level is dictated by the pump and syringe specifications.

SMART PUMPS

As technology has advanced, some syringe pumps have incorporated advanced computer technology, leading to their identification as "smart pumps." Smart pumps have built-in software that is capable of being programmed to include drug libraries with standard drug concentrations, minimum and maximum infusion rates, and checks for dosing errors. Smart pumps may be specifically programmed for each institution's patient population, common drugs, standard concentrations, and infusion rates. More advanced models are capable of integrating with other institution computer systems and allow for wireless data updates, electronic prescribing, bar-code administration, and electronic medical recording.

Pharmacy personnel not only play a vital role in the decision-making process for selecting smart pump technology for an institution, but also are usually responsible for programming and updating the drug libraries and alerts.[93,94] Standard concentrations for each drug must be chosen for each unit within an institution as well as minimum and maximum dosages and infusion rates.[93,95] Smart pumps are also capable of calculating and checking weight-based drug dosing for children to prevent medication dosing errors. Alert limits may be programmed to notify the user when specified dose limits are exceeded. "Soft limits" are displayed on the pumps, but may be overridden, whereas "hard limits" cannot be overridden.

Although the use of smart pumps has been shown to significantly reduce medication administration errors,[96–98] these devices are not foolproof. Data entry errors, such as entering the wrong patient weight or selecting the wrong concentration from the library, can still occur, which can have substantial implications for pediatric patients. The user can also override soft limits and has the ability to manually program an infusion. In addition, any errors that are made during the initial system setup can obviously have a unit-wide impact. [93,99,100]

Medication Safety Issues

Medication errors are of primary concern in the pediatric population. Unfortunately, medication errors involving intravenous medications are the most common and result in the most devastating results in an institution.[1,2] Multidisciplinary teams should work together to develop policies and procedures for preventing medication errors.[4,101,102]

In addition to developing standard concentrations and infusion guidelines for IV drugs, the medication order process and labeling of IV medications should be standardized. Although computerized physician order entry (CPOE) is preferred for medication ordering to reduce the potential for medication errors, preprinted order sets for medication orders may serve as another means to avoid prescribing errors and pharmacy interpretation errors.[4] Along with the standard requirements for medication orders, those for children should always include the patient weight (kg), weight-based dose (mg/kg/dose), final calculated dose, and route of administration.[4,101,102] Organizations should adopt the ISMP guidelines for preparing labels for IV syringes,[103] and all labels for IV medications in children should clearly state the final concentration of the medication within the syringe, the volume to be delivered, the priming volume (if indicated), and the route of administration. Including the route of administration is important because many oral medications for children may also be dispensed in syringes.

Lastly, pediatric-specific drug references that provide dosing and administration information for IV drugs should be readily available to all personnel prescribing, preparing, and administering medications to children. Among the valuable resources are *Teddy Bear Book: Pediatric Injectable Drugs*,[104] *Pediatric and Neonatal Dosage Handbook*,[105] and *Neofax*.[106]

Conclusion

Preparing CSPs for pediatric patients requires knowledge of equipment and safety considerations for this patient population. Understanding of the types of toxicities that can occur secondary to aluminum contamination and preservatives is an example of the unique considerations that must be accounted for in pediatric preparations. Pediatric CSPs require a different set of preparation techniques than are typically used for adult CSPs, such as drug dilutions. All personnel involved in the preparation process must be familiar with these types of techniques and be able to perform them with accuracy. Further, understanding administration limitations with pediatric patients is an important aspect of compounding sterile preparations. Because of the increased potential for medication errors in this type of patient population, institutions and those involved in the preparation and verification processes must implement practices and procedures to ensure the sterility and accuracy of all CSPs administered to pediatric patients.

Review Questions

1. Describe why dilutions are needed for parenteral drugs administered to pediatric patients.
2. List the factors that influence the selection of standard concentrations for use in infants and young children.
3. Which toxicities have been attributed to benzyl alcohol and propylene glycol in pediatric patients?
4. What is DEHP? Describe the toxicities associated with DEHP exposure.
5. Describe the advantages of drug administration via a central venous catheter in pediatric patients.
6. Explain why dead space can have a significant impact on the drug dose delivery in pediatric patients.
7. What are the advantages of small-volume pumps and smart pumps for use in children?
8. List measures to improve medication safety in the preparation and administration of parenteral medications in infant and children.

CASE STUDY

While working the night shift in the inpatient pharmacy, you receive an order for a dopamine infusion for an infant in the pediatric intensive care unit. The order states:

Dopamine 5 mcg/kg/min; maximally concentrated

You call the unit and speak to the infant's nurse to determine the infant's weight, which she tells you it is 4.9 kg. She also mentions that she is having difficulty infusing all of medications in this patient, who has one peripheral IV and a central line with a single lumen.

1. Which of the following considerations is important in determining which concentration to prepare for administration to the infant?
   a. Age of infant
   b. Site of infusion
   c. Duration of infusion
   d. Rate of infusion
2. What is the risk or concern if dopamine were to be infused through a peripheral line in this infant?
   a. Precipitation
   b. Line occlusion
   c. Extravasation
   d. Incompatibility
3. Calculate the rate of infusion of dopamine (mL/hr) for this patient, assuming that this medication is to be infused through the central line at a concentration of 6400 mcg/mL.
   a. 0.03 mL/hr
   b. 0.23 mL/hr
   c. 5 mL/hr
   d. 24.5 mL/hr
4. Which type of pump should the nurse use to infuse the dopamine?
   a. Syringe pump
   b. Large-volume pump
   c. Pump is not necessary
5. Which size of syringe should be prepared for the dopamine infusion?
   a. 5 mL
   b. 10 mL
   c. 20 mL
   d. 60 mL

References

1. Doherty C, McDonnell C. Tenfold medication errors: 5 years' experience at a university affiliated pediatric hospital. *Pediatrics.* 2012;129:916–924.

2. Crowley E, Williams R, Cousins D. Medication errors in children: a descriptive summary of medication error reports submitted to the United States Pharmacopeia. *Curr Ther Res.* 2001;26;627–640.

3. Institute for Safe Medication Practices. Proceedings from the ISMP sterile preparation compounding safety summit: guidelines for SAFE preparation of sterile compounds. Available at: http://www.ismp.org/Tools/guidelines/IVSummit/IVCGuidelines.pdf. Accessed May 10, 2013.

4. Levine SR, Cohen MR, Blanchard NR, Frederico F, et al. Guidelines for preventing medication errors in pediatrics. *J Pediatr Pharmacol Therap.* 2001;6:426–442.

5. Joint Commission on Accreditation of Healthcare Organizations. JCAHO approves national patient safety goals for 2003. *JCAH Perspect.* 2002;22:1.

6. National patient safety goals. In: *2006–2007 comprehensive accreditation manual for home care.* Oakbrook Terrace, IL: The Joint Commission; 2006:chap 9.

7. American Society of Health-System Pharmacists. Organization and delivery of services, 0807: standardization of intravenous drug concentrations. Available at: http://www.ashp.org/DocLibrary/BestPractices/policypositions2010.aspx. Accessed May 10, 2013.

8. Institute for Safe Medication Practices, Vermont Oxford Network. Standard concentrations of neonatal drug infusions, 2011. Available at: http://www.ismp.org/Tools/PediatricConcentrations.pdf. Accessed May 10, 2013..

9. Phillips MJ. Standardizing IV infusion concentrations: national survey results. *Am J Health-Sys Pharm.* 2011;68:2176–2182.

10. Proceedings of a summit on preventing patient harm and death from i.v. medication errors. *Am J Health-Syst Pharm.* 2008;65:2367–2379.

11. LeBel M, Ferron L, Masson M, et al. Benzyl alcohol metabolism and elimination in neonates. *Dev Pharmacol Ther.* 1988;11:347–356.

12. Gershanik J, Boecler B, Ensley H, et al. The gasping syndrome and benzyl alcohol poisoning. *N Engl J Med.* 1982;307:1384–1388.

13. Brown WJ, Buist NR, Gipson HT, et al. Fatal benzyl alcohol poisoning in a neonatal intensive care unit. *Lancet.* 1982;1:1250.

14. Anderson CW, Ng KJ, Andresen B, Cordera L. Benzyl alcohol poisoning in a premature newborn infant. *Am J Obstet Gynecol.* 1984;148:344–346.
15. Menon PA, Thach BT, Smith CH, et al. Benzyl alcohol toxicity in a neonatal intensive care unit: incidence, symptomatology, and mortality. *Am J Perinatol.* 1984;1:288–292.
16. American Academy of Pediatrics Committee on Fetus and Newborn and Committee on Drugs. Benzyl alcohol: toxic agent in neonatal units. *Pediatrics.* 1983;72(3):356–358.
17. Hiller JL, Benda GI, Rahatzad M, et al. Benzyl alcohol toxicity: impact on mortality and intraventricular hemorrhage among very low birth weight infants. *Pediatrics.* 1986;77:500–506.
18. Benda GI, Hiller JL, Reynolds JW. Benzyl alcohol toxicity: impact on neurologic handicaps among surviving very low birth weight infants. *Pediatrics.* 1986;77:507–512.
19. Jardine DS, Rogers K. Relationship of benzyl alcohol to kernicterus, intraventricular hemorrhage, and mortality in preterm infants. *Pediatrics.* 1989;83:153–160.
20. Anonymous. Benzyl alcohol may be toxic to newborns. *FDA Drug Bull.* 1982;12:10–11.
21. American Academy of Pediatrics Committee on Drugs. "Inactive" ingredients in pharmaceutical products: update. *Pediatrics.* 2004;99:268–278.
22. Nahata MC. Safety of "inert" additives or excipients in paediatric medicines. *Arch Dis Child Fetal Neonatal Ed.* 2009;94(6):F392–F393.
23. Louis S, Kutt H, McDowell F. The cardiocirculatory changes caused by intravenous Dilantin and its solvent. *Am Heart J.* 1967;74:523–529.
24. York RC, Coleridge ST. Cardiopulmonary arrest following intravenous phenytoin loading. *Am J Emerg Med.* 1988;6:255–259.
25. Owen SC, Weller PJ. Propylene glycol. In: Rowe RC, Sheskey PJ, Owen SC, eds. *Handbook of pharmaceutical excipients.* 5th ed. London, UK: Pharmaceutical Press; 2006:521–523.
26. Arulanantham K, Genel M. Central nervous system toxicity associated with ingestion of propylene glycol. *J Pediatr.* 1978;93:515–516.
27. Martin G, Finberg L. Propylene glycol: a potentially toxic vehicle in liquid dosage form. *J Pediatr.* 1970;77:877–878.

28. MacDonald MG, Getson PR, Glasgow AM, et al. Propylene glycol: increased incidence of seizures in low birth weight infants. *Pediatrics.* 1987;79:622–625.

29. Rasmussen LR, Ahflors CE, Wennberg RP. The effect of paraben preservatives on albumin binding of bilirubin. *J Pediatr.* 1976;89(3):475–478.

30. de Oliveira SR, Bohrer D, Garcia SC, et al. Aluminum content in intravenous solutions for administration to neonates: role of product preparation and administration methods. *J Parenter Enteral Nutr.* 2010;34:322–328.

31. Bohrer D, do Nascimento PC, Binotto R, Pomblum SC. Influence of the glass packing on the contamination of pharmaceutical products by aluminum. Part I: salts, glucose, heparin and albumin. *J Trace Elem Med Biol.* 2001;15:95–101.

32. Bohrer D, do Nascimento PC, Binotto R, et al. Contribution of the raw material to the aluminum contamination in parenterals. *J Parenter Enteral Nutr.* 2002;26:382–388.

33. Aluminum in large and small volume parenterals used in total parenteral nutrition—FDA. Proposed rule. *Fed Regist.* 1998;63:176–185.

34. Aluminum in large and small volume parenterals used in total parenteral nutrition. *Fed Regist.* 2011;21:89–90.

35. American Academy of Pediatrics Committee on Nutrition. Aluminum toxicity in infants and children. *Pediatrics.* 1986;78:1150–1154.

36. Koo WW. Parenteral nutrition–related bone disease. *J Parenter Enteral Nutr.* 1992;16:386–394.

37. Weir H, Kuhn RJ. Aluminum toxicity in neonatal parenteral nutrition: what can we do? *Ann Pharmacother.* 2012;46:137–140.

38. FDA Public Health Notification. Safety assessment of di(2-ehtyl-hexyl) phthalate (DEHP) released from PVC medical devices. Available at: http://www.fda.gov/downloads/MedicalDevices/.../UCM080457.pdf. Accessed May 10, 2013.

39. Sjöberg PO, Bondesson UG, Sedin EG, Gustafsson JP. Exposure of newborn infants to plasticizers: plasma levels of di-(2-ethylhexyl)

phthalate and mono-(2-ethylhexyl) phthalate during exchange transfusion. *Transfusion.* 1985;25(5): 424–428.

40. Pearson S, Trissel L. Leaching of diethylhexylphthalate from polyvinyl chloride containers by selected drugs and formulation components. *Am J Health-Syst Pharm.* 1993;50:1405–1409.

41. Smistad G, Waaler T, Roksvaag PO. Migration of plastic additives from soft polyvinyl chloride bags into normal saline and glucose infusions. *Acta Pharm Nord.* 1989;1:287–290.

42. Loff S, Kabs F, Witt K, et al. Polyvinylchloride infusion lines expose infants to large amounts of toxic plasticizers. *J Pediatr Surg.* 2000;35(12):1775–1781.

43. Crocker J, Safe S, Acott P. Effects of chronic phthalate exposure on the kidney. *J Toxicol Environ Health.* 1988;23:433–444.

44. Davis BJ, Maronpot RR, Heindel JJ. Di-(2-ethylhexyl) phthalate suppresses estradiol and ovulation in cycling rats. *Toxicol Appl Pharmacol.* 1994;128:216–223.

45. Gray LE, Wolf C, Lambright C, et al. Administration of potentially antiandrogenic pesticides (procymidone, linuron, iprodione, chlozolinate, p,p'-DDE, and ketoconazole) and toxic substances (dibutyl- and diethylhexyl phthalate, PCB 169, and ethanedimethane sulphonate) during sexual differentiation produces diverse profiles of reproductive malformations in threat. *Toxicol Indust Health.* 1999;15:94–118.

46. Huber WW, Grasl-Kraupp B, Schulte-Hermann R. Hepatocarcinogenic potential of DEHP in rodents and its implications on human risk. *Crit Rev Toxicol.* 1996;26:365–481.

47. Roth B, Herkenrath P, Lehmann HJ, et al. DEHP: a plasticizer in PVC respiratory tubing systems: indications of hazardous effects on pulmonary function in mechanically ventilated, preterm infants. *Eur J Pediatr.* 1988;147:41–46.

48. Latini G, Avery G. Materials degradation in endotracheal tubes: a potential contributor to bronchopulmonary disease. *Acta Paediatr.* 1999;88:1174–1175.

49. Center for the Evaluation of Risks to Human Reproduction. NTPCERHR Expert Panel update on the reproductive and developmental toxicity of di(2-ethylhexyl) phthalate. Available

at: http://cerhr.niehs.nih.gov/chemicals/dehp/DEHP__Report_fi nal.pdf. Accessed May 10, 2013.

50. Calafat A, Needham L, Silva M, Lambert G. Exposure to di(2-ethylhexyl) phthalate among premature neonates in a neonatal intensive care unit. *Pediatrics.* 2004;113:e429–e434.

51. Shea K. Pediatric exposure and potential toxicity of phthalate plasticizers. *Pediatrics.* 2003;111:1467–1474.

52. Green R, Hauser R, Calafat A, et al. Use of di(2-ethylhexyl) phthalate–containing medical products and urinary levels of mono(2-ethylhexyl) phthalate in neonatal intensive care unit infants. *Environ Health Perspect.* 2005;113:1222–1225.

53. FDA Public Health Notification. PVC devices containing the plasticizer DEHP. Available at: http://www.fda.gov/MedicalDevices/Safety/AlertsandNotices/PublicHealthNotifications/ucm062182.htm. Accessed May 10, 2013.

54. Lininger RA. Pediatric peripheral IV insertion success rates. *Pediatr Nurs.* 2003;29:351–354.

55. Hartzog TH, Eldridge DL, Larsen PG, et al. *Putting in the pediatric IV: does confidence and competence make a difference?* Paper presented at American Academy of Pediatrics 2008 National Conference & Exhibition; October 11–14, 2008; Boston, MA.

56. Intravenous Nurses Society. Position paper: midline and midclavicular catheters. *J Intraven Nurs.*1997;20:175–178.

57. American Academy of Pediatrics. *Pediatric nutrition handbook.* Elk Grove Village, IL: American Academy of Pediatrics; 1998.

58. Hoffmann E. A randomised study of central venous versus peripheral intravenous nutrition in the perioperative period. *Clin Nutr.* 1989;8(4):179–180.

59. Isaacs JW, Millikan WJ, Stackhouse J, et al. Parenteral nutrition of adults with 900-milliosmolar solution via peripheral vein. *Am J Clin Nutr.* 1977;30:552–559.

60. A.S.P.E.N. Board of Directors and the Clinical Guidelines Task Force. Guidelines for the use of parenteral and enteral nutrition in adult and pediatric patients. *J Parenter Enteral Nutr.* 2002;1SA.

61. Pereira-da-Silva L, Henriques G, Videira-Amaral JM, et al. Osmolality of solutions, emulsions and drugs that may have high

osmolality: aspects of their use in neonatal care. *J Matern Fetal Neonatal Med.* 2001;11(5):333–338.

62. Ernst JA, Williams JM, Glick MR, Lemmons JA. Osmolality of substances used in the intensive care nursery. *Pediatrics.* 1983;72:347–352.

63. Stanz M. Adjusting pH and osmolarity levels to fit standards and practices. *J Vasc Access Device.* 2002;7:12–17.

64. Kuwahara T, Asanami S, Tamura T, Kaneda S. Effects of pH and osmolality on phlebitic potential of infusion solutions for peripheral parenteral nutrition. *J Toxicol Sci.* 1998;23:77–85.

65. Fonkalsrud EW, Pederson BM, Murphy J, Beckerman JH. Reduction of infusion thrombophlebitis with buffered glucose solutions. *Surgery.* 1968;63:280.

66. Maki DG, Ringer M. Risk factors for infusion-related phlebitis with small peripheral venous catheters: a randomized controlled trial. *Ann Intern Med.* 1991;114:845–854.

67. Macklin D. What's physics got to do with it? *J Vasc Access Devices.* 1999;4(2):7–11.

68. Conn C. The importance of syringe size when using implanted vascular access devices. *J Vasc Access Networks.* 1993;3(1):11–18.

69. Shah PS, Kalyn A, Satodia P, et al. A randomized, controlled trial of heparin versus placebo infusion to prolong the usability of peripherally placed percutaneous central venous catheters (PCVCs) in neonates: the HIP (Heparin Infusion for PCVC) study. *Pediatrics.* 2007;119:e284–e291.

70. Shah P, Shah V. Continuous heparin infusion to prevent thrombosis and catheter occlusion in neonates with peripherally placed percutaneous central venous catheters. *Cochrane Database Syst Rev.* 2008(2):CD002772.

71. Hadaway L. Heparin locking for central venous catheters. *J Assoc Vasc Access.* 2006;II(4):224–231.

72. Randolph A, Cook D, Gonzales C, Andrew M. Benefit of heparin in central venous and pulmonary artery catheters: a meta-analysis of randomized controlled trials. *Chest.* 1998;113:165–171.

73. Rosetti VA, Thompson BM, Miller J, et al. Intraosseous infusion: an alternative route of pediatric intravascular access. *Ann Emerg Med.* 1985;14(9):103–106.

74. Macht DI. Studies on intraosseous injections of epinephrine. *Am I Physiol.* 1943;38:269–272.

75. Macht DI. Absorption of drugs through the bone marrow. *P Soc Exp Biol Med.* 1941;47:299–305.

76. Goult T, Roberts RJ. Therapeutic problems arising from the use of intravenous route of drug administration. *J Pediatr.* 1979;95:465–471.

77. Roberts RJ. Intravenous administration of medication in pediatric patients. *Pediatr Clin North Am.* 1981;28(1):23–34.

78. Koren G. Therapeutic drug monitoring principles in the neonate. *Clin Chem.* 1997;43(1):222–227.

79. Lovich MA, Doles J, Peterfreund RA. The impact of carrier flow rate and infusion set dead-volume of dynamics of intravenous drug delivery. *Anesth Analg.* 2005;100:1048–1055.

80. Bartels K, Moss DR, Peterfreund RA. An analysis of drug delivery dynamics via a pediatric central venous infusion system: quantification of delays in achieving intended doses. *Anesth Analg.* 2009;109:1156–1161.

81. Lovich MA, Peterfreund GL, Sims NM, Peterfreund RA. Central venous catheter infusions: a laboratory model shows large differences in drug delivery dynamics related to catheter dead volume. *Crit Care Med.* 2007;35:2792–2798.

82. American Society of Hospital Pharmacists. ASHP statement on the pharmacist's role with respect to drug delivery systems and administration devices. *Am J Hosp Pharm.* 1993;50:1724–1725.

83. Apkon M, Leonard J, Probst L, et al. Design of a safer approach to intravenous drug infusions: failure mode effects analysis. *Qual Saf Health Care.* 2004;13:265–271.

84. Berman WJ, Whitman V, Marks KH. Inadvertent overadministration of digoxin to low birthweight infants. *J Pediatr.* 1978;92:1024–1025.

85. Zenke KE, Anderson S. Improving the accuracy of min-volume injections. *Infusion.* 1982;6:7–11.

86. Schmidt N, Saez C, Seri I, Matana A. Impact of syringe size on the performance of infusion pumps at low flow rates. *Pediatr Crit Care Med.* 2010;1:282–286.

87. Neal DA, Lin JA. The effect of syringe size on reliability and safety of low flow infusions. *Pediatr Crit Care Med.* 2009;10:592–596.

88. Neff SB, Neff TA, Gerber S, Weiss MM. Flow rate, syringe size and architecture are critical to start-up performance of syringe pumps. *Eur J Anaesthesiol.* 2007;24:602–608.

89. Aubel F, Bernstein T, Fuentes C. Variations in effective volume delivery using a continuous infusion syringe pump at low flow infusion rates. *E-PAS.* 2006;59:4850.217.

90. Weiss M, Hug MI, Neff T, Fischer J. Syringe size and flow rate affect drug delivery from syringe pumps. *Can J Anaesth.* 2000;47:1031–1035.

91. Rakza T, Richard A, Lelieur AC, et al. Factors altering low-flow drug delivery using syringe pumps: consequences on vasoactive drug infusion in preterm infant. *Arch Pediatr.* 2005;12: 548–554.

92. Kim DW, Steward DJ. The effect of syringe size on the performance of an infusion pump. *Paediatr Anaesth.* 1999;9:335–337.

93. Institute for Safe Medication Practices. Proceedings from the ISMP summit on the use of smart infusion pumps: guidelines for safe implementation and use. Available at: http://www.ismp .org/tools/guidelines/smartpumps/printerVersion.pdf. Accessed May 10, 2013.

94. American Society of Hospital Pharmacists. ASHP statement on the pharmacist's role with respect to drug delivery systems and administration devices. *Am J Hosp Pharm.* 1993;50:1724–1725.

95. Manrique-Rodriguez S, Sanchez-Galindo A, Fernandez-Llamazares CM, et al. Developing a drug library for smart pumps in a pediatric intensive care unit. *Artif Intell Med.* 2012;54:155–161.

96. Rothschild JM, Keohane CA, Cook EF, et al. A controlled trial of smart infusion pumps to improve medication safety in critically ill patients. *Crit Care Med.* 2005;33:533–540.

97. Larsen GY, Parker HB, Cash J, et al. Standard drug concentrations and smart pump technology reduce continuous medication infusion error in pediatric population. *Pediatrics.* 2005;116(1):e21–e25.

98. Murdoch LJ, Cameron VJ. Smart infusion technology: a minimum safety standard for intensive care? *Br J Nurs.* 2008;17(10);630–636.

99. Tourel J, Delage E, Lebel D, et al. Smart pump use in pediatrics. *Am J Health-Sys Pharm.* 2012;69:1628–1629.

100. Manrique-Rodriguez S, Sanchez-Galindo A, Fernandez-Llamazares CM, et al. Smart pump alerts: all that glitters is not gold. *Int J Med Informatics.* 2012;81:344–350.

101. Fortescue E, Kaushal R, Landrigan CP, et al. Prioritizing strategies for preventing medication errors and adverse drug events in pediatric inpatients. *Pediatrics.* 2003;111(4 Pt 1):722–729.

102. American Academy of Pediatrics Committee on Drugs and Committee on Hospital Care. Prevention of medication errors in pediatric inpatient setting. *Pediatrics.* 2003;112:431–436.

103. Institute for Safe Medication Practices. Principles for designing a medication label for injectable syringes for patient specific, inpatient use. Available at: http://www.ismp.org/tools/guidelines/labelFormats/Injectable.asp. Accessed May 10, 2013.

104. Phelps SJ, Hak EB, Crill CM. In: Phelps SJ, Hak EB, Crill CM, eds. *Teddy bear book: pediatric injectable drugs.* 9th ed. Bethesda, MD: American Society of Health-System Pharmacists; 2010.

105. Taketomo CK, Hodding JH, Kraus DM, eds. *Pediatric and neonatal dosage handbook.* 19th ed. Hudson, OH: Lexi-Comp; 2012.

106. Young TE, ed. *Neofax.* 24th ed. Montvale, NJ: Thomson Reuters; 2011.

CHAPTER **11**

Quality Assurance and Quality Control for Sterile Compounding

Patricia C. Kienle

 Where this icon appears, visit http://go.jblearning.com /OchoaCWS to view the corresponding video.

Chapter Objectives

1. Distinguish between quality control and quality assurance.
2. Identify the key areas of quality systems when compounding sterile preparations.
3. List the main elements monitored in the sterile compounding facility.
4. Describe the three simulation tests required for personnel who compound sterile preparations.
5. Cite the requirements for end-product testing.

Key Terminology

Endotoxin
Primary engineering control
Pyrogen
Particulate matter
Personal protective equipment
Clean room

Colony-forming units (CFU)
Risk management
Policies and procedures
Facility
Growth media
Classified space

Overview

Establishing and maintaining quality are essential when preparing compounded sterile preparations (CSPs). Each compounding facility must have a robust quality control and quality assurance program to promote patient safety. Quality cannot be "tested" into a finished CSP; it must be built into the system.

Quality control generally refers to those processes that can be measured as the CSP is being produced. It includes elements, such as use of FDA-approved components, to ensure that the facility meets the specifications required for certification and competence of personnel. Quality assurance generally involves evaluation of the final preparation and the facility in which it is compounded, such as monitoring of the CSPs, facility, and use of specific personnel tests to simulate conditions commonly encountered during compounding.

Elements of Quality Assurance and Quality Control

Quality assurance is an important aspect of ensuring that proper standards are maintained for CSPs and related processes. United States Pharmacopeia (USP) Chapter <797> provides information that can serve as a general guide to the types of practices that should be involved in quality assurance systems related to sterile compounding. Specific elements should be observed, inspected, and tested as part of a quality assurance program, including the following measures:[1]

- Testing of air quality and routine disinfection processes
- Donning of personal protective equipment (PPE)

- Review of orders and packages of ingredients for identity and accuracy
- Inspection of CSPs for absence of particulate matter and leakages
- Inspection of CSPs for thoroughness of labeling

Institutions should develop formal quality assurance programs using at least these elements as the basis for the program. The emphasis of the program should be on maintaining and improving the quality of systems for compounding as well as improving the provision of patient care. Specific aspects of the program can be delegated to individuals who are knowledgeable and able to support consistency of the program. The program should have the following characteristics:[1]

- Formal and written
- Considerate of all aspects of preparations and dispensing, including environmental testing and verification results
- Descriptive of specific activities relating to monitoring and evaluation
- Descriptive of how results of monitoring will be reported and evaluated
- Includes thresholds or limits for evaluations and outlines appropriate follow-up mechanisms
- Effectively addresses risk management

In addition to identifying important quality assurance characteristics as part of a quality assurance program, aspects of quality control should be specified. Given that quality control focuses on testing and measuring, it is helpful for institutions to have written descriptions of the specifics of the quality controls that will be evaluated. For example, written descriptions should be developed specifically for training and performance evaluation of personnel involved in compounding.

Outlining the specifics of a quality assurance program and effective quality control is an important step in preventing patient harm and ensuring safe and accurate CSPs.

ALERT: *Always remember that the CSP you compound is a critical element in a patient's care.*

Education and Training

Personnel expectations are defined in USP Chapter <797> and are supplemented by state regulations related to compounding and the pharmacy's orientation and training program. USP Chapter <797> is a federally enforceable standard that defines the minimum levels required for education and training; it is not just a guideline. It applies to all personnel who compound sterile preparations—pharmacists, pharmacy technicians, students, physicians, nurses, and other personnel—and in all places where CSPs are prepared. To meet the USP Chapter <797> standard, institutions need to establish and follow a quality plan, based on the scope of sterile compounding performed. Appropriate orientation and training are required for anyone who compounds CSPs.

ELEMENTS OF TRAINING

Employees and students new to an institution must be introduced to the facility's CSP processes by a compounding supervisor or designee. The compounding supervisor is the person who coordinates the orientation, training, observation, competence assessment, facility control and monitoring, and assurance of quality.

Education and training should consist of some or all of the following elements:

- Access to policies and procedures
- Knowledge of types of medications that will be handled, including hazardous drugs
- Didactic instruction, which may be live or video
- Instruction, observation, and return demonstration of procedures
- Written evaluations

- Completion of practical evaluations that demonstrate aseptic preparation of CSPs
- Guidance in completion of steps in the quality plan

Individuals who will be mixing CSPs for patients need to complete all portions of the quality plan that apply.

Regulatory Agencies and Accreditation Organizations

Each pharmacy has specific standards that must be followed. In addition, many states have specific compounding regulations. Pharmacies with a business focus on compounding can undergo voluntary accreditation by organizations such as the Pharmacy Compounding Accreditation Board (PCAB) or specialty organizations such as the Accreditation Commission for Health Care (ACHC), which accredits home care pharmacies.

Hospitals and health systems are held to additional standards that are based on patient safety and maintenance of quality systems. Federal regulations include those promulgated by the Centers for Medicare and Medicaid Services (CMS) in its Hospital Conditions of Participation,[2] which are used to certify hospitals. Most health systems are also accredited by an accrediting organization, such as The Joint Commission,[3] DNV Healthcare,[4] Healthcare Facilities Accreditation Program (HFAP),[5] or the Center for Improvement in Healthcare Quality.[6]

All of these certification and accreditation processes are intended to ensure that the pharmacies and other healthcare institutions protect patients and develop and maintain quality systems. Establishment of robust practices promotes assurance of quality. All of these components are designed to limit risk to the patient, personnel, and facility.

Major Tenets of Quality

Three major components must be controlled when evaluating quality in sterile compounding: facilities, personnel, and monitoring.

> **ALERT:** *The three major areas of quality control and assurance are the compounding facility, the competence of compounding personnel, and monitoring of personnel, facilities, and CSPs.*

- Facilities: Proper facilities must be well designed and operate based on established criteria as defined in USP Chapter <797> and equipment manufacturers' instructions. Primary engineering controls (PECs), commonly referred to as "hoods," are complex engineering controls that require proper use and maintenance to ensure facilities' quality systems are operating as expected.
- Personnel: The most important element in compounding sterile preparations is the competence of the personnel. Individuals must be carefully trained and meticulous in following aseptic procedures.
- Monitoring: Monitoring both personnel and facilities is key to the quality process. Individuals must demonstrate competence in the ability to aseptically garb, clean the processing areas, and aseptically compound sterile preparations. Pharmacies and other facilities must be monitored for environmental conditions (temperature, humidity, light, and sound), elements required of a cleanroom (particle count, air changes, pressure, and HEPA filtration), and freedom from contamination (including bacteria or fungi).

CSPs are most often prepared from manufactured sterile products, such as commercially prepared IV bags and FDA-approved drugs. Those facilities that compound sterile preparations from non-sterile ingredients and solutions requiring terminal sterilization prior to patient use require an even more robust quality process to ensure safety.

All three areas—facilities, personnel, and monitoring—contribute to the quality system necessary to safely compound sterile preparations.

Facility Control

There are three facets to control of the facility: the design of the sterile compounding area, the daily monitoring required by pharmacy personnel, and the periodic certification by a professional who specializes in evaluating pharmacy sterile compounding facilities.

DESIGN OF THE STERILE COMPOUNDING AREA

The facility must be designed to adequately support the CSPs that will be compounded. A commonly used design includes the following elements:

- An ante-area, which serves as the transition area between the main pharmacy and the cleanroom
- A positive-pressure buffer area, where nonhazardous CSPs are mixed
- A negative-pressure buffer area, where hazardous CSPs, such as chemotherapy for oncology patients, are mixed[7]

The PECs must be placed in the buffer areas. Ideally, the buffer area and the ante-area will be separate rooms, but USP Chapter <797> allows for a single ante/buffer room that is appropriately divided, provided that CSPs are only prepared from commercially manufactured drugs and solutions. If any sterile compounding involves use of non-sterile ingredients, the ante-area and buffer area must be in separate rooms.[1] For safety of personnel, the PEC used for preparation of hazardous drugs should be located in a separate room. The ante-area, buffer area, and PEC area are collectively considered the cleanroom.

In some cases, a PEC may be found in an area outside a clean room; this space is called a segregated compounding area. This arrangement may occur in a hospital that does not have a cleanroom that complies with USP Chapter <797>, or it may be encountered in a specialty area for critical patients, such as an intensive care unit or surgical suite.

"Classified space" refers to areas that must be monitored for particle counts, freedom from contamination, use by personnel who have demonstrated competency in aseptic preparation, and related requirements. These are the main areas that must be monitored as part of the institution's quality plan.

CSPs occasionally need to be mixed in an urgent patient care situation, such as when a patient is experiencing cardiac arrest. Given that these solutions are made outside of the cleanroom or segregated compounding area, the areas in which they are prepared are considered "unclassified space."

The cleanroom and related space require daily monitoring of environmental factors to ensure that everything is "in control"— that is, within the parameters for safe mixing of CSPs. Pharmacy staff should be assigned to monitor and record these parameters, including the following:

- Temperature of the storage areas outside the cleanroom
    o When parenteral drugs and solutions are approved by the FDA, a temperature range is assigned. Generally, these specifications include controlled room temperature, refrigeration, or freezing (**Table 11-1**). The temperature of the storage areas must be monitored to ensure that the components used for CSPs remain within the defined parameters.
- Temperature of the ante-area and buffer area
    o USP Chapter <797> suggests a temperature not to exceed 20°C.
- Airflow patterns
    o The ante-area and buffer room operate on a process of pressure differences. These differences apply when the buffer area and ante-area are separate rooms. For nonhazardous CSPs, the buffer room must be a positive-pressure; in other words, the pressure in the room must exceed that of the surrounding area. This design prevents particles and other contaminants from coming into the room when the door is opened. The positive pressure will result in air being directed out of the

room. For hazardous preparations, negative pressure is required; it prevents any hazardous drug contamination from entering the surrounding areas. The pressure of the rooms must be monitored to ensure that airflow patterns are correct.

o In a combined ante/buffer area, no pressure difference is possible, because both components are located in the same room. USP Chapter <797> allows for a process of displacement airflow, where the air from the buffer area sweeps across a line of demarcation in the room. The displacement airflow must be monitored.

▪ Humidity, light, and sound levels

o While these levels are not required to be monitored by USP Chapter <797>, many institutions include them in their daily monitoring. Humidity should be maintained between 35% and 65%. A lower humidity may lead to static electricity, which is uncomfortable for personnel and potentially dangerous for equipment. A higher humidity could promote microbial growth, which must be avoided in aseptic areas. Light and sound levels are determined by the equipment manufacturer, as well as federal, state, and local regulations. If required by regulation or institutional policy, they must be monitored.

If any of these established parameters are outside the defined range, the pharmacy's policy must be followed for adjustment, remonitoring, reporting, and escalation of the issue if it is unresolved.

Table 11-1   USP Temperature Ranges

	Degrees Centigrade	**Degrees Fahrenheit**
Controlled room temperature	20 to 25	68 to 77
Refrigerated	2 to 8	36 to 46
Frozen	−25 to −10	−13 to 14

Source: Data from U.S. Pharmacopeial Convention. Chapter <797>: pharmaceutical compounding: sterile preparations. *United States Pharmacopeia 36/National Formulary 31.* Rockville, MD: U.S. Pharmacopeial Convention; 2013.

CERTIFICATION OF THE PRIMARY AND SECONDARY ENGINEERING CONTROLS

As described in the *Primary and Secondary Engineering Controls* chapter, primary engineering controls are areas in which direct compounding occurs, while secondary engineering controls are the surrounding areas, such as the buffer area and ante-area. In addition to the daily monitoring by pharmacy personnel, a professional who evaluates pharmacy cleanrooms must certify the primary and secondary controls at least every 6 months.

The Controlled Environment Testing Association (CETA) provides industry guidance for evaluating and certifying pharmacy cleanrooms. Individuals who certify pharmacy cleanrooms should use the CETA guidance documents, which detail elements to be monitored and explain how to certify the devices and rooms.[8] Additionally, some certifiers complete a specialized course and national examination, which evaluates their competency in assessing sterile compounding facility compliance, based on USP Chapter <797> and the CETA *Certification Guide for Sterile Compounding Facilities*. Certifiers who have successfully completed this examination are designated as a Registered Cleanroom Certification Professional in Sterile Compounding (RCCP-SC).[9]

Certification of Sterile Compounding Facilities

The certifier must examine each of the PECs and all of the secondary engineering controls during the semiannual certification process. The certifier should subsequently validate the monitoring that is performed by pharmacy personnel, providing an independent check of the parameters monitored daily, such as temperature, pressure, and humidity. The certifier then should evaluate the devices and other controls in the cleanroom.

The institutional evaluation performed by the certifier includes evaluation of each PEC, including checks of HEPA filter integrity, airflow patterns, and particle counts. Calibrated equipment is used to perform these tests. All PECs must be evaluated and certified at least every 6 months, whether or not they are placed in a cleanroom or a segregated compounding area.

The secondary engineering controls must be evaluated for two types of issues: nonviable and viable parameters. Nonviable monitoring is related to particle counts in the room, and includes HEPA filter integrity, airflow patterns, and air exchanges per hour. Viable monitoring is related to potential microbial contamination. Such testing requires electronic air sampling of air from the clean room. The device draws in air over the culture medium, which is then incubated. Different culture media are used for detection of bacterial and fungal contaminants. Viable monitoring can be done by hospital personnel such as those individuals deemed competent from the laboratory, infection prevention, facilities departments, the professional certifier, or personnel from another company that specializes in monitoring healthcare environments.

Microbial growth appears as colony-forming units (CFUs) on an agar plate. The growth must be identified at least to the genus level. USP Chapter <797> includes recommended action levels if microbial growth is identified. If the CFUs exceed the action levels, the situation must be remediated.[1] The necessary steps include recleaning the area, retraining staff, and retesting to ensure that these actions were adequate to resolve the issue.

Policies and Procedures

One key principle underlying a quality system is standardization of processes. Policies and procedures are required to ensure that all personnel are aware of the requirements for compounding sterile preparations, maintaining quality systems, and reporting elements that are out of control based on parameters set to maintain quality processes.

ALERT: *Individuals should not perform a procedure until a written policy is in place and, if equipment is involved, only after the equipment has been certified as operating within expected ranges.*

Cleaning the Sterile Compounding Area

The quality plan must include specific policies and procedures to clean the sterile compounding area. USP Chapter <797> defines minimum cleaning frequencies (**Table 11-2**). Cleaning solution components and dilutions must be approved by the institution's Infection Control Committee if the pharmacy is part of a health system or by the consultant infection preventionist if the facility is not part of a health system.

Organizational policy varies on the issue of allowing an outside department, such as Environmental Services, or a contracted cleaning company to clean the cleanroom. If such practices are permitted, institutional policies must outline those areas that must be cleaned by pharmacy personnel. Only pharmacy personnel may clean the PECs. Responsibility for cleaning the floors, walls, and ceilings can be shared with the Environmental Services department if permitted by policy and if those individuals have documented competency in cleaning sterile compounding areas.

Cleaning the PECs throughout the workday is generally performed with sterile 70% isopropyl alcohol and sterile water. Sterile alcohol is used because filtration removes, and gamma-radiation kills, any spores that might be in the alcohol. A germicidal/sporicidal detergent should be used on at least a daily basis.

Table 11-2   Minimum Frequency of Cleaning Sterile Compounding Areas

Minimum Frequency	Area
Immediately	After spills and whenever contamination is known or suspected
Daily	PECs: at the beginning of each shift, before each batch, and every 30 minutes during compounding
	Counters and easily cleanable work surfaces
	Floors
Monthly	Walls
	Ceilings
	Storage shelving

Source: Data from U.S. Pharmacopeial Convention. Chapter <797>: pharmaceutical compounding: sterile preparations. *United States Pharmacopeia 36/National Formulary 31.* Rockville, MD: U.S. Pharmacopeial Convention; 2013.

Cleaning hazardous drug areas involves additional steps, including decontamination and deactivation of the hazardous drugs. No single product is capable of removing all hazardous drugs, so the FDA-approved labeling for each agent used must be consulted for specific information on its scope of use. If no information is available, most facilities use a combination of sodium hypochlorite (bleach) and sodium thiosulfate. The thiosulfate is necessary both to inactivate some hazardous drugs and to neutralize the bleach so pitting of the stainless steel surfaces on the PECs does not occur.

Personnel Monitoring

The key element in sterile compounding is the competence of the personnel who mix the CSPs. The quality plan must document the orientation, training, and ongoing competence of each individual who compounds sterile preparations.

ORIENTATION AND INITIAL TRAINING

Individuals who compound sterile preparations must always be vigilant and attentive to detail, have the ability to follow policies, be able to physically manipulate the devices and equipment, and demonstrate willingness to escalate concerns to an appropriate level. Once selected to perform tasks in the sterile compounding area, personnel must be adequately trained by a qualified instructor.

The compounding supervisor must oversee didactic and practical training. Training and documentation of competence must occur even if personnel have compounded sterile preparations at another institution. Competence involves both the skill needed to safely and efficiently prepare CSPs and a thorough knowledge of the institution's policies and procedures.

Training and competency documentation includes completion of didactic instruction, assessment of the facility's specific policies and procedures, written tests, return demonstration with oversight by an experienced compounder, and successful completion of three specific tests defined by USP Chapter <797>: media fill, gloved fingertip, and surface sampling.

Media Fill Test

A media fill test simulates mixing of CSPs, simulating the most complex preparation that personnel would be expected to compound. A variety of tests are available, one of which uses a vial and bag containing liquid culture media instead of drugs. For this particular test (such as the one developed by Q.I. Medical), personnel remove 1 mL of media from the vial and inject it into the bag, repeating the process 20 times. A new needle is utilized with each withdrawal from the vial; however, the port of the bag and the rubber closure of the vial are disinfected only once, at the beginning of the process. If personnel successfully compound a preparation that is free of microbial growth, then the media contained in the vial and the bag will remain clear after incubating them at a temperature of 20–25°C, or at a temperature of 30–35°C for at least 14 days.[10] **Figure 11-1** and **Figure 11-2** illustrate tests that are negative (i.e., free from microbial growth) and tests that are positive for growth. Media fill tests must be successfully completed prior to compounding for patients, and then at least every 12 months for

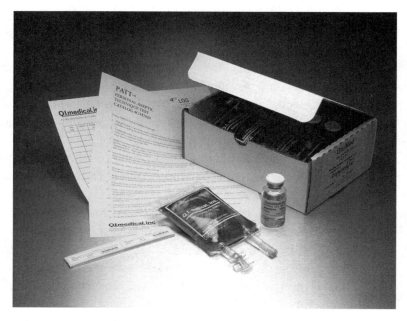

Figure 11-1   Media Fill Kit
Courtesy of QI Medical.

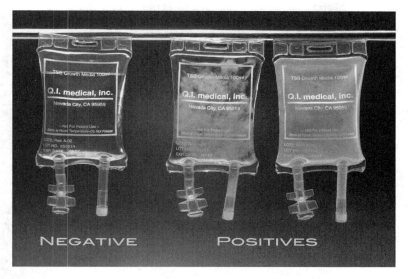

Figure 11-2 Negative and Positive Media Fill Test Results
Courtesy of QI Medical.

facilities where only low- and medium-risk preparations (which use only sterile commercially manufactured drugs and solutions) are mixed, or at least every 6 months for facilities where high-risk preparations (from non-sterile drugs or solutions) are prepared.[1]

 ## Gloved Fingertip Test

The gloved fingertip test demonstrates that an individual can garb without contamination. After garbing, but prior to applying alcohol to the sterile gloves, the individual places each finger and thumb in a plate of contrast media. Two plates are used for each person—one for each hand. An example of a gloved fingertip test is shown in **Figure 11-3**. After initial training, this test must be successfully completed three times with no evidence of growth prior to mixing CSPs for patients. The test needs to be completed every 12 months in facilities that prepare only low- and medium-risk CSPs and at least every 6 months in facilities that prepare high-risk CSPs. USP Chapter <797> defines suggested action limits for the annual or semiannual recertification, but no growth is still the expected result.

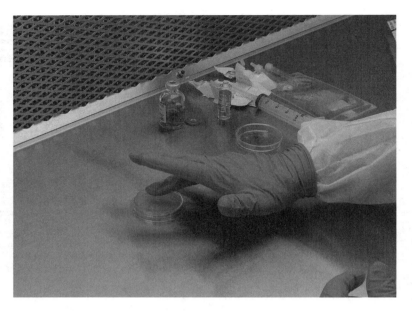

Figure 11-3 Gloved Fingertip Testing
Courtesy of CriticalPoint, LLC.

SURFACE SAMPLING

Surface sampling is a test used to evaluate two quality domains: personnel's ability to properly clean the work area and assurance of the proper solutions and dilutions for cleaning. The facility's compounding supervisor, in consultation with the infection preventionist, should develop a sampling map of areas in the sterile compounding suite that will be routinely tested (**Figure 11-4**). This allows for trending, which is useful in the event that microbial growth occurs. Repeated growth in the same area, growth of the same organism in different areas, or growth of pathogenic organisms provides clues to the source of the growth.

Surface sampling tests are performed by compounding personnel who use media plates and swabs to collect samples from assigned areas based on the sampling map. USP Chapter <797> requires this test to be done "periodically,"[1] although most institutions perform it monthly or quarterly. If growth is found, the frequency of the test must be increased.

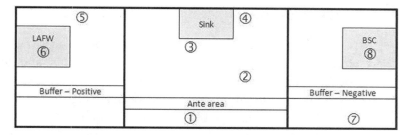

Figure 11-4   Sample Map to Monitor Surface Sampling

> **ALERT:** *Two types of monitoring are used to ensure freedom from microbial growth: (1) periodic surface sampling and (2) electronic air sampling at least every 6 months.*

Labeling

Prior to dispensing, all CSPs must be visually checked for elements such as the identity of all ingredients, appropriate appearance of the CSP, and the label. Organizational policy dictates the format and elements of the label. In addition, federal and state requirements and the patient's status as either an inpatient in an institution or an outpatient determine many components of the label. CSP-specific elements include a listing of all active ingredients, the quantity or strength of the compound, beyond-use date and time, directions for use, and any applicable instructions to the patient or caregiver to maintain the potency of the CSP through its beyond-use date. Labels alert personnel administering the CSP as to the contents and instructions for administration, as well as the patient for whom the CSP is intended. The label is also important for the verification step, in which the right patient, right drug, right dose, right route, and right time are assessed. All diluents, expiration dates of products and admixtures, and instructions for use must also be verified from the labeling and signed off by a pharmacist.

End-Product Testing

CSPs need to contain the labeled strength of the drug, need to be free of unintended additives or other components, and need to be free from microbial contamination.

Low- and medium-risk CSPs are made only from commercially available manufactured products, such as FDA-approved drugs and IV solutions. Low- and medium-risk CSPs labeled with the beyond-use date (BUD) limits defined in USP Chapter <797> do not require testing, although institutional policy may require it.

In contrast, low- and medium-risk CSPs that exceed the USP Chapter <797> BUD limits must be tested for the stability of the CSP. Due to the expense of testing, and the increased risk of either instability or contamination of the CSP, most institutions limit the BUDs to those listed in USP Chapter <797>.

Assignment of BUDs requires evaluation of both the stability of the drug and other components (including the diluent and container) and the sterility limits. The BUD must be the *shorter* of the stability or sterility limits.

High-risk CSPs made in batches of more than 25 require sterility testing[11] (**Table 11-3**). Knowledge and application of additional USP chapters are essential when compounding high-risk CSPs, because creating a CSP that began as a non-sterile compound is far more difficult than maintaining sterility with use of commercially available sterile products. USP provides standards that must be followed, including:

Table 11-3   Sterility Test Requirements

	Within USP <797> BUDs	Exceeding USP <797> BUDs
Low- and medium-risk CSPs	Not required	Required
High-risk CSPs of 25 or fewer units	Not required	Required
High-risk CSPs of more than 25 units	Required	Required

Source: Data from U.S. Pharmacopeial Convention. Chapter <797>: pharmaceutical compounding: sterile preparations. *United States Pharmacopeia 36/National Formulary 31.* Rockville, MD: U.S. Pharmacopeial Convention; 2013.

- USP <71>: Sterility Tests[11]
- USP <85>: Bacterial Endotoxins Test[12]
- USP <1211>: Sterilization and Sterility Assurance of Compendial Articles[13]

Compounding high-risk CSPs is far more complex than compounding with only commercially available sterile products and devices. The process to create a sterile preparation (versus maintaining sterility, as is done with low- and medium-risk CSPs) includes robust processes that must be validated to ensure safety:

- Facilities and equipment specifically designed to safely work with powders, raw chemicals, concentrated solutions, containers, and container closures
- Examination and understanding of the Certificate of Analysis that accompanies non-sterile components to ensure compliance with FDA, USP, or other industry standards
- Peer-reviewed literature to support the clinical use of the CSP and the assigned BUD
- Use of a certified laboratory to provide end-product testing to validate strength, potency, purity, and freedom from contaminants (including endotoxins)

Those personnel who compound high-risk preparations must be competent in the operation and monitoring of the equipment used for these special preparations. Autoclaves are the most common type of device used to terminally sterilize high-risk CSPs. Compounding personnel must be able to demonstrate that they can safely operate the autoclave, and can appropriately place and monitor the biological indicators that are used for each autoclave cycle to ensure that the sterilization has been completed.

Filtration may be used for terminal sterilization of heat-labile CSPs. In such a case, the filter must be chemically and physically stable for the compound used, and must be tested for integrity after use, based on the manufacturer-recommended filter integrity test.

Documentation of Elements of the Quality Plan

All the components of quality control and quality assurance are part of the facility's quality plan. The quality plan identifies and documents the elements determined to be needed to develop, maintain, and compound CSPs:

- Facility issues, such as semiannual certification status of all PECs and all ante-areas and buffer areas, and any remediation that occurred
- Routine facility monitoring, such as daily temperature, humidity, and pressure results, and action taken if any readings are out of range
- Personnel competence documentation, including state certification (if required), initial and annual testing, and the status of all personnel who mix CSPs
- Viable monitoring, including both periodic surface sampling by personnel and semiannual electronic air monitoring, and identification of any growth and action taken
- Daily calibration of any equipment such as automated compounding devices, repeater pumps, or robotic devices
- Other applicable data, such as the number of CSPs dispensed, and any testing or recalls of those items

ALERT: *The quality plan should list all elements that contribute to safe and effective CSP processes.*

Conclusion

Institutions maintain a responsibility for the patients whom they care for. While protecting the patient from harm should be a responsibility of each individual involved in the preparation process, overarching checks and balances must also be in place.

Many factors must be considered in developing quality assurance programs, and many characteristics of quality control must be established. Effective quality assurance programs provide the education and tools needed for compounding personnel to compound sterile preparations safely and effectively. Quality control allows the opportunity to verify equipment, environment, and practices.

One of the most important activities of compounding is the ability to safely and effectively compound sterile preparations. It involves a skill set that must be learned and competency that must be maintained. Quality needs to be built into the processes used to compound sterile preparations. The quality control used in the process, and the triad of personnel, facilities, and robust policies and procedures, become the quality assurance practices that promote patient safety.

Review Questions

1. Which of the following USP chapters provides guidance on the testing for bacterial endotoxins?
   a. <797>
   b. <85>
   c. <1211>
   d. <71>

2. Describe the difference between quality control and quality assurance.

3. Which of the following is a main element that is monitored in the sterile compounding facility?
   a. Donning of PPE
   b. Temperature
   c. Aseptic technique
   d. Hand cleanliness

4. List the three simulation tests required for personnel who compound sterile preparations.

5. Which of the following require sterility testing?
   a. Low-risk CSPs
   b. Medium-risk CSPs
   c. High-risk CSPs
   d. High-risk CSPs made in batches of more than 25 units

6. Given that a PEC has not been moved and is not suspected to be compromised, how often should PECs and secondary engineering controls be certified?

7. A compounding employee performs a media fill test. After the proper amount of time for incubation of the media, a positive result is noted. Based on this observation, which of the following is the most reasonable explanation?
   a. The employee did not don PPE in the proper sequence
   b. The employee did not perform effective aseptic technique and/or hand hygiene
   c. The air quality in the room was poor
   d. The employee used a new needle with each transfer

8. An employee was recently hired to compound sterile preparations. The employee undergoes training for this responsibility, including didactic instruction and assessment of institutional policies and procedures. Which other requirements must be met before the new employee can compound sterile preparations for patients?

9. A new facility is beginning to compound sterile preparations. Supervisors have completed all the required steps, including implementing new policies and procedures. Certifiers have visited the facility and the results are pending. Can personnel begin compounding in the new facility?
   a. Yes
   a. No

10. List two types of monitoring that are used to ensure freedom from microbial growth.

CASE STUDIES *Case 1*

Lauren, a P2 pharmacy student, has recently started work as a technician at General Hospital. She has made IVs before at another hospital. Her co-workers are anxious for her to begin working in the IV room during her first weekend. Lauren asks Kurt, the pharmacy supervisor, if she can do that. What is his response?

Kurt provides Lauren with the hospital-applicable didactic and video training and is pleased with her progress. The next weekend while she works, Kurt reviews the initial training materials, answers Lauren's questions, and observes her technique. Both agree that Lauren is ready to take the required personnel tests required by USP Chapter <797>. What are these tests and what do they demonstrate?

When can Lauren begin mixing IVs for patients?

Case 2

Jason is responsible for monitoring the temperatures of all refrigerators, freezers, warmers, and incubators at Harris Compounding Pharmacy. The temperature of the cleanroom refrigerator is 10°C at 11 a.m. one morning.

Is any action necessary?

What is the appropriate next step?

Which actions should be taken if the temperature is still out of range?

What if the temperature is now within range?

References

1. U.S. Pharmacopeial Convention. Chapter <797>: pharmaceutical compounding: sterile preparations. *United States Pharmacopeia 36/National Formulary 31*. Rockville, MD: U.S. Pharmacopeial Convention; 2013.

2. Centers for Medicare and Medicaid Services. Hospital conditions of participation, Rev 84 06-07-13. Available at: http://cms.hhs.gov/Regulations-and-Guidance/Guidance/Manuals/downloads/som107ap_a_hospitals.pdf. Accessed January 28, 2014.

3. The Joint Commission. Available at: http://www.jointcommission .org. Accessed August 25, 2013.

4. DNV Healthcare. Available at: http://www.dnvaccreditation .com. Accessed August 25, 2013.

5. Healthcare Facilities Accreditation Program. Available at: http://www.hfap.org. Accessed August 25, 2013.

6. Center for Improvement in Healthcare Quality. Available at: http://www.cihq.org. Accessed August 25, 2013.

7. Department of Health and Human Services. NIOSH list of anti-neoplastics and other hazardous drugs in healthcare settings 2012. Publication 2012-150. June 2012. Available at: http://www .cdc.gov/niosh/docs/2012-150/pdfs/2012-150.pdf. Accessed August 25, 2013.

8. Controlled Environment Testing Association. Available at: http://www.cetainternational.org. Accessed August 25, 2013.

9. CETA National Board of Testing. Available at: http://www .cetaboardoftesting.org. Accessed August 25, 2013.

10. Q.I. Medical. Available at: http://qimedical.com/pricelist.htm. Accessed August 25, 2013.

11. U.S. Pharmacopeial Convention. Chapter <71>: sterility tests. *United States Pharmacopeia 36/National Formulary 31*. Rock-ville, MD: U.S. Pharmacopeial Convention; 2013.

12. U.S. Pharmacopeial Convention. Chapter <85>: bacterial endo-toxins test. *United States Pharmacopeia 36/National Formulary 31*. Rockville, MD: U.S. Pharmacopeial Convention; 2013.

13. U.S. Pharmacopeial Convention. Chapter <1211>: sterilization and sterility assurance of compendial articles. *United States Pharmacopeia 36/National Formulary 31*. Rockville, MD: U.S. Pharmacopeial Convention; 2013.

Glossary

2-in-1 admixture: a solution that contains amino acids, dextrose, and micronutrients; injectable lipid emulsions are not contained within the final preparation, but are administered as a separate piggyback infusion.

Absorption: the permeation of one substance into another; when drug molecules in a solution permeate into the container.

ACPE: Accreditation Council for Pharmacy Education.

Admixture: the result of mixing a medication or other additive with a diluent, as with the mixture of two liquids or a solid and a liquid.

Adsorption: the process in which chemicals from the contents within a container adhere to the inner surface of the container.

Alligation: a calculation used to determine the number of parts of two products with stronger and weaker concentrations required to achieve the desired concentration.

Amorphous: the state of a drug or solid whose atomic-scale structure is not a crystalline structure.

Ante-area: area preceding the buffer area; an ISO Class 8 environment must be maintained in this area; area in which hand washing, donning personal protective equipment, and other approved activities occur.

Asepsis: a state that is free of microorganisms or contamination related to microorganisms.

Aseptic technique: methods of manipulating parenteral supplies and equipment during the compounding process in such a way as to prevent contamination of the final preparation.

ASHP Technical Assistance Bulletins: extensive recommendations provided by American Society of Health-System Pharmacists; they address equipment and work practices for hazardous drug compounding, so they are most applicable to pharmacy personnel.

Automated compounding device (ACD): a machine that has multiple incoming lines to which multiple bags or bottles of large-volume additives, such as dextrose, are attached; it can be programmed to deliver a set volume from the large-volume products into the final preparation.

Auxiliary label: a label used in addition to the main labels that contains specific alerts and instructions that should be highlighted.

Batch compounding: preparing multiple products, either for multiple patients or for a single patient, during one extended preparation process.

Benzyl alcohol: a common preservative agent in parenteral drugs, which may be toxic to infants and young children.

Beyond-use date: date and time beyond which a sterile compounded preparation should not be administered to a patient and should be discarded appropriately.

Biological safety cabinet (BSC): a ventilated cabinet for compounded sterile products. It has an open front with inward airflow for personnel protection, downward HEPA-filtered laminar airflow for product protection, and HEPA-filtered exhausted air for environmental protection.

Buffer area: area in which primary engineering controls are located; air quality must be of ISO Class 7.

Central venous catheter (CVC): an intravenous catheter inserted such that the tip of the catheter ends in the superior vena cava or right atrium of the heart; used for delivering parenteral solutions to the central circulation.

Chemotherapy spill kit: a kit that includes the following items: (1) supplies to absorb a spill of about 1000 mL; (2) appropriate personal protective equipment, including two pairs of disposable chemotherapy gloves, chemotherapy gowns, shoe covers, and face shield; (3) absorbent, plastic-backed sheets or spill pads; (4) disposable toweling; (5) at least two sealable, thick-plastic hazardous waste disposal bags; (6) one disposable scoop for collecting glass fragments; (7) one puncture-resistant container for glass fragments; and (8) a decontamination supply.

Classified space: areas that must be monitored for particle counts, freedom from contamination, use by personnel who have demonstrated competency in aseptic preparation, and related requirements.

Clean room: an area in which airborne particles are controlled to meet specifications for cleanliness based on airborne particulate concentrations; may include buffer areas and ante-areas.

Clean zone: an area within the workbench in which first air is distributed; the area in which manipulations take place.

Closed system: a system that does not allow free passage of air in and out of the container secondary to a closure system.

Closed-system vial-transfer device (CSTD): a device that mechanically prohibits the escape of a hazardous drug or vapor into the environment during drug-transferring processes.

Colony-forming units (CFU): a measure of viable cells or a cluster of cells containing two or more of the same organism growing together.

Compounding aseptic containment isolator (CACI): a ventilated isolator designed to prevent toxic materials processed inside the unit from escaping to the surrounding environment. This type of isolator is used for compounding hazardous drugs.

Compounded sterile preparation (CSP): a preparation that is free of microorganisms and is processed using sterile supplies, equipment, and technique from manufactured sterile products.

Coring: a process in which a piece of rubber is carved out from the rubber vial closure during penetration with a needle; results from improper entry into the vial.

Critical sites: areas on the syringe and needle that, if touched, are associated with contamination of the final product; critical sites must always be in contact with first air.

Crystallization: the formation of crystals within a saturated solution; occurs as solid–liquid separation in which crystals form within a solution.

Crystalloid solutions: solutions containing small molecules that can pass through vascular spaces, allowing them to move through intracellular spaces; used for hydration and electrolyte replenishment (as with sodium chloride).

Dead space: reservoirs for drug volume within an intravenous infusion set in which drug can be trapped or unaccounted for during infusions. Common reservoirs include needles, stopcocks, ports, and filters.

Decarboxylation: a chemical reaction that results in the loss of a carboxyl group from a compound and forms carbon dioxide.

DEHP: di-ethylhexyl phthalate; a chemical used to make polyvinyl chloride (PVC) plastic soft and flexible, which may cause toxicity in infants, particularly in relation to the reproductive system.

Depyrogenation: the process of removing pyrogens.

Diaphragm: a rubber closure, as with a vial or entry port on a bag.

Diluent: an aqueous solution that is used to dilute a medication or other solution; used for reconstitution of powder medications.

Dilution control: a method of providing airflow by mixing existing air with HEPA-filtered air, thereby diluting any airborne contaminates.

Direct compounding area: an ISO Class 5 environment where critical site exposure takes place within a primary engineering control.

Displacement volume: the volume occupying additional space as a result of expansion from reconstitution.

Effervescence: the formation of gas or bubbles in a solution; often the result of a chemical reaction of parenteral products.

Endotoxin: a toxin that is contained in bacteria cell walls and is released when the bacteria disintegrate.

Environment control: the design of and requirements for the room (area) where hazardous drugs are stored and compounded. Major environment controls for the room for compounding hazardous drugs include ventilation, negative pressure, and particulate count.

Epimerization: formation of an epimer; the result of a reaction in which the center is altered in an optically active compound with two or more asymmetric centers.

Extravasation: leakage of a vesicant drug being infused intravenously out of the vein and into the surrounding tissues; it results in damage to the surrounding tissues.

Facility: a pharmacy or other area in which compounding occurs.

Filter needle: a needle containing a filter within its hub; the filter prevents particulate matter from being passed into or out of the syringe.

First air: clean air; air that undergoes filtration and exits the HEPA filter; air that has been cleansed of particulate matter greater than 0.3 micron and microorganisms; the first air to exit a HEPA filter.

Flow control: a method of providing HEPA-filtered air in a unidirectional pattern, intended to eliminate particles from the work zone by sweeping them away from the compounding area.

Fomite: an inanimate object that can be contaminated with bacteria, fungi, or viruses and can participate in the transmission of infectious organisms.

Garb: personal protective equipment; clothing and other equipment worn during compounding that protects the operator from the preparation and protects the preparation from the operator.

Gauge: numerical reference indicating the size of the needle lumen or bore.

Geometric dilution: process in which a small drug dose is diluted with a larger volume of base solution (diluent) to form a solution containing a lower concentration of the drug.

Gravimetric analysis: verification process to ensure the accuracy of the final admixture; uses the weights of additives, based on the volumes to be added, to determine a theoretical final weight, which is then compared to the actual weight of the final preparation.

Growth media: liquid or gel substances containing essential elements needed for the growth of microorganisms.

Hazardous agent/drug: a drug or agent that may cause genotoxicity, carcinogenicity, teratogenicity, fertility impairment, and serious organ or other toxicity at low doses, in either animal models or treated patients.

Hypertonic: more concentrated than normal saline; results in osmosis of water out of cells and into extracellular space.

Hypotonic: less concentrated than normal saline; results in osmosis of water into cells.

Incompatibility: an undesirable reaction that can occur between two drug substances, a drug substance and an excipient used in the drug product, or a drug substance or excipient with the container used in drug product storage.

Infiltration: leakage of the solution being infused intravenously out of the vein and into the surrounding tissues; it may cause damage to the affected tissues.

Injectable lipid emulsion (ILE): a component of parenteral nutrition that provides nutrition as lipids (fats) and is formulated as an emulsion.

Intraosseous (IO) catheter: an intravenous catheter that is inserted into the anteromedial surface of the tibia in emergency situations in infants and young children. IO catheters provide access to the central circulation for parenteral drug administration.

ISO classification: International Organization for Standardization numerical categories that differentiate environments based on particle counts in room air.

ISO class number: International Organization for Standardization numbers that denote the classification of air cleanliness. For hazardous drug compounding, the primary engineering control must be put in an ISO Class 7 air quality room, and ISO Class 5 air quality must be maintained within the primary engineering control.

Isotonicity: relating to the tonicity of a solution; isotonic solutions are those that have the same tonicity (or number of particles in the solution) as blood, tears, and normal saline.

Large-volume pump: a computer-controlled infusion pump that is used to deliver IV fluids, total parenteral nutrition, and intermittent drug doses in children. Rates of infusion range from 0.1 to 999 mL/hr.

Leaching: the process in which chemicals, such as plasticizers and other polymer additives, come out from plastic and enter the contents of a container.

Macrobore tubing: standard intravenous tubing set with a large internal diameter and high volume capacity (approximately 17 mL).

Maillard reaction: a chemical reaction between intravenous dextrose and certain amino acids, such as lysine, resulting in a brown color for the final preparation.

Methylparaben: a common preservative agent in parenteral drugs, which may be toxic to infants and young children.

Microbore tubing: intravenous tubing set with a small internal diameter and low volume capacity (0.3–0.4 mL).

Micron: a metric unit of measure of length; one micron is one-millionth of a meter.

Milking: the exchange of air and solution in and out of a vial to remove a specified volume of solution from the vial.

Milliosmoles per liter (mOsm/L): a representation of the number of osmotically active particles in 1 liter of solution; the unit used to express the concentrations of parenteral preparations.

Negative-pressure room: a room that is at a lower atmospheric pressure than the adjacent spaces, so that the net flow of air is into the room. The purpose of compounding hazardous drugs in a negative-pressure room is to prevent the escape of airborne contaminates into the workplace.

Normal saline (NS): a solution containing 0.9% sodium chloride. This isotonic solution is used for fluid replacement as a large-volume parenteral product; as a small-volume parenteral solution, it is used for reconstitution and dilution of parenteral products.

Open system: a system that allows free passage of air in and out of the container.

Osmolarity: solute concentration represented in a fluid-to-fluid ratio of milliosmoles per liter.

Osmoles (Osm): the number of moles multiplied by the number of particles present when dissolved in water.

Parenteral nutrition (PN): the provision of nutritional supplementation through a parenteral route in patients unable to tolerate nutrition through the gastrointestinal tract.

Particulate matter: dust and other particles that influence air quality and/or contaminate preparations.

Pathogen: any bacterium, virus, or microorganism that is capable of inducing disease.

Percentage strength: concentration expressed as the number of parts per 100, as with w/w, w/v, and v/v.

Percutaneous central venous catheter (PCVC): a central venous catheter that is inserted in a peripheral vein (usually in the upper arm) and threaded such that the tip of the catheter ends in the superior vena cava or right atrium.

Personal protective equipment (PPE): garb; special attire that is worn when compounding and in controlled environments. It includes items such as gloves, gowns, respirators, goggles, shoe covers, face masks, and face shields that protect individual workers from hazardous physical or chemical exposure and protect the final preparation from operator-related contamination.

PhaSeal: a type of closed-system vial-transfer device used during hazardous drug compounding and administration.

Phase separation: the result of physical instability in which the contents of a compounded sterile preparation separate into two phases or layers.

Phlebitis: inflammation of a vein.

Photochemical degradation: chemical breakdown by light.

Piggyback: a secondary medication added for infusion along with a primary infusion; an injection added through a medication port while a solution or medication is infusing.

Policies and procedures: formal documents that are developed by institutions to guide decisions and outline steps for consistency and quality purposes.

Powder volume: the volume that a powder takes up once it is reconstituted.

Precipitate: a solid substance within a solution.

Precipitation: the formation of precipitates; the result of a chemical reaction between two substances resulting in the formation of a solid within a solution.

Primary engineering control (PEC): a device or room for sterile preparations. Such devices include, but are not limited to, laminar airflow workbenches, biological safety cabinets, compounding aseptic isolators, and compounding aseptic containment isolators.

Propylene glycol: a common solvent found in parenteral drugs, which can be toxic in young children.

Pyrogen: a substance released by bacteria that induces fever; it can be found as a contaminant of compounded sterile preparations.

Pyrogenicity: relating to the presence of pyrogens.

Radiopharmaceutical: a radioactive drug that is used for diagnostic or therapeutic purposes.

Reconstitute: to add a solvent to a lyophilized or freeze-dried powder to make a liquid formulation prior to withdrawing it from a vial.

Reconstitution: the process of adding a diluent to a vial containing dry powder to make a solution.

Refractometry: a verification technique that can establish whether a parenteral nutrition formulation was prepared correctly; it compares measured refractive indices to known refractive indices of nutrients.

Risk levels: low, medium, and high risk categories into which compounded sterile products are classified based on risk of contamination of the final preparation.

Risk management: strategies that identify, eliminate, minimize, and control for unacceptable risks.

Small-volume pump: a computer-controlled infusion pump that is used to deliver intermittent and continuous infusion medications in infants and young children. Rates of infusion range from 0.01 to 10 mL/hr.

Smart pump: a small-volume pump with built-in software capable of being programmed to include drug libraries with standard drug concentrations, minimum and maximum infusion rates, and checks for dosing errors.

Sodium hypochlorite solution: a deactivating agent for many hazardous drugs; used in cleaning, disinfection, and decontaminating of hazardous drug compounding areas.

Solubility: the amount or quantity of a drug or substance that can dissolve in a given amount or quantity of solvent; the ability of a drug or substance to dissolve in a solvent.

Solution: the liquid formulation of a solute dissolved in a solvent.

Solution: a mixture of two or more substances; references liquid formulations involving a solvent.

Spike: a dispensing pen; a means to puncture a rubber closure; a plastic needle-like apparatus.

Stability: retention of product characteristics and properties from the time of manufacturing and throughout the product's shelf-life; conversely, instability relates to loss of product characteristics or properties over time.

Standard concentration: an established concentration of a parenteral drug adopted by an institution.

Sterility: relating to a sterile preparation; free of microorganisms.

Thrombophlebitis: swelling of a vein secondary to a blood clot.

Tonicity: a measure of the relative number of particles in a solution; associated with the concentration of a solution.

Total nutrient admixture (TNA): a 3-in-1 or all-in-one admixture; contains amino acids, dextrose, micronutrients, and injectable lipid emulsions.

United States Pharmacopeia: a national organization that sets standards for the purity, quality, identity, and strength, of medicines, food ingredients, and dietary supplements, including compounded sterile preparations.

USP Chapter <797>: Chapter 797 from the United States Pharmacopeia, which sets out standards for pharmaceutical compounding in sterile preparations. A section of the chapter is specific to hazardous drug compounding. USP <797> is an enforceable standard.

Vesicant: a type of drug that causes blistering and other tissue damage that may result in tissue necrosis.

v/v: volume in volume; used in percentage strength calculations.

Workbench: a hood; a term that describes the entire structure for primary engineering controls, such as a horizontal laminar airflow hood or biological safety cabinet.

Work surface: the flat, bottom-most portion of the workbench; the area in which manipulations occur.

w/v: weight in volume; used in percentage strength calculations.

w/w: weight in weight; used in percentage strength calculations.

Zones of turbulence: areas in which laminar airflow within the workbench is disrupted, often as a result of improper placement of objects; objects in these areas are at increased risk of contamination.

Index

Note: Page numbers followed by *f* and *t* indicate material in figures and tables respectively.

A